Clinical Guide to
Cardiovascular Disease

Vincent E. Friedewald

Clinical Guide to Cardiovascular Disease

Volume 2

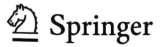 Springer

Vincent E. Friedewald
Division of Cardiology
UT Health Science Center at Houston Division of Cardiology
Houston, Texas, USA

ISBN 978-1-4471-7291-8   ISBN 978-1-4471-7293-2   (eBook)
DOI 10.1007/978-1-4471-7293-2

Library of Congress Control Number: 2016960003

Printed on acid-free paper

This Springer imprint is published by Springer Nature
The registered company is Springer-Verlag London Ltd.
The registered company address is: 236 Gray's Inn Road, London WC1X 8HB, United Kingdom

To our patients – our best teachers, when we listen

Preface

The *Clinical Guide to Cardiovascular Disease* culminates over 70 years of disease data collection, begun by my father, Vincent E. Friedewald, Sr. M.D., when he was awarded patent rights for the first medical computer – a mechanical index card-sorting machine – for differential diagnosis and other elements of medical decision support (Figs. 1 and 2). Today these data reside within the largest medical relational database in the world,[1] comprising a unified lexicon of thousands of confirmed clinical manifestations of human disease. This massive collection of information is the foundation for the *Clinical Guide to Cardiovascular Disease* and the preceding *Clinical Guide to Bioweapons and Chemical Agents* (Friedewald VE, Springer-Verlag, 2006).

Unlike traditional books, the *Clinical Guide* is specifically designed for rapid access to disease information, segregated into keyword data elements organized under 20 separate headings relevant to clinical care. In addition, external links are provided for supplemental and updated information.

The bulk of content in the *Clinical Guide* is focused on information essential to correct disease diagnosis, for good reason. According to the Institute of Medicine (IOM),[2] *"diagnosis—and, in particular, the occurrence of diagnostic errors—has been largely unappreciated in efforts to improve the quality and safety of health care. The result of this inattention*

---

[1] COR Medical Technologies, Inc. https://www.cormedicaltechnologies.com/landing.aspx.

[2] National Academies of Sciences, Engineering, and Medicine. *Improving diagnosis in health care*. Washington: The National Academies Press; 2015.

is significant: The committee concluded that most people will experience at least one diagnostic error in their lifetime, sometimes with devastating consequences." The IOM report further points out that:

- Five percent of adults in the USA seeking outpatient care experience a diagnostic error.
- Diagnostic errors contribute to 10 % of deaths.
- 6–17 % of adverse hospital events are due to diagnostic errors.
- Diagnostic errors are the leading cause of malpractice claims in the USA.

The *Clinical Guide* directly addresses the challenges of diagnostic accuracy with eight sections of information relevant to diagnosis in every disease chapter:

- Signs and Symptoms
- Predisposing/Comorbid Conditions
- Differential Diagnosis
- ECG
- Genomics
- Imaging
- Laboratory
- Other Tests

While the main emphasis of the *Clinical Guide* content is on diagnosis, treatment is presented in a more generic form. The reasons for this less-granular information about treatment are threefold:

1. Treatment recommendations are extremely dynamic, constantly changing as new outcome studies for current treatments are completed and as new modalities emerge, thereby greatly reducing the shelf life of treatment information.
2. Treatment is more and more being personalized according to individual patient preferences, circumstances, comorbidities, and other factors, all of which cannot be accommodated in one book.

3. Treatment recommendations are exquisitely defined and openly accessed in major Guidelines – especially those written by the American College of Cardiology/American Heart Association and by the European Society of Cardiology; they are linked to each disease in the *Clinical Guide* when they exist and are relatively current.

In addition to diagnostic and treatment information, other information that is often important to patient management is included in separate sections, such as demographics, pathophysiology, and clinical course. The style of the *Clinical Guide* is designed for easy use on mobile devices, as well for rapid access in its print form. This design includes extensive use of abbreviations, keywords, short phrases, and external links to both professional and patient information.

All of the content in the *Clinical Guide* was made possible by thousands of researchers worldwide via their contributions to the many excellent cardiovascular and general medical journals we are fortunate to have at our disposal. To them, I offer my deepest thanks, and an apology: because this book is so content-rich, it would take a second book just to accommodate standard referencing, and even then many of these primary authors would likely be slighted. Thus, I have chosen to list only a relatively few, select articles in the section Professional Information, along with their links, that I encourage readers to access for additional information.

I acknowledge and thank the many authors of major Guidelines, especially Guidelines written by the American College of Cardiology and American Heart Association, and by the European Society of Cardiology. Such Guidelines are remarkable documents – in my opinion, far too underutilized by practitioners – and a rich source of information for this book. In places, I have gone so far as to extract exact language from Guidelines, with the source specified.

I thank some of the many persons who assisted in compiling the *Clinical Guide* information, especially Doctor Patrick Finnigan, Mr. Ryan Carbone, my daughter Natalie Nieto, and the cardiology Fellows at The Cleveland Clinic, selected for me by my friend and colleague, Doctor James Young. Those Fellows are Doctor Mohammed B. Elshazly, Doctor Samuel Horr, Doctor Manju Pai, Doctor Grant Reed, Doctor Brett Sperry, and Doctor Amanda Vest.

As further testament to the digital age, I thank Mr. John Scott – who does not even pretend to understand a word in this book, nor do I have even the most remote notion of what he does – for building the software program that so greatly facilitated writing this book.

Finally, I offer a great big Texas-size mountain of gratitude to my publisher at Springer-Verlag, Mr. Grant Weston, for his patience, which is a vanishing virtue.

Houston, TX, USA   Vincent E. Friedewald
                                              MD, FACC, FACP

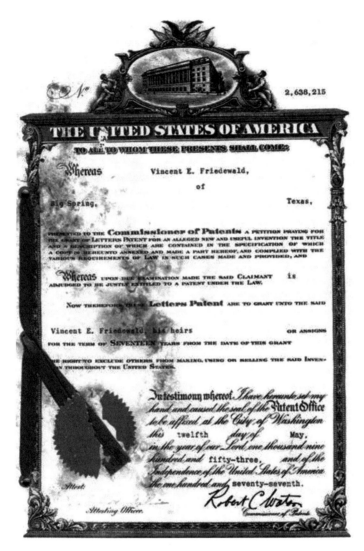

FIG. I United States patent award in 1953 to Vincent E. Friedewald, Sr, M.D., for the first medical computer

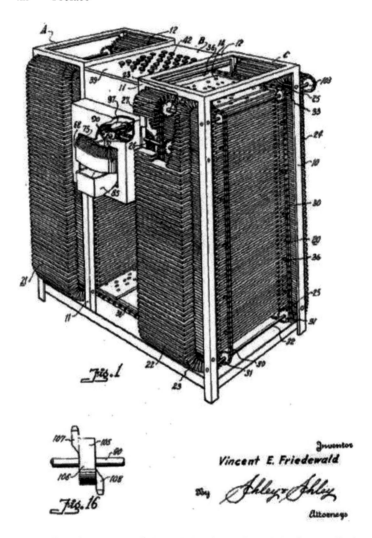

FIG. 2 Exterior of Dr. Friedewald, Sr's, invention of the first medical computer. Note the keys at the top center of the machine, where clinical information such as signs and symptoms were entered for differential diagnosis

Abbreviations

A2	Aortic valve second heart sound
AAA	Abdominal aortic aneurysm
AATS	American Association for Thoracic Surgery
ABD	Abdominal
ACC	American College of Cardiology
ACCF	American College of Cardiology Foundation
ACCP	American College of Chest Physicians
ACEI(S)	Angiotensin converting enzyme inhibitor(s)
ACS	Acute cardiac syndrome
AED	Automated external defibrillator
AF	Atrial fibrillation
AHA	American Heart Association
AMI	Acute myocardial infarction
ANT	Anterior
AOS	Aneurysms-osteoarthritis syndrome
APOB	Apolipoprotein B
AR	Aortic regurgitation
ARB(S)	Angiotensin receptor blocker(s)
ARVD	Arrhythmogenic right ventricular dysplasia
AS	Aortic stenosis
ASA	Aspirin, acetylsalicylic acid
ASD	Atrial septal defect
AT	Atrial tachycardia
ATP	Adenosine triphosphate
ATVR	Atrioventricular
AV	Aortic valve
A-V	Arterio-venous
AVN	Atrioventricular node

AVNRT	Atrioventricular node reentry tachycardia
AVR	Aortic valve replacement
AVRT	Atrioventricular reentry tachycardia
AVSD	Atrioventricular septal defect
BBB	Bundle branch block
BP	Blood pressure (arterial)
BPM	Beats per minute
BS	Breath sounds
BUN	Blood urea nitrogen
BVH	Biventricular hypertrophy
CABG	Coronary artery bypass graft surgery
CAD	Coronary artery disease
CAS	Carotid artery stenosis
CAF	Coronary arteriovenous fistula
CAV	Cardiac allograft vasculopathy
CCA	Circumflex coronary artery
CCB(S)	Calcium channel blocker(s)
CKD	Chronic kidney disease
CKMB	Ck-Mb fraction
CMRI	Cardiac magnetic resonance imaging
COA	Coarctation of aorta
CONT	Continuous
COPD	Chronic obstructive pulmonary disease
CPAP	Continuous positive airway pressure
CPR	Cardiopulmonary resuscitation
CPVT	Catecholaminergic polymorphic ventricular tachycardia
CRT	Cardiac resynchronization therapy
CT	Computed tomography
CVA	Cerebrovascular accident
CVD	Cardiovascular disease
CXR(S)	Chest X-ray(s)
DCM	Dilated cardiomyopathy
DECR	Decreased
DEPR	Depression(s)
DESC	Descending
DIAS	Diastolic, diastole
DIL	Dilation, dilated

DM	Diabetes mellitus
DSA	Digital subtraction angiography
DVT	Deep vein (venous) thrombosis
DYSRHY	Dysrhythmia
ECG	Electrocardiogram
ECHO	Echocardiogram (includes Doppler, transesophageal)
ECMO	Extracorporeal membrane oxygenation
EF	Ejection fraction
EG	For Example
ELEV	Elevation(s)
EMB	Endomyocardial biopsy
EMF	Endomyocardial fibrosis
EMG	Electromyogram
EP	Electrophysiology test
ERS	Early repolarization syndrome
ESC	European Society of Cardiology
ESP	Especially
EXT	External
FFR	Fractional flow reserve
FMC	First medical contact
FMD	Fibromuscular dysplasia
GCM	Giant cell myocarditis
GDMT	Guideline directed medical therapy
HB	Heart block
HCM	Hypertrophic cardiomyopathy
HDL-C	High-density lipoprotein cholesterol
HEFH	Heterozygous familial hypercholesterolemia
HF	Heart failure
HFpEF	Heart failure preserved ejection fraction
HFrEF	Heart failure reduced ejection fraction
HIV	Human immunodeficiency virus
HOCM	Hypertrophic obstructive cardiomyopathy
HOEF	Homozygous familial hypercholesterolemia
HR	Heart rate
HTN	Hypertension
IART	Intraatrial reentrant tachycardia
ICD(S)	Implantable cardiac defibrillator(s)

ICD-10	International Classification of Diseases, Tenth Revision
ICS	Intercostal space
IOC	Iron overload cardiomyopathy
IE	Infective endocarditis
INCR	Increased
INF	Inferior
INSP	Inspiration
INT	Internal
IST	Inappropriate sinus tachycardia
IV	Intravenous
IVC	Inferior vena cava
IVS	Interventricular septum
JVP	Jugular venous pulse/pulsation
L	Left
LA	Left atrium
LAA	Left atrial appendage
LAD	Left anterior descending coronary artery
LAT	Lateral
LBB(B)	Left bundle branch (block)
LCA	Left coronary artery
LDL-C	Low-density lipoprotein cholesterol
LE	Lower extremity
LEAD	Lower extremity artery disease
LGE	Late gadolinium enhancement
LLQ	Lower left quadrant
LMWH	Low molecular weight heparin
LQTS	Long QT syndrome
L-R	Left to right
LSB	Left sternal border
LUQ	Left upper quadrant
LV	Left ventricle
LVAD	Left ventricular assist device
LVEDP	Left ventricular end-diastolic pressure
LVEDV	Left ventricular end-diastolic volume
LVH	Left ventricular hypertrophy
LVOT	Left ventricular outflow tract
LVSV	Left ventricular stroke volume
M1	Mitral valve first heart sound

MACE	Major adverse cardiovascular/cerebrovascular events
MALE	Major adverse limb events
MAP	Mean arterial pressure
MPI	Myocardial perfusion imaging
MR	Mitral regurgitation
MRA	Magnetic resonance angiography
MRI	Magnetic resonance imaging
MS	Mitral stenosis
MUR	Murmur
MV	Mitral valve
MVP	Mitral valve prolapse
MYOCARD	Myocardial, myocardium
NA	Not applicable
NEG	Negative
NO	Nitric oxide
NS	Nonspecific/no specific
NSTEMI	Non ST segment elevation myocardial infarction
NSVT	Nonsustained ventricular tachycardia
O2	Oxygen
OSA	Obstructive sleep apnea
P2	Pulmonic valve second heart sound
PA	Pulmonary artery
PAC(S)	Premature atrial contraction(s)
PAD	Peripheral arterial disease
PAH	Pulmonary arterial hypertension
PAROX	Paroxysmal
PAT	Paroxysmal atrial tachycardia
PCI	Percutaneous coronary intervention
PCR	Polymerase chain reaction
PDA	Patent ductus arteriosus
PET	Positron emission tomography
PFT	Pulmonary function test
PH	Pulmonary hypertension
PHEO	Pheochromocytoma
PPCM	Peripartum cardiomyopathy
PPV	Positive pressure ventilation
PRESS	Pressure

PROX	Proximal
PS	Pulmonary stenosis
PSVT	Paroxysmal supraventricular tachycardia
PTCA	Percutaneous transluminal coronary angioplasty
PV	Pulmonary valve
PVC(S)	Premature ventricular contraction(s)
PVR	Pulmonary vascular resistance
QOL	Quality of life
QTC	Corrected QT interval
RA	Right atrium
RAA	Right atrial appendage
RAAS	Renin aldosterone angiotensin system
RAS	Renal artery stenosis
RBB(B)	Right bundle branch (block)
RCA	Right coronary artery
RCM	Restrictive cardiomyopathy
RF	Radiofrequency
RHF	Right heart failure
R-L	Right to left
RLQ	Right lower quadrant
RSB	Right sternal border
RUQ	Right upper quadrant
RV	Right ventricle
RVEDP	Right ventricular end-diastolic pressure
RVEDV	Right ventricular end-diastolic volume
RVH	Right ventricular hypertrophy
RVOT	Right ventricular outflow tract
S/S	Signs and symptoms
S1	First heart sound
S2	Second heart sound
S3	Third heart sound (gallop)
S4	Fourth heart sound (gallop)
SAH	Systemic arterial hypertension
SCD	Sudden cardiac death
SD	Sudden death
SIHD	Stable ischemic heart disease
SLE	Systemic lupus erythematosus

SQTS	Short QT syndrome
STEMI	ST segment elevation myocardial infarction
SubAS	Subvalvular aortic stenosis (discrete)
SVA	Sinus of Valsalva aneurysm
SVAS	Supravalvular aortic stenosis
SVC	Superior vena cava
SVT	Supraventricular tachycardia
SX(S)	Sign(s)
SYMP(S)	Symptom(s)/symptomatic
SYS	Systolic, systole
T1	Tricuspid valve first heart sound
TAVR	Transcatheter aortic valve replacement
TEE	Transesophageal echocardiogram
TG(S)	Triglyceride(s)
TGA	Transposition of great arteries
TIA	Transient ischemic attack
TIC	Tachycardia-induced cardiomyopathy
TIMI	Thrombolysis in myocardial infarction
TNF	Tumor necrosis factor
TNG	Tri-nitroglycerin
TOF	Tetralogy of Fallot
TR	Tricuspid regurgitation
TS	Tricuspid stenosis
TSH	Thyroid stimulating hormone
TTE	Transthoracic echocardiogram
TV	Tricuspid valve
TVP	Tricuspid valve prolapse
UA	Unstable angina, urinalysis
UE	Upper extremity
UTI	Urinary tract infection
VF	Ventricular fibrillation
VAD	Ventricular assist device
VMA	Vanillylmandelic acid
VSD(S)	Ventricular septal defect(s)
VT	Ventricular tachycardia
WHO	World Health Organization
WPW	Wolff-Parkinson-White syndrome
WS	Williams syndrome

Contents

Chapter 51
Giant Cell Myocarditis

ICD-10 Code

I40.1

Alternate Names/Abbreviation

GCM

Description/Etiology [12]

Nonischemic, rapidly progressive necrosis of cardiac myocytes with multinucleated giant cell, lymphocytic, and
eosinophilic inflammatory infiltrate

Generally presumed an autoinflammatory disease, sometimes
associated with and preceded by other chronic inflammatory disorders (see COMORBID CONDITIONS)

Comorbid Conditions [1] [2]

ALOPECIA TOTALIS VITILIGO
ARRHYTHMOGENIC RIGHT VENTRICULAR
DYSPLASIA

V.E. Friedewald, *Clinical Guide to Cardiovascular Disease*,   665
DOI 10.1007/978-1-4471-7293-2_51,
© Springer-Verlag London 2016

ASYMMETRIC SEPTAL HYPERTROPHY
CHRONIC HEPATITIS
CROHN DIS
CRYOFIBRINOGENEMIA
DIABETES MELLITUS [INSULIN-DEPENDENT]
DRUG HYPERSENSITIVITY [3]
FIBROMYALGIA
HASHIMOTO THYROIDITIS
HEART TRANSPLANT [10]
HYPERTHYROIDISM
HYPOTHYROIDISM
LYMPHOMA
MYASTHENIA GRAVIS
OPTIC NEURITIS
ORBITAL MYOSITIS
PARVOVIRUS B19 INFECTION
PERNICIOUS ANEMIA
RHEUMATOID ARTHRITIS
SJOGREN SYNDROME
SYSTEMIC LUPUS ERYTHEMATOSUS
TAKAYASU ARTERITIS
THYMOMA [4]
ULCERATIVE COLITIS
WEGENER GRANULOMATOSIS

Demography

Age of clinical onset (mean) 42 years [5]
All ethnicities
Gender equal

Pathophysiology

LV myocardial necrosis and fibrosis causing LV dysfunction and atrioventricular heart block

EMB histology:

> Eosinophils
> Giant cells (early)
> Interstitial Fibrosis
> Lymphocytes

Signs/Symptoms

BREATHING – DIFF (DYSPNEA)
BREATHING   –   DIFF,   RECLINING   FLAT
  (ORTHOPNEA)
CHEST – PAIN [7] [8]
CHEST – PALPITATIONS
CONSCIOUSNESS – LOSS, SUDDEN (SYNCOPE)
EXTREM, LOWER, BILAT – EDEMA
FATIGUE

Differentiation

AMI [8]
Cardiac Sarcoidosis
Other causes of Myocarditis/Cardiomyopathy/HF
Other causes of heart block

Complications

Cardiac rupture/hemopericardium
Complete heart block [7]
HF [7] [12]
Infections
Renal failure [11]
Sudden death
VT [6] [7]

Laboratory

BLOOD, TROPONIN, CARD – INCR

ECG

AV COND – 1ST DEGREE BLOCK
AV COND – 3RD DEGREE BLOCK
DYSRHYTHMIAS – VENTRICULAR (PVCS/ OTHERS) [9]
EPSILON WAVE
Q WAVE – ABN [8]

Imaging

IVS, THICKNESS – INCR (SEPTAL HYPERTROPHY)
LV, CHAMBER, SIZE – INCR
LV, EF – DECR
LV, MYOCARD, WALL THICKNESS – INCR (HYPERTROPHY)
LV, WALL THICKNESS, SEG – INCR
MYOCARD – FIBROSIS
RV, CHAMBER, SIZE – INCR

Other Tests

EMB

Treatment: Nonpharmacologic

NS

Treatment: Pharmacologic

Immunosuppression

Treatment: Surgical/Invasive [12]

LVAD
Cardiac transplant

Course

HF with cardiac transplant within 1 year of diagnosis often
  required
Post-cardiac transplant survival: about 70 % at 5 years
Recurrence common for several years after initial
  diagnosis

Notes

[1] Most cases not associated with other conditions; some
  conditions listed based on single case reports
[2] Some conditions, eg, Inflammatory Bowel Disease, may
  precede onset of GCM by several years
[3] Many drug classes reported, including antiinfectives,
  antiepileptics, vaccines, antihypertensives
[4] Also reported post-thymoma resection
[5] All ages reported, from infancy to >85 years
[6] Often sustained and refractory
[7] May be initial clinical manifestation
[8] Chest pain syndrome resembling AMI may occur
[9] Especially VT
[10] Many reports in transplants replacing GCM hearts and
  isolated reports of GCM in transplants for other causes
[11] Due to HF/chronic calcineurin use

[12] Excerpted from ACCF/AHA 2013 Guidelines for Management of Heart Failure (J Am Coll Cardiol 2013;62:e147-e239):

"Sec 5.6.1 Myocarditis

Giant cell myocarditis is a rare form of myocardial inflammation characterized by fulminant HF, often associated with refractory ventricular arrhythmias and a poor prognosis. Histologic findings include diffuse myocardial necrosis with numerous multinucleated giant cells without granuloma formation. Consideration for advanced HF therapies, including immunosuppression, mechanical circulatory support (MCS), and transplantation, is warranted."

Guidelines

2013 ACCF/AHA guideline for the management of heart failure
J Am Coll Cardiol. 2013;62:e147–239. http://content.onlinejacc.org/article.aspx?articleid=1695825.
ESC Guidelines for the diagnosis and treatment of acute and chronic heart failure 2012
Eur Heart J. 2012;33:1787–847. http://eurheartj.oxfordjournals.org/content/ehj/33/14/1787.full.pdf.

Patient Information

Myocarditis Foundation

http://www.myocarditisfoundation.org/about-giant-cell-myocarditis/.

Mayo Clinic

http://www.mayoclinic.org/diseases-conditions/myocarditis/basics/definition/con-20027303.

Medlineplus

ENGLISH
    http://www.nlm.nih.gov/medlineplus/ency/article/000149.htm.
ESPANOL
    http://www.nlm.nih.gov/medlineplus/spanish/ency/article/000149.
    htm.

NORD

https://rarediseases.org/rare-diseases/giant-cell-myocarditis/.

Professional Information

Review

Herz. 2012;37:632–6. http://www.ncbi.nlm.nih.gov/pubmed/22930389
    ?dopt=Abstract.

Drug Hypersensitivity

Cardiovasc Path. 2000;8:287–91. http://www.sciencedirect.com/sci-
    ence/article/pii/S1054880700000491.

EMB/Immunosuppression

Circ Heart Failure. 2013;6:15–22. http://circheartfailure.ahajournals.
    org/content/6/1/15.long.

ECG Epsilon Waves: Case Report

Eur Heart J. 2014;35:9. http://eurheartj.oxfordjournals.org/
    content/35/1/9.

Imaging: MRI

Circulation. 2014;129:e467–9. http://circ.ahajournals.org/content/129/17/e467.full.

Immunosuppression

Am J Cardiol. 2008;102:1535–9. http://www.ncbi.nlm.nih.gov/pmc/articles/PMC2613862/.

Long-Term Follow-Up

Am J Cardiol. 2015;115:1733–8. http://www.ajconline.org/article/S0002-9149(15)00978-9/abstract.

Myocardial Gene Expression Profiling

Eur Heart J. 2014;35:2186–95. http://eurheartj.oxfordjournals.org/content/35/32/2186.

Natural History/Treatment

N Engl J Med. 1997;336:1860–6. http://www.nejm.org/doi/full/10.1056/NEJM199706263362603.

VT as Presenting Manifestation

Heart. 2007;93:119–21. http://heart.bmj.com/content/93/1/119.extract.

Updates and More

https://clinicalguidecvd.com/gcm

Chapter 52
Heart Failure (CHF/ Congestive Heart Failure)

Management Keys

Consider reversible causes, including:

Acute Myocarditis
Cardiomyopathy – Peripartum
Cardiomyopathy – Tachycardia-Induced
Cardiomyopathy – Takotsubo
Cardiomyopathy – Toxic (eg, Cobalt) [58]
Hypocalcemia/Hypomagnesemia [62]

Consider treatment with ICD for primary prevention if LVEF ≤35 % in non-ischemic DCM; or ischemic heart disease at least 40 days post-AMI with EF ≤30 % (NYHA I) or ≤35 % (NYHA II-IV)

Diagnose specific stage/treat specific cause if identified

Diagnose/treat comorbid conditions (both CV and non-CV)

Early diagnosis/treatment of asymptomatic patients with LVEF <40 % [33]

Evaluate for cardiac transplantation/mechanical circulatory support for select patients with stage D HF

Provide multidisciplinary specialist services to enhance QOL and survival while simultaneously decreasing hospital readmissions up to 30–50 %

Provide prompt diagnosis/treatment of decompensated HF including hospitalization

V.E. Friedewald, *Clinical Guide to Cardiovascular Disease*, 673
DOI 10.1007/978-1-4471-7293-2_52,
© Springer-Verlag London 2016

- Treat with Aldosterone antagonists to decrease morbidity and mortality in NYHA class II-IV pts with LVEF ≤35 % or with LVEF ≤40 % post-AMI or Diabetes Mellitus (with acceptable creatinine/potassium blood levels)
- Treat with Angiotensin-Converting Enzyme Inhibitors or Angiotensin-II Receptor Blockers in patients with HFrEF to decrease morbidity and mortality
- Treat with 1 of 3 specific Beta-blockers (carvedilol, metoprolol, bisoprolol) to decrease morbidity and mortality in patients with HFrEF [67]
- Treat with LCZ696 to reduce risk of CV death/HF hospitalization
- Treat with CRT if LVEF ≤35 % with sinus rhythm, LBBB and QRS ≥150 ms
- Treat with hydralazine combined with isosorbide dinitrate in African-Americans with HFrEF (NYHA Class III-IV) to decrease morbidity and mortality in addition to other guideline-recommended drugs
- Treat with caution when using long-term continuous or intermittent IV inotropes, which are potentially harmful and not recommended (other than bridging to definitive treatment/palliative care)
- Consider exercise training therapy for patients with HFrEF [25]

ICD-10 Code

I50.22 (Chronic Systolic)
I50.32 (Chronic Diastolic)

Alternate Names/Abbreviation

HF
Congestive heart failure (CHF)
Ischemic Cardiomyopathy (ICM)
Left ventricular failure

Left ventricular diastolic dysfunction
Left ventricular systolic dysfunction (LVSD)
Non-ischemic Cardiomyopathy (NICM)
HFrEF: abnormal systolic function with reduced EF ($\leq$40 %); also termed "systolic heart failure" [7]
HFpEF: abnnormal diastolic function with preserved EF ($\geq$50 %); also termed "diastolic heart failure" [7]

Description/Etiology

Clinical syndrome caused by structural or functional cardiac impairment; recognized by characteristic pattern of hemodynamic, renal, and neurohumoral responses
All forms of heart disease can result in HFrEF in advanced stages
Causal categories:

Ischemic heart disease, including:

AMI [66]
Myocardial "stunning"
Myocardial "hibernation"
Ventricular remodeling post-AMA

Cardiomyopathies, including:

Acquired
Inherited

Myocarditis, including:

Infectious
Infiltrative
Inflammatory
Toxic

Increased ventricular pressure load, including:

Aortic Stenosis – Valvular
Aortic Stenosis – Subvalvular
Aortic Stenosis – Supravalvular
Hypertension – Systemic Arterial

Increased ventricular volume load, including:

Aortic Regurgitation – Acute
Aortic Regurgitation – Chronic
Arteriovenous fistula (including Peripheral Extremity Arteriovenous Fistula)
Intracardiac shunts/congenital heart disease
Mitral Regurgitation – Acute
Mitral Regurgitation – Chronic

Restrictive pericardial disease, including

Pericardial effusion
Pericarditis – Constrictive

Restrictive myocardial function, including:

Decreased myocardial dispensability
Endocardial fibroelastosis
Restrictive myocardial disease

Electrical abnormalities, including:

Tachycardias (including Cardiomyopathy – Tachycardia-Induced)
Ventricular dyssynchrony

High output states, including:

Anemia
Beriberi
Hyperthyroidism and Graves Disease
Paget Disease
Peripheral Arteriovenous Fistula

AHA Stages:

A. High risk for HF without structural heart disease or HF symptoms
B. Structural Heart disease without HF signs/symptoms
C. Structural Heart disease with prior or current HF symptoms
D. Refractory HF requiring specialized interventions

NYHA Functional Classification:

I.   No limitation of physical activity; ordinary activity does not cause HF symptoms
II. Slight limitation of physical activity; comfortable at rest, but ordinary activity causes HF symptoms
III. Marked limitation of physical activity; comfortable at rest, but < ordinary activity causes HF symptoms
IV. Unable to carry on any physical activity without HF symptoms, or HF symptoms at rest

Common triggers of acute decompensation/HF progression:

Acute infections (eg, viral illnesses, pneumonia)
Acute Kidney Injury/decreased renal function
Alcohol use (heavy)
Anemia
AF
Brady/tachyarrhythmias
Fluid retention caused by noncardiac medication (eg, NSAID)
Hypertension – Systemic Arterial
Hyperthyrodism and Graves Disease
Hypoxia
Myocardial ischemia

Nonadherence with medications/diet

Comorbid Conditions [42]

MOST COMMON

ACUTE MYOCARDIAL INFARCTION [66]
ALZHEIMER DISEASE/DEMENTIA
ANEMIA [54]
ARTHRITIS
ASTHMA [AGE <65 years]
ATHEROSCLEROSIS IN OTHER CV AREAS

ATRIAL FIBRILLATION [52] [AND OTHER CAUSES OF RAPID VENTRIC RATE]
CARDIOMYOPATHY – DILATED [IDIOPATHIC, INCL FAMILIAL]
CEREBROVASCULAR DISEASE
CHRONIC KIDNEY DISEASE
CHRONIC OBSTRUCTIVE PULMONARY DISEASE (EMPHYSEMA)
CORONARY ARTERY DISEASE [AND OTHER FORMS OF ATHEROSCLEROTIC DIS]
DEPRESSION
DIABETES MELLITUS [49]
DYSLIPIDEMIA
DYSRHYTHMIAS – VENTRICULAR [63]
FUNCTIONAL MITRAL REGURGITATION [32]
HYPERTENSION – SYSTEMIC ARTERIAL
METABOLIC SYNDROME
PERIPHERAL ARTERY DISEASE
VALVULAR HEART DISEASE

OTHERS

ACROMEGALY
ALCOHOL USE/EXCESS
ARRHYTHMOGENIC RIGHT VENTRICULAR DYSPLASIA/CARDIOMYOPATHY
AUTOIMMUNE/CONNECTIVE TISSUE DISEASE
CARDIAC AMYLOIDOSIS
CARDIAC SARCOIDOSIS
CARDIOMYOPATHY – DANON DISEASE
CARDIOMYOPATHY – HIV
CARDIOMYOPATHY – HYPERTROPHIC
CARDIOMYOPATHY – IRON OVERLOAD
CARDIOMYOPATHY – NONCOMPACTION
CARDIOMYOPATHY – PERIPARTUM
CARDIOMYOPATHY – RESTRICTIVE
CARDIOMYOPATHY – TAKOTSUBO
CARDIORENAL SYNDROME
CHAGAS DISEASE

COCAINE
CONGENITAL HEART DISEASE [72] [73]
DRUGS: CANCER THERAPY [CARDIOTOXICITY]
[50] [51]
ENDOMYOCARDIAL FIBROSIS
FABRY DISEASE
GROWTH HORMONE DEFICIENCY
HEMOCHROMATOSIS
HIV
HYPERTHYROIDISM
HYPOMAGNESEMIA
HYPOTHYROIDISM
MITOCHONDRIAL DISEASE
MUSCULAR DYSTROPHY
MYOCARDITIS [INCL VIRAL, EOSINOPHILIC,
GIANT CELL]
NUTRITIONAL DEFICIENCIES
OBESITY [70]
OBSTRUCTIVE SLEEP APNEA [68]
OSTEOPOROSIS
RELAPSING   CATASTROPHIC   ANTIPHOS
PHOLIPID ANTIBODY SYNDROME
STORAGE DISORDERS
TOXINS

Demography

Varies with etiology
CAD and DM increasingly prevalent etiology; hyperten-
sion and valve disease have become less common
causes in more economically advanced societies
Increased risk with age: 20 % lifetime risk in persons age
>40 year
Highest incidence in USA: non-Hispanic black males
Mortality: 50 % within 5 years of diagnosis (except revers-
ible forms)

Patients with HFpEF more often:

> Female
> Less likely to have CAD
> More likely to have Systemic Arterial Hypertension and AF
> Obese
> Older age

Pathophysiology

HF is a highly complex syndrome, comprising many physiological abnormalities, including:

1. Abnormal systolic/diastolic cardiac pump function to:
   Meet body's metabolic demands, with associated neuroendocrine compensatory changes (eg, fluid retention)
   Accommodate venous return

2. Ventricular remodeling: spherical LV with decreased contractility comprising numerous myocardial functional/structural functions; begins with hypertrophy in response to wall stress

3. Neurohormone activation:
   Arginine vasopressin
   Endothelin-1
   Natriuretic peptides (ANP, BNP)
   Nitric oxide
   RAAS
   Sympathetic nervous system (earliest response to decreased card output)

4. Myocardial fibrosis

5. Ketone bodies: significant fuel source for oxidative ATP production in hypertrophied and failing heart as cardiac capacity to utilize fatty acids (chief fuel in normal hearts) diminishes

Signs/Symptoms [73]

ABDOMEN – DISTENSION
ABDOMEN – FLUID (ASCITES) [8]
ABDOMEN – FULLNESS
ABDOMEN – PAIN [ESP RUQ] [34]
APPETITE – DECR (ANOREXIA)
APPETITE, SATIETY – EARLY [34]
ARTERIAL PRESSURE, UPRIGHT – DECR (ORTHOSTATIC HYPOTENSION) [11]
ARTERIAL PRESSURE, VALSALVA RESPONSE – ABN
ARTERIAL PULSE PRESSURE – DECR [38]
ARTERIAL PULSE, AMP – ALTERNATING (PULSUS ALTERNANS) [37]
ARTERIAL PULSE, AMP – DECR/ABS
BEHAVIOR – BIZARRE/CHANGED [1]
BLOOD PRESSURE, ARTERIAL – INCREASED/ELEVATED
BODY, APPEARANCE – WASTING (CACHEXIA) [9]
BODY, GEN – EDEMA (ANASARCA)
BOWEL MOVEMENTS – DIARRHEA
BREATH SOUNDS – CRACKLES (RALES) [10]
BREATH SOUNDS – DECR
BREATH SOUNDS – WHEEZES
BREATH SOUNDS, BASILAR – DECR
BREATHING – DIFF (DYSPNEA)
BREATHING – DIFF, NOCTURNAL (DYSPNEA, NOCT)
BREATHING – DIFF, RECLINING FLAT (ORTHOPNEA) [8]
BREATHING – RAPID (TACHYPNEA)
BREATHING – RHYTHMIC CHANGES (CHEYNE-STOKES)
BREATHING, NOCT – PAUSES (SLEEP APNEA)
CAPILLARY REFILL – SLUGGISH
CHEST – PAIN [4]

CHEST – PALPITATIONS
CHEST, ANT – MURMUR, SYS
COGNITION – DEFECT, NS
CONSCIOUSNESS – LOSS, SUDDEN (SYNCOPE)
COUGH
COUGH – NOCT [35]
EXTREM, LOWER, BILAT – EDEMA [5] [8]
EXTREM, LOWER, BILAT – FATIGUE
EXTREM, LOWER, TEMP – DECR [12]
EXTREM, UNILAT – EDEMA
EYES – PROMINENT (EXOPHTHALMOS/
    PROPTOSIS) [2]
EYES/SKIN – YELLOW (JAUNDICE)
FATIGUE
GENITALS, SCROTUM – SWOLLEN (EDEMA)
HEADACHE
HEART, LV, APEX, IMP – DISPLACED, INF
HEART, LV, APEX, IMP – DISPLACED, LAT
HEART, P2, INTENSITY – INCR
HEART, RATE – RAPID (TACHYCARDIA)
HEART, RHYTHM – IRREG [3]
HEART, S3 LV
HEART, S3 RV
HEART, S4 LV
HEART, S4 RV
HEART, SOUNDS, INTENSITY – DECR
HYPOTENSION (BLOOD PRESSURE –
    DECREASED/LOW)
LIVER – ENLARGED (HEPATOMEGALY)
LIVER – TENDER
MENTATION – CONFUSION [1]
MENTATION – WEAKNESS (MALAISE)
MOOD – DEPRESSED
MUSCLES – ATROPHY
MUSCLES – WEAK
NAUSEA [34]
NECK, JVP – ABDOMINOJUGULAR REFLUX [36]

NECK, JVP – ELEV [8] [36]
SKIN – ITCHING (PRURITUS)
SKIN, COLOR – BLUE (CYANOSIS)
SKIN, COLOR – PALE (PALLOR)
SLEEP – DISTURBED (INSOMNIA)
SLEEP – DISTURBED (INSOMNIA)
SPLEEN, SIZE – INCR (SPLENOMEGALY)
SPUTUM – BLOOD (HEMOPTYSIS)
URINATION – NIGHTTIME (NOCTURIA) [35]
VOMITING (EMESIS) [34]
WEIGHT – INCREASED/GAIN [8]

Differentiation

Other causes of abdominal pain
Other causes of dyspnea
Other causes of leg edema
Pulmonary Hypertension

Complications

Acute pulmonary edema
Acute Pulmonary Embolism
Cachexia
Cardiogenic shock
Congestive hepatopathy
Deep Vein Thrombosis – Lower Extremity
Dysrhythmias – atrial (esp AF)
Dysrhythmias – ventricular
Functional MR [32]
Pericardial effusion
Peripheral arterial embolism
Pleural effusion
Pneumonia
Pulmonary Hypertension

Renal failure
Stroke – Ischemic
Sudden death [69]

Laboratory [39]

BLOOD, BILIRUBIN – INCR
BLOOD, BUN – INCR [6]
BLOOD, CHOLESTEROL, TOTAL – DECR
BLOOD, CREATININE – INCREASED
BLOOD, GALECTIN-3 – INCR [56]
BLOOD, GLUCOSE – DECR (HYPOGLYCEMIA)
BLOOD, GLUCOSE – INCR (HYPERGLYCEMIA) [65]
BLOOD, HGB/HCT – DECR (ANEMIA) [54]
BLOOD, LIVER ENZYMES – INCREASED
BLOOD, NT-PROBNP – INCR [13] [14]
BLOOD, SODIUM – DECR (HYPONATREMIA)
BLOOD, ST2 – INCR [57] [SEE APPENDIX A]
BLOOD, TROPONIN – INCR
BLOOD, URIC ACID – INCR [53]
URINE, PROTEIN – INCR (PROTEINURIA)

ECG

DYSRHYTHMIAS – ATRIAL (PACS/OTHERS) [52]
    [especially AF]
DYSRHYTHMIAS – VENTRICULAR (PVCS/
    OTHERS)
HEART, RATE, VARIABILITY – DECR [64]
NS/VAR PER COMORBIDITY(S)
QRS – LVH PATTERN

Imaging [16]

CARDIOMEGALY [15]
LA, CHAMBER, SIZE – INCR [41]
LV, CHAMBER, SIZE – INCR [15] [41]

LV, DIAS – DYSF [7]
LV, EF – DECR [7]
LV, FILLING – DECR/RESTRICTED HFpEF
LV, MYOCARD, WALL THICKNESS – INCR (HYPERTROPHY) [ESP WHEN PRECEDED BY LVH] [19]
LV, SYS – DYSF [7]
LV, WALL MOTION – DECR
LV, WALL MOTION, SEG – DECR/AKINETIC [18]
LV, WALL THICKNESS – DECR [ESP WHEN PRECEDED BY DIL CARDIOMYOPATHY]
MV, FLOW – DECR
MV, FLOW – REGURG [20]
PA, MAIN, SIZE – INCR [17]
PERICARD – FLUID
PLEURA – FLUID
PUL, VASCULARITY – INCR [40]
PUL, VEINS – CONGESTED
RA, CHAMBER, SIZE – INCR [41]
RV, CHAMBER, SIZE – INCR [41]
RV, WALL MOTION – DECR
RV, WALL MOTION, SEG – DECR/AKINETIC
TV, FLOW – REGURG

Genomics

NS

Other Tests

Exercise test [69]
Right heart catheterization: to resolve specific clinical or therapeutic question (routine use to guide therapy not effective)
Left heart catheterization and coronary angiography: to determine ischemic versus non-ischemic etiology, and subsequently for possible coronary revascularization (eg, angina/ischemia-related LV dysfunction) [4]

EMB: when specific cause is suspected that would influence therapy (eg, suspect Giant Cell Myocarditis in new onset acute HF)

Pulmonary artery pressure wireless monitoring

Treatment: Nonpharmacologic [21]

Alcohol restriction/avoidance

Cocaine, amphetamine avoidance

CPAP when Obstructive Sleep Apnea present

Dietary sodium restriction [22]

Exercise training [25]

Self-care education (e.g., diet, symptom/weight monitoring, medication adherence, exercise)

Social support

Treatment: Pharmacologic [30]

Adjuvant parenteral therapy in selected decompensated patients

Aldosterone Antagonists, including eplerenone [28] [47]

ACEIs/ARBs [26] [43] [47]

Antithrombotics [48]

BP control (especially patients with HFpEF)

Beta-Blockers [23] [44] [45] [46] [67]

Calcium/magnesium replacement when Hypocalcemia/Hypomagnesemia present [62]

Digoxin if already receiving guideline-directed therapy [29] or control of ventricular rate in AF when beta-blocker insufficient

Diuretics, including furosemide and hydrochlorothiazides [27]

Fluid restriction: select patients

Hospital management of decompensated HF including:

Diuretics and other fluid management strategies

Deep Vein Thrombosis prophylaxis

Hydralazine and isosorbide for self-described African American patients or patients intolerant of RAAS inhibitors

Influenza vaccination [55]

Ivabradine [31]

LCZ696 (angiotensin receptor-neprilysin inhibitor) [61]

Non-dihydropyridine CCBs contraindicated with HFrEF

Omecamtiv mecarbil (investigational)

Omega-3 fatty acids

Other drug avoidance:

> NSAIDS
> Antiarrhythmics except amiodarone and dofetilide
> IV inotropes
> Thiazolidinediones

Prompt diagnosis/treatment of decompensated HF including hospitalization

Serelaxin (acute HF) (investigational)

Statins (Hx of CAD or hyperlipidemia; no indication for HF alone)

Ularitide (acute HF) (investigational)

Treatment: Surgical/Invasive (Consult Current Guidelines for Specific Indications)

Coronary revascularization

CRT

ICD [24]

Mechanical circulatory support, including [59]:

> Intra-aortic balloon pump
> Durable pulsatile or continuous flow VAD
> ECMO
> Temporary percutaneous VAD
> Total artificial heart

MV repair

> Surgical

Transcatheter

Heart transplant
Aquapharesis (investigational)
Bariatric surgery (investigational) [71]
Gene Therapy (investigational)
Stem cell/Regenerative (investigational)
Unidirectional L-R interatrial shunting (investigational)

Prevention

Control atherosclerosis risk factors
Control blood pressure
Control lifestyle risk factors [60]
Early diagnosis and GDMT of Cardiomyopathies, Valvular Heart disease, CAD, Congenital heart disease to prevent progression from stage A or B HF

Course

Variable per cause
Prognosis worse with:

Advanced NYHA functional class
Anemia
Cachexia
Decreased cholesterol
Decreased LVEF
Decreased systolic BP
High dose diuretics
Hyperuricemia
Hyponatremia
Increased relative lymphocyte count
Ischemic etiology

Notes

[1] Especially elderly, patients with low cardiac output

[2] Due to chronically increased venous pressure

[3] From AF or multiple PVCs

[4] Chest pain may occur in absence of demonstrable CAD; coronary angiography may be indicated in select patients

[5] Peripheral edema absent in many patients with volume overload, especially younger persons; may be due to peripheral causes, especially obesity and age-related venous insufficiency

[6] May be due to low cardiac output or venous congestion

[7] Most patients have combination of systolic and diastolic dysfunction; HF with EF 40–50 % considered intermediate group

[8] Along with vital signs, should be assessed at every encounter for volume status, especially JVP

[9] Indicates poorer prognosis

[10] Rales often absent in chronic HF

[11] May indicate volume depletion

[12] May indicate inadequate cardiac output

[13] Useful for:

> Diagnostic uncertainty
> Gauging HF severity
> Prognosis and when HF dx uncertain
> (Use for monitoring controversial)

[14] Other causes of increased natriuretic peptides:

Cardiac:

> AF
> Acute coronary syndrome
> Cardiac surgery
> Cardioversion
> LVH

Myocardial disease
Pericardial disease
Valvular heart disease

Non-cardiac:

Advanced age
Anemia
Bacterial sepsis
Burns (severe)
Critical illnesses
Pulmonary disease
Renal failure
Toxins (cancer chemotherapy, envenomation)

[15] May be normal size on CXR
[16] 2D echo: most useful diagnostic test for HF and should be performed as part of initial evaluation for LV function and associated cardiac conditions and serially with proper clinical indications, such as for LV remodeling
    MRI/CT/radionuclide ventriculography: useful in select cases, especially when echo is suboptimal
[17] Pulmonary artery dilation suggests Pulmonary Hypertension, a common consequence of LV dysfunction; primary PAH may also result in secondary RHF
[18] Suggests ischemic cardiomyopathy
[19] Suggests LVH-related HF, especially secondary to Systemic Arterial Hypertension or to infiltrative cardiomyopathy
[20] Functional MV regurgitation common in HF with ventricular dilatation; in absence of significant dilatation or when regurgitation is severe, other causes should be considered (eg, papillary muscle dysfunction, primary valve disease)
[21] Including recommendations for patients in stages A and B with goal of preventing progression to overt HF
[22] Not universal recommendation as evidence for efficacy indefinite and may worsen neurohormonal profile
[23] Caution when starting beta-blockers in decompensated patients, as can cause clinical deterioration; start at very

low dose and up-titrate gradually toward target dose as tolerated by symptoms

[24] For patients with LVEF ≤35 % in non-ischemic dilated or ischemic cardiomyopathy, at least 40 days post-AMI, EF ≤30 % (NYHA class I) or ≤35 % (NYHA class II–III), if already receiving appropriate medical therapy and have reasonable expectation of survival >1 year

[25] Safe with multiple benefits, including improvements in mortality, functional capacity, exercise duration, QOL, decreased hospitalizations

[26] ACEIs first choice but ARBs considered reasonable alternative

[27] All patients with fluid retention, with close monitoring of electrolytes and renal function; loop diuretics (furosemide, torsemide, bumetanide) are first-line, with second line intermittent use of thiazide "boosters" (metolazone, chlorothiazide)

[28] Aldosterone antagonists recommended to decrease morbidity and mortality in NYHA class II–IV with LVEF ≤35 % or with LVEF ≤40 % post-AMI or in DM (providing acceptable blood creatinine and potassium); blood creatinine and K should be closely monitored

[29] Use digoxin with caution including close monitoring of electrolytes and appearance of dysrhythmias, heart block, GI symptoms, neurological changes; reduce hospitalizations but not mortality, which may actually increase with its use

[30] Except for BP control, drug treatment for HFpEF not efficacious, with no proven strategies to decrease mortality

[31] EF ≤35 %, HR ≥70 bpm, persistent symptoms, despite beta-blockers and RAAS-inhibition or when beat-blockers not tolerated

[32] Occurs in >50 % of patients with LVEF <40 % and severity correlates with survival; invasive management remains controversial; also common in patients with HFpEF

[33] Early medical treatment can slow HF progression

[34] Suggests liver congestion

[35] Fluid redistribution while recumbent

[36] Measure of RA pressure that correlates with PCWP; should not be used as a marker of PCWP in AMI-related HF

[37] Highly indicative of decreased cardiac output

[38] Proportional pulse pressure (systolic BP minus diastolic BP/systolic BP) <25 % correlates with cardiac index <2.2 L/min by RH catheterization; decreased pulse pressure associated with poor prognosis in HFrEF but less correlation with prognosis in HFpEF

[39] In addition to this list: cardiac enzyme measurement indicated if ACS suspected; special tests when underlying disease suspected (eg thyroid disease, connective tissue disease, Hemochromatosis); chemistries for monitoring HF treatment (eg, serum K with use of RAAS inhibitors)

[40] Also on CXR: cephalization, interstitial/alveolar edema, Kerley B lines

[41] 4-chamber dilatation suggests possible non-ischemic etiology

[42] About 50 % of HF readmissions due to comorbid conditions; comorbidities may occur more often with HFpEF

[43] Mildly increased blood K, mild decrease in renal function and BP expected; should be carefully monitored but do not require changing therapeutic course; ACEIs and ARBs similar for these effects

[44] Beta-blockers vary greatly in efficacy for HF, and special attention should be paid to GDMT for this class: only 1 of carvedilol, metoprolol, bisoprolol should be prescribed for HF

[45] Decreased BP, bradycardia, lethargy, depression exacerbation, impotence may occur with beta-blockers and occurrence may require down-titration to maximally tolerated dose if possible before discontinuation; when beta-blocker termination needed, should not be abrupt

[46] Beta-blockers in HF patients with:

DM: equal benefit in patients with/without DM

COPD: most patients tolerate well, but use caution with bronchospasm including slow titration and close monitoring

Peripheral vascular disease: may worsen limb ischemia but usually tolerated well

[47] Efficacy/safety of combining ARBs/ACEIs/aldosterone antagonists not supported by evidence and carries added risk of hyperkalemia

[48] No randomized trial data for guidance in absence of AF/history of thromboembolic event/recent AMI/ventricular thrombus

[49] Increased 2 year mortality by up to 70 %

[50] Anthracyclines (most severe; eg, doxorubicin), mitoxantrone, cyclophosphamide, mitomycin, trastuzumab, alemtuzumab, sorafenib, imatinib, paclitaxel, docetaxel

[51] Anthracycline-induced form may occur early during treatment (within 1 year) in acute form or delayed 10–20 years post-initial exposure; delayed form has very poor prognosis

[52] AF: both a trigger for and predictor of HF progression; occurs in >50 % of patients with HF

[53] Especially males and African-Americans hospitalized for worsening HFrEF

[54] Anemia associated with increased mortality/length of hospitalization: greater in patients with HFpEF than HFrEF

[55] May be associated with decreased mortality

[56] Galectin-3: associated with myocardial fibrosis/increased risk of HF/HF mortality

[57] ST2: cardiac biomarker assay; useful for prognosis; may be superior to galectin-3 for risk stratification; also increased in other CV conditions, including:

Acute Myocardial Infarction
Aortic Stenosis --Valvular
Arterial Hypertension --Systemic

Cardiomyopathy --Dilated
Diabetes Mellitus
Kawasaki Disease
Mitral Regurgitation --Chronic
Peripheral artery disease
Pulmonary Arterial Hypertension
Stable Ischemic heart disease
ST2 also increased in many non-CV conditions

[58] Cobalt toxicity should be considered in patients with prosthetic (metal-on-metal) hip replacement; removal of prosthesis has been associated with improvement/ reversal of cardiac dysfunction; other manifestations include:

Hypothyroidism
Neuropathy
Polycythemia

[59] In USA, current CMS criteria should be consulted for LVAD implant

[60] Most common lifestyle risk factors associated with decreased risk of HF:

Modest alcohol intake
Obesity avoidance
Physical activity
Tobacco avoidance

[61] FDA-approved indication for LCZ696: chronic heart failure (NYHA Class II–IV) and reduced EF

[62] Hypocalcemia as a reversible cause of HF should especially be considered in patients with QT prolongation and paresthesias; and in settings known to predispose to hypoparathyroidism, such as post-thyroidectomy; hypomagnesemia must also be taken into account in such patients

[63] Frequent PVCs associated with decreased LVEF, increased incidence of HF, and increased mortality

[64] Increased HR range (as measured by ambulatory ECG) associated with better prognosis

[65] Dysglycemia: common and is associated with increased risk of adverse CV outcomes
[66] AMI: HF frequent complication of first AMI, both during acute phase and shortly after hospital discharge
[67] Beta-blockers: tolerability comparable in HFrEF and HFpEF; short-term efficacy greater in HFrEF
[68] Sleep-Disordered Breathing: moderate-severe form common in patients with HF (prevalence >45 % in SchlaHF Registry); associated with:

> Age
> BMI
> Male sex
> Symptom severity/LV function

[69] Exercise test in patients with HFrEF: strong predictors of death including decreased:

> Peak Vo2
> Exercise duration
> % ppVo2

[70] Obesity: compared with subjects with normal BMI, obese patients may have up to 2× risk of HF, especially HFpEF
[71] Bariatric surgery: may be associated with decreased HF exacerbation rate in obese HF patients
[72] Heart Failure due to Congenital Heart Disease (from AHA Scientific Statement: Chronic Heart Failure in Congenital Heart Disease, J Am Coll Cardiol 2008;52:e143–e263):

> Major cause of late death (>30 days) in children after pediatric cardiac surgery, contributing to 27 % of deaths and occurring at median age of 5.2 years
> Leading cause of death in adults with CHD, described in 26 % of all deaths in a national registry of >8000 adults with CHD, with similar findings in other reports
> One study demonstrated that adults with CHD admitted with HF had fivefold increase in mortality compared with those who were not admitted;

also showed 1- and 3- year mortality rates of 24 and 35 % after a first HF admission

[73] Clinical presentation of adult HF patient with congenital heart disease may vary significantly by defect or age; patients can have classic symptoms of fatigue, dyspnea, and exercise intolerance but may manifest more subtle signs of malnutrition, growth failure, or cachexia

Guidelines

2013 ACCF/AHA guideline for the management of heart failure
J Am Coll Cardiol. 2013;62:e147–239. http://content.onlinejacc.org/article.aspx?articleid=1695825.

ESC guidelines for the diagnosis and treatment of acute and chronic heart failure 2012
Eur Heart J. 2012;33:1787–847. http://eurheartj.oxfordjournals.org/content/ehj/33/14/1787.full.pdf.

NICE: implantable cardioverter defibrillators and cardiac resynchronisation therapy for arrhythmias and heart failure
http://www.nice.org.uk/guidance/ta314.

Patient Information

AHA

Circulation.   2014;129:e293–4.   http://circ.ahajournals.org/content/129/3/e293.full.

Heart Diagrams

http://www.nlm.nih.gov/medlineplus/ency/imagepages/1056.htm.
http://www.nlm.nih.gov/medlineplus/ency/imagepages/1097.htm.
http://www.nlm.nih.gov/medlineplus/ency/imagepages/19387.htm.

General

http://www.nlm.nih.gov/medlineplus/ency/article/000158.htm.

General: Heart Failure

ENGLISH
  http://www.cardiosmart.org/~/media/Documents/Fact%20
  Sheets/en/tb1488.ashx.
ESPANOL
  http://www.cardiosmart.org/~/media/Documents/Fact%20
  Sheets/es-US/tb1488.

ACE Inhibitors

ENGLISH
  http://www.cardiosmart.org/~/media/Documents/Fact%20
  Sheets/en/zp3950.ashx.
ESPANOL
  http://www.cardiosmart.org/~/media/Documents/Fact%20
  Sheets/es-US/zp3950.ashx.

Aldosterone Receptor Antagonists

ENGLISH
  http://www.cardiosmart.org/~/media/Documents/Fact%20
  Sheets/en/tb1728.ashx.
ESPANOL
  http://www.cardiosmart.org/~/media/Documents/Fact%20
  Sheets/es-US/tb1728.ashx.

ARBS

ENGLISH
   http://www.cardiosmart.org/~/media/Documents/Fact%20
   Sheets/en/zp3959.ashx.
ESPANOL
   http://www.cardiosmart.org/~/media/Documents/Fact%20
   Sheets/es-US/zp3959.ashx.

Daily Weights

ENGLISH
   http://www.cardiosmart.org/~/media/Documents/Fact%20
   Sheets/en/zp3773.ashx.
ESPANOL
   http://www.cardiosmart.org/~/media/Documents/Fact%20
   Sheets/es-US/zp3773.ashx.

Digoxin

ENGLISH
   https://www.cardiosmart.org/~/media/Documents/Fact%20
   Sheets/en/zp3974.ashx.
ESPANOL
   https://www.cardiosmart.org/~/media/Documents/Fact%20Sheets/
   es-US/zp3974.ashx.

Diuretics

ENGLISH
   http://www.cardiosmart.org/~/media/Documents/Fact%20
   Sheets/en/tb1708.ashx.
ESPANOL
   http://www.cardiosmart.org/~/media/Documents/Fact%20
   Sheets/es-US/tb1708.ashx

Heart Rhythm Disturbances

ENGLISH
> https://www.cardiosmart.org/~/media/Documents/Fact%20Sheets/
> en/tb1476.ashx.

ESPANOL
> https://www.cardiosmart.org/~/media/Documents/Fact%20Sheets/
> es-US/tb1476.ashx

How Is Heart Failure Diagnosed?

ENGLISH
> http://www.cardiosmart.org/~/media/Documents/Fact%20
> Sheets/en/tb1491.ashx.

ESPANOL
> http://www.cardiosmart.org/~/media/Documents/Fact%20
> Sheets/es-US/tb1491.ashx.

How to Limit Fluids

ENGLISH
> http://www.cardiosmart.org/~/media/Documents/Fact%20
> Sheets/en/tb1470.ashx.

ESPANOL
> http://www.cardiosmart.org/~/media/Documents/Fact%20
> Sheets/es-US/tb1470.ashx.

How to Limit Sodium

ENGLISH
> http://www.cardiosmart.org/~/media/Documents/Fact%20
> Sheets/en/zp3754.ashx.

ESPANOL
> http://www.cardiosmart.org/~/media/Documents/Fact%20
> Sheets/es-US/zp3754.ashx.

Leg Edema

http://www.nlm.nih.gov/medlineplus/ency/imagepages/19607.htm.

Living with Heart Failure

ENGLISH
> http://www.cardiosmart.org/~/media/Documents/Fact%20
> Sheets/en/zp3778.ashx.

ESPANOL
> http://www.cardiosmart.org/~/media/Documents/Fact%20
> Sheets/es-US/zp3778.ashx.

Lifestyle Changes

ENGLISH
> http://www.cardiosmart.org/~/media/Documents/Fact%20
> Sheets/en/zp3781.ashx.

ESPANOL
> http://www.cardiosmart.org/~/media/Documents/Fact%20
> Sheets/es-US/zp3781.ashx.

Managing Other Diseases

ENGLISH
> http://www.cardiosmart.org/~/media/Documents/Fact%20
> Sheets/en/tb1482.ashx.

ESPANOL
> http://www.cardiosmart.org/~/media/Documents/Fact%20Sheets/
> es-US/tb1482.ashx.

Medicines that Slow Heart Failure

ENGLISH
> http://www.cardiosmart.org/~/media/Documents/Fact%20Sheets/
> en/tb1485.ashx.

ESPANOL
> http://www.cardiosmart.org/~/media/Documents/Fact%20Sheets/
> es-US/tb1485.ashx.

Medicines to Avoid

ENGLISH
http://www.cardiosmart.org/~/media/Documents/Fact%20Sheets/en/tb1467.ashx.
ESPANOL
http://www.cardiosmart.org/~/media/Documents/Fact%20Sheets/es-US/tb1467.ashx.

Shortness of Breath

Circulation.   2014;129:e447–9.   http://circ.ahajournals.org/content/129/15/e447.full.

Sleep APNEA

ENGLISH
http://www.cardiosmart.org/~/media/Documents/Fact%20Sheets/en/tb1479.ashx.
ESPANOL
http://www.cardiosmart.org/~/media/Documents/Fact%20Sheets/es-US/tb1479.ashx.

Understanding Heart Failure Symptoms

ENGLISH. http://www.cardiosmart.org/~/media/Documents/Fact%20Sheets/en/tb1494.ashx.
ESPANOL. http://www.cardiosmart.org/~/media/Documents/Fact%20Sheets/es-US/tb1494.ashx.

Vasodilators

ENGLISH. http://www.cardiosmart.org/~/media/Documents/Fact%20Sheets/en/zp3967.ashx.
ESPANOL. http://www.cardiosmart.org/~/media/Documents/Fact%20Sheets/es-US/zp3967.ashx.

Professional Information

AHA scientific statement: chronic heart failure in congenital heart disease.

Circulation. 2016;133:770–801. http://circ.ahajournals.org/content/133/8/770.full.

AHA scientific statement: transitions of care.

Circulation Heart Fail. 2015;8:384–409. http://circheartfailure.ahajournals.org/content/8/2/384.full.

AHA/HFSA scientific statement: care in skilled nursing facilities.

Circulation Heart Fail. 2015;8:655–87 http://circheartfailure.ahajournals.org/content/8/3/655.full.

History

Circulation Heart Fail. 2008;1:63–71.
http://circheartfailure.ahajournals.org/content/1/1/63.full.

Review

J Nurse Pract. 2013;9:634–42.
http://www.sciencedirect.com/science/article/pii/S1555415513005357.

Review

Cleveland   clinic   center   for   continuing   education. http://www.clevelandclinicmeded.com/medicalpubs/diseasemanagement/cardiology/heart-failure/#references.

Review: Acute HF in Africa

Heart 2013;99:1317-1322. http://heart.bmj.com/content/99/18/1317.abstract

Review: ARB/Neprilysin Inhibitor

J Am Coll Cardiol. 2015;65:1029–41. http://content.onlinejacc.org/article.aspx?articleID=2194884.

Review: Cardiomyopathies

J Nurse Pract. 2007;3:248–58. http://www.sciencedirect.com/science/article/pii/S1555415507000189.

Review: Classification and Pathophysiology

Med. 2010;38:467–72. http://www.sciencedirect.com/science/article/pii/S1357303910001519.

Review: Drugs

JAMA. 2015;313:1052–3. http://jama.jamanetwork.com/article.aspx?articleid=2190983.

Review: from Acute Decompensated to Chronic Heart Failure

Am J Cardiol. 2014;114:1923–9. http://www.sciencedirect.com/science/article/pii/S000291491401861X.

Review: Gene Therapy

Cardiovascular Res. 2015;108:4–20. http://cardiovascres.oxfordjournals.org/content/108/1/4.full.

Review: HFpEF Phenotypes

J Am Heart Assoc. 2016;5:e002477. http://jaha.ahajournals.org/content/5/1/e002477?etoc.

Review: LCZ696/Entresto (Opinion)

Ann Intern Med. 2016;164:125–6. http://annals.org/article. aspx?articleID=2478160.

Review: LVAD

J Am Coll Cardiol. 2015;65:2542–55. http://content.onlinejacc.org/ article.aspx?articleID=2319402.

Review: Management Mechanisms

Heart.2016;102:707–11.http://heart.bmj.com/content/102/9/707?etoc.

Review: Pharmacotherapy

Eur Heart J Cardiovasc Pharmacother. 2015;1:10–2. http://ehjcvp. oxfordjournals.org/content/1/1/10.full.

Review: Stem Cell/Regenerative RX

Philos Trans R Soc Lond B Biol Sci. 2015 19;370(1680):20140373. doi: 10.1098/rstb.2014.0373. http://rstb.royalsocietypublishing. org/content/370/1680/20140373.long.

Review: Treatment

J Nurse Pract. 2013;9:224–32. http://www.sciencedirect.com/science/ article/pii/S1555415513005357.

ACE Inhibitors

JAMA. 1995;273:1450–6. http://jama.jamanetwork.com/article. aspx?articleid=388358.

Acute Myocardial Infarction

J Am Heart Assoc. 2016;5:e002667. http://jaha.ahajournals.org/content/5/1/e002667.full.

Acute Myocardial Infarction

Heart Fail Clin. 2012;8:43–51. http://www.sciencedirect.com/science/article/pii/S1551713611000961.

Alcohol/Mortality

Am J Cardiol. 2014;114:1065–8. http://www.sciencedirect.com/science/article/pii/S0002914914014490.

Alcohol/Risk

Circulation: Heart Fail.2015;8:422–7. http://circheartfailure.ahajournals.org/content/8/3/422.full#ref-26.

Alcohol/Risk

Eur Heart J. 2015. doi: http://dx.doi.org/10.1093/eurheartj/ehu514. http://eurheartj.oxfordjournals.org/content/early/2015/01/17/eurheartj.ehu514

Aldosterone Antagonism (Spironolactone): Topcat Study

Circulation. 2015; 131:34–42. http://circ.ahajournals.org/content/131/1/34.abstract?etoc.

Anemia and Outcomes: HFpEF Versus HFrEF

Am J Cardiol. 2014;114:1850–4. http://www.ajconline.org/article/S0002-9149(14)01852-9/abstract.

Angiotensin: Neprilysin Inhibition

N Engl J Med. 2014;371:993–1004. http://www.nejm.org/doi/full/10.1056/NEJMoa1409077#t=articleResults

Angiotensin: Neprilysin Inhibition

Circulation. 2015;131:54–61. http://circ.ahajournals.org/content/131/1/54.abstract?etoc.

Anthracycline

Circulation. 2015;131:1981–8. http://circ.ahajournals.org/content/131/22/1981.full.

Anthracycline

J Am Coll Cardiol. 2010;55:213–20. http://content.onlinejacc.org/article.aspx?articleID=1140340.

Aquapharesis Versus Diuretics

J Am Coll Cardiol HF. 2016;4:95–105. http://heartfailure.onlinejacc.org/article.aspx?articleID=2467229.

ARBS

Br J Cardiol. 2010;17:s10–2. http://bjcardio.co.uk/2010/05/arbs-in-chronic-heart-failure/.

Atrial Fibrillation

Circulation. 2016;133:484–92. http://circ.ahajournals.org/content/133/5/484.abstract.

Atrial Fibrillation

Eur Heart J. 2015;36:3250–7. http://eurheartj.oxfordjournals.org/content/36/46/3250.full?etoc.

Atrial Fibrillation

Circulation. 2009;119:2516–25. http://circ.ahajournals.org/content/119/18/2516.full?sid=f0fae08f-980b-474f-bee3-1561b90af589.

Atrial Fibrillation (New Onset): HF Progression

Am J Med. 2014;127:963–71. http://www.sciencedirect.com/science/article/pii/S0002934314004793.

Atrial Fibrillation: Rhythm Control

J Am Coll Cardiol. 2014;64:710–21. http://content.onlinejacc.org/article.aspx?articleID=1895477.

Atrial Fibrillation: Rhythm Versus Rate Control

N Engl J Med. 2008;358:2667–77. http://www.nejm.org/doi/full/10.1056/NEJMoa0708789.

Bariatric Surgery

Circ Heart Fail. 2016;9:e002260. doi: 10.1161/CIRCHEART FAILURE.115.002260.
http://circheartfailure.ahajournals.org/content/9/3/e002260.abstract.

Bariatric Surgery

J Am Coll Cardiol. 2016;67:895–903. http://content.onlinejacc.org/article.aspx?articleID=2492944.

Beta-Blockers

Mayo Clin Proc. 2009;84:718–29. http://www.ncbi.nlm.nih.gov/pmc/
articles/PMC2719525/.

Beta-Blockers: Tolerability/Feasibility in HFrEF Vs HFpEF

J Am Coll Cardiol HF. 2016;4:140–9. http://heartfailure.onlinejacc.
org/article.aspx?articleID=2475067.

BNP: Guided Treatment

Eur Heart J. 2014;35:1559–67. http://eurheartj.oxfordjournals.org/
content/35/23/1559.

BNP: Predictor of Worsening HF

J Am Coll Cardiol HF. 2014;2:148–58. http://heartfailure.onlinejacc.
org/article.aspx?articleid=1857471.

BNP: Prognosis IN LVrEF/LVpEF HF

J Am Coll Cardiol. 2013;61:1498–506. http://content.onlinejacc.org/
issue.aspx?journalid=101&issueid=926685.

CAD (Commentary)

Am J Med. 2014;127:574–8. http://www.sciencedirect.com/science/
article/pii/S0002934314001430.

Cardiohepatic Interactions

J Am Coll Cardiol. 2013;61:2397–405. http://content.onlinejacc.org/
article.aspx?articleID=1696807.

Cardiorenal Syndrome

J Am Coll Cardiol. 2008;52:1527–39. http://content.onlinejacc.org/article.aspx?articleID=1187963.

Central Sleep APNEA

J Am Coll Cardiol. 2015;65:72–84. http://content.onlinejacc.org/article.aspx?articleid=2087923.

Cobalt Toxicity/Hip Prosthesis

Circulation Cardiovascular Imaging. 2015;8:e003352. http://circimaging.ahajournals.org/content/8/6/e003352.extract?.

Comorbidities

J Am Coll Cardiol HF. 2015;3:542–50. http://heartfailure.onlinejacc.org/article.aspx?articleID=2375103.

Comorbidities (Multimorbidity)

Am J Med. 2015;128:38–45. http://www.sciencedirect.com/science/article/pii/S0002934314007906.

Comorbidities: Non-cardiac in HFrEF

J Am Coll Cardiol. 2014;64:2281–93. http://content.onlinejacc.org/article.aspx?articleID=1974825.

Cognitive Impairment

Am J Med. 2013;126:120–6. http://www.sciencedirect.com/science/article/pii/S000293431200558X.

COPD

Eur Heart J. 2013;34:2795–807. http://eurheartj.oxfordjournals.org/content/34/36/2795.

CPAP

N Engl J Med. 2005;353:2025–33. http://www.nejm.org/doi/full/10.1056/NEJMoa051001.

CRT

Circulation. 2013;128:2407–18. http://circ.ahajournals.org/content/128/22/2407.full.

CRT

Eur Heart J. 2013;34:1396–403. http://eurheartj.oxfordjournals.org/content/34/19/1396.

CRT

J Cardiovasc Electrophysiol. 2012; 23:163–8. http://onlinelibrary.wiley.com/doi/10.1111/j.1540-8167.2011.02144.x/abstract.

CRT: RV Function/Outcomes

Heart. 2013;99:722–8. http://heart.bmj.com/content/99/10/722.abstract.

CRT: Response/QRS Widening

Am J Cardiol. 2015;115:214–9. http://www.sciencedirect.com/science/article/pii/S0002914914020128.

CRT-D: Survival

N Engl J Med. 2014;370:1694–701. http://www.nejm.org/doi/
full/10.1056/NEJMoa1401426.

Depression

Am J Cardiol. 2012;109:768–72. http://www.sciencedirect.com/sci-
ence/article/pii/S0002914911032139.

Diabetes Mellitus: Effect on Outcomes

Circulation. 2015;132:923–31. http://circ.ahajournals.org/content/
132/10/923.abstract.

Diabetes Mellitus

Diabetes Care. 2004;27:1879–84. http://care.diabetesjournals.org/
content/27/8/1879.long.

Diet: Sodium

Circulation. 2012;126:479–85. http://circ.ahajournals.org/content/
126/4/479.full?sid=8b7664b2-3963-4266-a017-be15b03de36e.

Digoxin: Increased Risk (Review/ Metaanalysis)

Eur Heart J. 2015 doi: http://dx.doi.org/10.1093/eurheartj/ehv143.
http://eurheartj.oxfordjournals.org/content/early/2015/04/30/eur-
heartj.ehv143

Digoxin

J Am Coll Cardiol. 2014;63:1823–32. http://content.onlinejacc.org/
article.aspx?articleID=1841453.

Digoxin

Am J Med. 2013;127:61–70. http://www.amjmed.com/article/
S0002-9343(13)00786-9/fulltext.

Digoxin

N Engl J Med. 1997;336:525–33. http://www.nejm.org/doi/
full/10.1056/NEJM199702203360801.

Diuretics

Eur Heart J. 2014;35:1284–93. http://eurheartj.oxfordjournals.org/
content/35/19/1284.

Diuretics

Am J Med. 1981;70:234–9. http://www.sciencedirect.com/science/
article/pii/0002934381907555.

Diuresis: Hemoconcentration-Directed

Am J Med. 2014;127:1154–9. http://www.sciencedirect.com/science/
article/pii/S0002934314004823.

Echo-dopper Hemodynamics

Circulation.   2015;131:1031–4.   http://circ.ahajournals.org/con-
tent/131/11/1031.full.

Economic Burden

J Am Coll Cardiol. 2014;63:1123–33. http://content.onlinejacc.org/
article.aspx?articleID=1828672.

Eplerenone: HF/Rehospitalization

Eur Heart J. 2015 36: 2310–7. http://eurheartj.oxfordjournals.org/content/36/34/2310.abstract?etoc.

Exercise Testing: Predictors of Death in HFrEF

J Am Coll Cardiol. 2016;67:780–9. http://content.onlinejacc.org/article.aspx?articleID=2491761.

Exercise Training

Circulation Heart Fail. 2015;8:209–20. http://circheartfailure.ahajournals.org/content/8/1/209.extract.

Exercise Training: HF-Action Trial

JAMA. 2009;301:1439–50. http://jama.jamanetwork.com/article.aspx?articleid=183708.

Exercise Training

BMJ. 2004:37938.645220.EE. http://www.bmj.com/content/early/2003/12/31/bmj.37938.645220.EE.

Galactin-3

J Am Coll Cardiol. 2012;60:1249–56. http://www.sciencedirect.com/science/article/pii/S0735109712023881.

Genetics: Causes

J Clin Invest. 2005;115:518–26. http://www.jci.org/articles/view/24351.

Heart Rate Range (Ambulatory ECG)/ Prognosis

Heart. 2016;102:223–9. http://heart.bmj.com/content/102/3/223.full.

Heart Rate: Prognostic Risk Factor

Eur Heart J. 2015;36:669–75. http://eurheartj.oxfordjournals.org/content/36/11/669.full?etoc.

Heart Rate at Time of Discharge: Risk for Death/Rehospitalization

J Am Heart Assoc. 2015;4:e001626. http://jaha.ahajournals.org/content/4/4/e001626.abstract.

HFpEF: Diabetes Mellitus

J Am Coll Cardiol. 2014;64:541–49. http://content.onlinejacc.org/article.aspx?articleid=1894685&resultClick=24.

HFpEF: Doppler Echo

Heart. 2014;100:68–76. http://heart.bmj.com/content/100/1/68.full.

HFpEF: Echo Evaluation of LV Diastolic Function

J Am Soc Echocardiogr. 2009;22:107–33. http://www.onlinejase.com/article/S0894-7317(08)00739-6/abstract.

HFpEF: Left Atrium

Circulation: Heart Fail. 2014;7:1042–9. http://circheartfailure.aha-journals.org/content/7/6/1042.extract?etoc.

HFpEF: Misconceptions

Am J Med. 2014;127:1144–7. http://www.sciencedirect.com/science/article/pii/S0002934314004847.

HFpEF: Mitral Regurgitation

J Cardiac Fail. 2011;117:806–12. http://www.sciencedirect.com/science/article/pii/S1071916411006257#.

HFpEF: Review

Eur Heart J. 2011;32:670–9. http://eurheartj.oxfordjournals.org/content/32/6/670.full?sid=a43135a3-ff6d-4b19-901c-6b3719f0c783.

HFpEF: Prevalence, Clinical Characteristics, Outcomes

Br J Cardiol. 2016;23:1. http://bjcardio.co.uk/2016/02/prevalence-clinical-characteristics-and-outcomes-of-hf-with-preserved-versus-reduced-ejection-fraction/.

HFpEF: RV Dysfunction

Circulation. 2014;130:2310–20. http://circ.ahajournals.org/content/130/25/2310.full.

HFpEF: RV Dysfunction

Eur Heart J. 2014;35:3452–62. http://eurheartj.oxfordjournals.org/content/35/48/3452.

HFpEF: Targeted Phenotypic Therapies

Eur Heart J. 2014;35:2797–815. http://eurheartj.oxfordjournals.org/content/35/40/2797

HFpEF: Trends

Circulation. 2012;126:65–75. http://circ.ahajournals.org/content/126/1/65.full?sid=f0fae08f-980b-474f-bee3-1561b90af589.

HFrEF: Mitral Regurgitation

Am J Cardiol. 2003;91:538–43. http://www.sciencedirect.com/science/article/pii/S0002914902033015.

High Output Failure: Renal Cell Carcinoma

Am J Med. 2014;127:22–4. http://www.sciencedirect.com/science/article/pii/S0002934313008474.

Histamine H2 Receptor Antagonists: Decreased HF Risk

J Am Coll Cardiol. 2016;67:1544–52. http://content.onlinejacc.org/article.aspx?articleID=2506358.

HIV

Circulation.   2014;129:1781–9.   http://circ.ahajournals.org/content/129/17/1781.full.

Hydralazine-Isosorbide Dinitrate in African-Americans

N Engl J Med. 2004;351:2049–57. http://www.nejm.org/doi/full/10.1056/NEJMoa042934.

Hydralazine-Isosorbide Dinitrate in African-Americans: Follow Up

Am J Cardiol. 2014;114:151–9. http://www.sciencedirect.com/science/article/pii/S0002914914009758.

Hyperglycemia

Circulation: Heart Fail. 2016;9:e002560. http://circheartfailure.ahajournals.org/content/9/1/e002560.abstract?etoc.

Hypocalcemia

J Emerg Med. 2005;28:155–9. http://www.sciencedirect.com/science/article/pii/S0736467904003269.

Hypocalcemia

N Engl J Med. 1982;307:869–72. http://www.nejm.org/doi/full/10.1056/NEJM198209303071407.

ICD: Adherence to Recommended Medications Before Implanation

J Am Coll Cardiol. 2016;67:1062–9. http://content.onlinejacc.org/article.aspx?articleID=2498352.

ICD

N Engl J Med. 1996;335:1933–40. http://www.nejm.org/doi/full/10.1056/NEJM199612263352601.

Imaging

J Am Coll Cardiol Img. 2010;3:429–39. http://imaging.onlinejacc.org/article.aspx?articleid=1109572.

Influenza Vaccination

J Am Coll Cardiol HF. 2016;4:152–8. http://heartfailure.onlinejacc.org/article.aspx?articleID=2479251.

Insomnia

Eur Heart J. 2014;35:1382–93. http://eurheartj.oxfordjournals.org/content/35/21/1382.

Intestinal Blood Flow

J Am Coll Cardiol. 2014;64:1092–102. http://content.onlinejacc.org/article.aspx?articleID=1902267.

Iron Deficiency

Heart. 2014;100:1414–20. http://heart.bmj.com/content/100/18/1414. abstract.

Iron Deficiency

Eur Heart J. 2013;34:816–29. http://eurheartj.oxfordjournals.org/ content/34/11/816.

Iron Therapy

Eur Heart J. 2015;36:657–68. http://eurheartj.oxfordjournals.org/ content/36/11/657.full?etoc.

Ivabradine

Lancet. 2010;376:11–7. http://www.sciencedirect.com/science/article/ pii/S0140673610611981.

Ivabradine: Collateral Coronary Circulation

Heart. 2014;100:160–6. http://heart.bmj.com/content/100/2/160. abstract.

Ivabradine: HR Rate Slowing Effect on Symptoms with HFpEF

Circulation. 2015;132:1719–25. http://circ.ahajournals.org/content/132/18/1719.full.

Ivabradine: LV Afterload Reduction

J Am Coll Cardiol. 2013;62:1977–85. http://content.onlinejacc.org/article.aspx?articleID=1725473.

Ivabradine: Outcomes

Eur Heart J. 2013;34:2263–70. http://eurheartj.oxfordjournals.org/content/34/29/2263.abstract.

Kidney Disease

Eur Heart J. 2012;33:2135–42. http://eurheartj.oxfordjournals.org/content/33/17/2135.full?sid=839f0731-0aed-4777-82df-afb57fa0c8b2.

Lifestyle Risk Factors

J Am Coll Cardiol HF. 2015;3:520–8. http://heartfailure.onlinejacc.org/article.aspx?articleID=2375099.

Liver Dysfunction

J Am Coll Cardiol. 2013;61:2253–61. http://content.onlinejacc.org/article.aspx?articleID=1677774.

LCZ696 (Angiotensin Receptor-Neprilysin Inhibitor)

Eur Heart J. 2015;36:434–9. http://eurheartj.oxfordjournals.org/content/36/7/434.

LCZ696 (Angiotensin Receptor-Neprilysin Inhibitor)

N Engl J Med. 2014;371:993–1004. http://www.nejm.org/doi/full/10.1056/NEJMoa1409077.

Left Atrial Function

Eur Heart J. 2015;36:733–42. http://eurheartj.oxfordjournals.org/content/36/12/733.full?etoc.

LVAD: Post-implant Management

Circulation. 2014;129:116–6. http://circ.ahajournals.org/content/129/10/1161.full.

Metabolic Impairment

J Am Coll Cardiol. 2014;64:1388–400. http://content.onlinejacc.org/article.aspx?articleID=1909592.

Metabolic Syndrome

Eur Heart J. 2015;36:2630–4. http://eurheartj.oxfordjournals.org/content/36/39/2630.

Minnesota Living with Heart Failure Questionnaire

Am Heart J. 1992;124:1017–25. http://www.sciencedirect.com/science/article/pii/0002870392909866.

Mitral Valve Flow Pattern in Diastolic Dysfunction

J Am Coll Cardiol. 1994;24:132–9. http://www.sciencedirect.com/science/article/pii/0735109794905533.

Mitral Valve Repair: Dilated Cardiomyopathies

Semin Thorac Cardiovasc Surg. 2012;24:51–8. http://www.ncbi.nlm.nih.gov/pubmed/22643662.

Monitoring: Remote

Heart. 2013;99:23:1717–26. http://heart.bmj.com/content/99/23/1717.full?sid=2c6e9ddc-dd65-4a0e-bdbc-cae580fe0825.

Monitoring: Wireless Pulmonary Artery Pressure

Lancet. 2011;377:658–66. http://www.thelancet.com/journals/lancet/article/PIIS0140-6736(11)60101-3/fulltext.

Monitoring: Wireless Pulmonary Artery Pressure in HFpEF

Circulation Heart Fail. 2014;7:935–44. http://circheartfailure.ahajournals.org/content/7/6/935.abstract?etoc.

Myocardial Fibrosis

J Am Coll Cardiol. 2016;67:251–60. http://content.onlinejacc.org/article.aspx?articleID=2481268.

Myocardial Interstitium

J Am Coll Cardiol. 2014;63:2188–98. http://content.onlinejacc.org/article.aspx?articleID=1847355.

Neurohormone/Sex Differences: Outcomes

Eur Heart J. 2013;34:2538–47. http://eurheartj.oxfordjournals.org/content/34/32/2538.

Obesity/Abdominal Adiposity/Overweight: Risk Factors

Circulation. 2016;133:639–49. http://circ.ahajournals.org/content/133/7/639.full.

Obesity: Paradox

J Am Coll Cardiol. 2014;64:2743–49. http://content.onlinejacc.org/article.aspx?articleID=2085758.

Obesity: Risk Factor

N Engl J Med. 2002;347:305–13. http://www.nejm.org/doi/full/10.1056/NEJMoa020245#t=article.

Obstructive Sleep Apnea

Arch Intern Med. 2006;166:1716–22. http://archinte.jamanetwork.com/article.aspx?articleid=410840.

Omecamtiv Mecarbil

J Am Coll Cardiol. 2016;67:1444–55. http://content.onlinejacc.org/article.aspx?articleID=2505134.

Outcomes: Stratified by Cardiomyopathy Etiology

J Am Coll Cardiol HF. 2015;3:906–16. http://heartfailure.onlinejacc.org/article.aspx?articleID=2451393.

Outcomes: Collaborative Care

Circulation. 2010;122:1806–14. http://circ.ahajournals.org/content/122/18/1806.full.pdf+html?sid=ebe93cdd-a461-4b98-b68d-7610b61b20cf

Outcomes: Readmission Rates/Predictors

Circulation Heart Fail. 2012;5:672–9. http://circheartfailure.ahajournals.org/content/5/6/672.full.pdf+html.

Outcomes: Rehospitalization Reduction Strategies

Circulation Cardiovasc Qual Out. 2013;6:444–50. http://circoutcomes.ahajournals.org/content/6/4/444.full.pdf+html.

Outcomes: Rehospitalization Reduction Strategies

J-Nurse Pract. 2013;9:224–32. http://www.sciencedirect.com/science/article/pii/S1555415513000275.

Pathophysiology

Cardiovasc Pathol. 2012;21:365–71. http://www.sciencedirect.com/science/article/pii/S1054880711001529.

Performance Measures: ACCF/AHA/ AMA- PCPI

Circulation.   2012;125:2382–401.   http://circ.ahajournals.org/content/125/19/2382.

Pericardial Effusion

Eur Heart J. 2013;34:1414–23. http://eurheartj.oxfordjournals.org/content/34/19/1414.

Phenotypes: Sex Differences

Circulation Cardiovasc Qual Out. 2015;8:S48–51. http://circoutcomes.ahajournals.org/content/8/2-suppl-1/S48.extract?etoc.

Pregnancy

Heart. 2014;100:231–8. http://heart.bmj.com/content/100/3/231.full.

Prevention

Circulation. 2008;117:2544–65. http://circ.ahajournals.org/content/117/19/2544.full?sid=f0fae08f-980b-474f-bee3-1561b90af589.

Pulmonary Hypertension

Eur Heart J. 2016;37:942–54. http://eurheartj.oxfordjournals.org/content/37/12/942.full?etoc.

Pulse Pressure Decrease: Prognosis in HFrEF Versus HFpEF

Eur Heart J. 2015 doi: http://dx.doi.org/10.1093/eurheartj/ehu490. http://eurheartj.oxfordjournals.org/content/early/2015/01/22/eur-heartj.ehu490.

PVCS: LVEF/HF/Mortality

J Am Coll Cardiol. 2015;66:101–9. http://content.onlinejacc.org/article.aspx?articleID=2383167.

QOL: Rural Patients

Circulation Heart Fail.2014;7:882–7. http://circheartfailure.ahajournals.org/content/7/6/882.full.

Rehospitalization

J Am Coll Cardiol. 2013;61:391–403. http://content.onlinejacc.org/article.aspx?articleID=1481163.

Rehospitalization: Risk Factors

J Am Coll Cardiol. 2013;61:635–42. http://content.onlinejacc.org/article.aspx?articleID=1567645.

Relapsing Catastrophic Antiphospholipid Antibody Syndrome (Case Report)

Am J Med. 2015;128:e13–4. http://www.sciencedirect.com/science/article/pii/S0002934314012200.

Remodeling

J Am Coll Cardiol Img. 2011;4:98–108. http://imaging.onlinejacc.org/article.aspx?articleid=1109830.

Remote Monitoring

Heart. 2013;99:1717–26. http://heart.bmj.com/content/99/23/1717.abstract.

Renal Dysfunction: Outcomes

Eur Heart J. 2014;35:455–69. http://eurheartj.oxfordjournals.org/content/35/7/455.

Renal Insufficiency: Treatment in HF

J Am Coll Cardiol. 2014;63:853–71. http://content.onlinejacc.org/article.aspx?articleID=1811652.

Scorpion Envenomation: Pulmonary Edema

Int J Cardiol. 2013;162:86–91. http://www.ncbi.nlm.nih.gov/pubmed/22075406?dopt=Abstract.

Seattle Heart Failure Model (Projected Survival Calculator)

http://depts.washington.edu/shfm/.

Serelaxin

Eur Heart J Cardiovasc Pharmacother. 2016;2:119–30. http://ehjcvp. oxfordjournals.org/content/2/2/119.full?etoc.

Serelaxin

Eur Heart J. 2014;35:431–41. http://eurheartj.oxfordjournals.org/ content/35/7/431.

Serelaxin

J Am Coll Cardiol. 2013;61:196–206. http://content.onlinejacc.org/ article.aspx?articleID=1500202.

Sinus Node Function: Remodeling

Circulation. 2004;110:897–903. http://circ.ahajournals.org/con- tent/110/8/897.full.

Skeletal Muscle Wasting

Eur Heart J. 2013;34:512–9. http://eurheartj.oxfordjournals.org/ content/34/7/512.

Sleep-Disordered Breathing

J Am Coll Cardiol HF. 2016;4:116–25. http://heartfailure.onlinejacc. org/article.aspx?articleID=2475324.

Socioeconomic Status/Outcomes

Circulation Heart Fail. 2015;8:473–80. http://circheartfailure.aha-journals.org/content/8/3/473.abstract?.

Spironolactone

N Engl J Med. 1999;341:709–17. http://www.nejm.org/doi/full/10.1056/NEJM199909023411001.

Sodium Nitrite Infusion

Circulation Heart Fail. 2015;8:565–71. http://circheartfailure.aha-journals.org/content/8/3/565.full.

Stem Cell/Regenerative RX: Metaanalysis

Circ Res. 2015;116:1361–77. http://circres.ahajournals.org/content/116/8/1361.abstract.

ST2 Assay

Am J Cardiol. 2015;115 Suppl:A1–8, 1B-80B. http://www.ajconline.org/issue/S0002-9149(15)X0003-8.

Strategies for Reducing Readmissions

J Nurse Pract. 2014;10:430–3. http://www.sciencedirect.com/science/article/pii/S1555415514002591.

Systemic Arterial Hypertension

Arch Int Med. 2011;171:384–94. http://archinte.jamanetwork.com/article.aspx?articleid=226833.

Thromboembolism Risk

Circulation. 2014;130:410–18. http://circ.ahajournals.org/content/130/5/410.full.

Transitional Care to Prevent Readmissions

Ann Intern Med. 2014;160:774–84. http://annals.org/article.aspx?articleid=1874735.

Tricuspid Regurgitation: Impact on Survival

Eur Heart J. 2013;34:844–52. http://eurheartj.oxfordjournals.org/content/34/11/844.

Ularitide

Eur Heart J. 2015;36:715–23. http://eurheartj.oxfordjournals.org/content/36/12/715.full?etoc.

Unidirectional L-R Interatrial Shunting

Lancet. 2016;387:1290–7. http://www.sciencedirect.com/science/article/pii/S0140673616005857.

Uric Acid

Semin   Nephrol.   2005;25:61–6.   http://www.ncbi.nlm.nih.gov/
pubmed/15660337.

Vagal Nerve Stimulation: Chronic Therapy for HFrEF

Eur Heart J. 2015 36:425–33. http://eurheartj.oxfordjournals.org/
content/36/7/425.

Valsalva Response

Am J Med. 2006;119:117–22. http://www.sciencedirect.com/science/
article/pii/S0002934305005668.

Updates and More

https://clinicalguidecvd.com/hf

Chapter 53
Systemic Arterial Hypertension (Essential Hypertension)

Management Keys

Consider secondary causes
Consider white coat syndrome [9]
Diagnose/treat target organ damage
Diagnose/treat co-existing CVD
Hospitalize for hypertension crisis [1]
Prescribe appropriate lifestyle modification [8]
Prescribe BP patient self-monitoring
Treat to target diastolic BP <90 mmHg in persons age <60 years
Treat to target sys BP <150 mmHg persons age >60 years

ICD-10 Code

I10

Alternate Names/Abbreviation

HTN
Essential hypertension

V.E. Friedewald, *Clinical Guide to Cardiovascular Disease*, 733
DOI 10.1007/978-1-4471-7293-2_53,
© Springer-Verlag London 2016

Description/Etiology

Diseases/conditions causing decreased intravascular compliance relative to circulating blood volume, leading to non-invasively measured systolic BP >140 mmHg/diastolic BP >90 mmHg

Genetic, environmental, lifestyle (eg, NaCl/K intake) factors, adiposity strongly influence development of primary HTN

Diagnosis: average of at least two readings obtained at three visits: 140/90 mmHg or greater

Secondary HTN occurs in up to 10 % of cases

Blood pressure increased risk for CVD beginning at 115/75 mmHg:

Linear
Continuous
Independent of/additive to other risk factors

Stages (JNC 7) (mm Hg):

Normal:	<120/80
Prehypertensive:	120/80–139/89
Stage 1:	140/90–159/99
Stage 2:	>159/110

Pseudohypertension: false BP elevation due to stiff, incompressible arteries [15]

White coat hypertension: increased office BP with normal home/ambulatory BP monitor [16]

Masked hypertension: normal office BP with increased BP at home/ambulatory BP monitoring [17]

Secondary hypertension causes: see predisposing/comorbid conditions; also suspect in patients with:

Drug-resistant HTN (>2 drugs at max doses)
New onset HTN age <25 years/>55 years
Severe vascular disease, including:
    Abdominal Aortic Aneurysm
    Aortic Dissection
    CAD

   Carotid Artery Stenosis
   Peripheral Artery Disease
   RAS
Resistant HTN: BP that remains above goal in spite of concurrent use of three antihypertensive agents of different classes; ideally, one of the three agents should be a diuretic and all agents should be prescribed at optimal doses [27] [28]

Predisposing/Comorbid Conditions [2] [6]

ACROMEGALY
ALDOSTERONISM
AMPHETAMINES
ATRIAL SEPTAL DEFECT, POST-CLOSURE
BRAIN TUMOR
BROMOCRYPTINE
CADMIUM TOXICITY
CHRONIC KIDNEY DISEASE
COARCTATION OF AORTA
COCAINE
CUSHING DISEASE
CYCLOSPORINE
DIABETES MELLITUS
DIABETIC NEPHROPATHY
DRUGS: CANCER THERAPY [13]
DRUGS: SYSTEMIC CORTICOSTEROIDS
DYSLIPIDEMIA
ECLAMPSIA
FIBROMUSCULAR DYSPLASIA
GLOMERULONEPHRITIS, ACUTE
GOUT
GUILLAIN-BARRE SYNDROME
HEART TRANSPLANT
HELLP SYNDROME
HEMANGIOPERICYTOMA
HYPERCALCEMIA
HYPERPARATHYROIDISM

HYPERTHYROIDISM
HYPERVISCOSITY SYNDROME
HYPOGLYCEMIA
HYPOKALEMIA
HYPOTHYROIDISM
LEAD POISONING
LICORICE
LIDDLE SYNDROME
METABOLIC SYNDROME
MITRAL ANNULAR CALCIFICATION
MULTIPLE ENDOCRINE NEOPLASIA
NEPHROTIC SYNDROME
NEUROBLASTOMA
NEUROFIBROMATOSIS
NONSTEROIDAL ANTIINFLAMMATORY DRUGS
OBESITY
OBSTRUCTIVE SLEEP APNEA
PHEOCHROMOCYTOMA
POLYCYSTIC KIDNEY DISEASE
POLYCYTHEMIA VERA
PREECLAMPSIA
PREGNANCY
QUADRIPLEGIA
RENAL ARTERY STENOSIS
RENAL EMBOLIZATION
RENAL FAILURE (UREMIA)
RENAL TRANSPLANT
SICKLE CELL DISEASE/TRAIT
TAKAYASU ARTERITIS
THALLIUM POISONING
TRANSFUSION
VASCULITIS, INTRARENAL
VON HIPPEL-LINDAU DISEASE

Demography

Age relation 40–70 years: each increment of 20 mmHg
systolic/10 mmHg diastolic doubles risk of CVD (in
range of 115/75–185/115 mmHg); risk increases

are higher in presence of other CV risk factors (eg, DM, CKD)

Populations: all

Location: global

Pathophysiology

Complex interplay of:

Aortic stiffness/fibrosis

Chronic intravascular volume expansion (largely due to excess salt intake)

Decreased vascular compliance

Increased vascular resistance

Multiple neurohormonal mechanisms, involved, including:

Increased RAAS activity

Increased sympathetic activity

Signs/Symptoms [5]

ARTERIAL PRESSURE – HIGHLY VARIABLE [26]

BLOOD PRESSURE, ARTERIAL – INCREASED/ ELEVATED

HEART, LV, APEX, IMP – FORCEFUL/SUSTAINED

HEART, S2, SPLIT – REVERSED (PARADOXICAL) [SEVERE HTN]

HEART, S4 LV

Differentiation [24]

Acromegaly

Acute Glomerulonephritis

Anemia

Anxiety

Aortic Dissection

Aortic Regurgitation – Chronic

Aortic rigidity (esp aging)
Atrioventricular Heart Block
Bath Salts – Recreation & Abuse
Beriberi
BZ Poisoning
Chlorine Poisoning
Chronic Nephritis
Coarctation Of Aorta
Cocaine
Collagen Vascular Disease
Congenital Adrenal Hyperplasia
Cushing Syndrome
Cyanide Poisoning
Diabetic Nephropathy
Drugs

  Amphetamines
  Anabolic steroids
  Antidepressants
  Appetite suppressants
  Caffeine
  Cocaine
  Cyclosporine
  Ecstasy
  Erythropoietin
  Ethanol
  Glucocorticoids
  Herbs

    Arnica
    Bitter orange
    Ephedra
    Gingko
    Gingseng
    Guarana
    Licorice
    Senna
    St Johns wort

  Ivabradine
  Mineralocorticoids

Monamine oxidase inhibitors
Nasal decongestants
NSAIDs
Oral contraceptives
Phenothiazines
Phenylephrine
Phenylcyclidine
Sympathomimetics
Tacrolimus
Tyramine

Dysautonomia
Elemental Mercury Poisoning – Acute
Erdheim-Chester Disease
Ethylene Glycol Poisoning
Extra adrenal chromaffin tumors
Fabry Disease
Fibromuscular Dysplasia
Guillain-Barre Syndrome
Hallucinogens – Recreation
Hydronephrosis
Hyperparathyroidism
Hypothyroidism
Lead Poisoning
Mineralocorticoid overproduction
Neurologic disorders
Nicotine Poisoning
Obstructive Sleep Apnea
Organophosphate Poisoning
Paget Bone Disease
Peripheral Extremity Arteriovenous Fistula
Pheochromocytoma
Polycystic Disease
Postoperative hypertension
Primary Aldosteronism
Quadriplegia
Renal Artery Stenosis
Renal parenchymal disease
Renal vascular disease
Sarin Poisoning

Takayasu Arteritis
Thallium Poisoning
VX Poisoning
Williams Syndrome
White Coat Syndrome

Complications

Atrial Fibrillation
Abdominal Aortic Aneurysm
Aortic Dissection
Cardiac arrhythmias
Cardiac hypertrophy
Carotid Artery Stenosis
Cerebral aneurysm
Cognitive changes [25]
Coronary artery disease
    AMI
    Stable Ischemic Heart Disease
Encephalopathy
HF
Intracerebral hemorrhage
Left ventricular hypertrophy
Nephropathy [4]
Peripheral Artery Disease
Renal failure [4]
Retinopathy
Stroke – Ischemic
Subarachnoid hemorrhage

Laboratory [7]

ASSESS FOR OTHER CAUSATIVE FACTORS, EG,
    ELECTROLYTES
ASSESS FOR TARGET ORGAN DAMAGE, EG,
    RENAL FUNCTION [4]
BLOOD, ST2 – INCR [22]

BLOOD, TROPONIN – INCR
BLOOD, URIC ACID – INCR
URINE, PROTEIN – INCR (PROTEINURIA)
  [NEPHROPATHY]

ECG

AV COND – BIFASCICULAR BLOCK [3]
DYSRHYTHMIAS – ATRIAL (PACS/OTHERS)
QRS – LBBB/LBBB PATTERN [3]
QRS – LVH PATTERN
QRS, AXIS – L

Imaging [10]

LA, CHAMBER, SIZE – INCR
LV, MYOCARD, WALL THICKNESS – INCR
  (HYPERTROPHY)
MYOCARD, THICKNESS – INCR

Genomics

ACCN3 [NOS3-PREGNANCY-INDUCED OMIM +163729]
APB1 [NOS3-PREGNANCY-INDUCED OMIM +163729]
KCNH2 [NOS3-PREGNANCY-INDUCED OMIM +163729]
NOS3 [NOS3-PREGNANCY-INDUCED OMIM +163729]
NR3C2 [EXACERBATION IN PREGNANCY]

Other Tests

Ambulatory BP monitoring – indications:

  Antihypertensive drug efficacy
  Diagnosis/treatment during pregnancy
  Early AM BP surge [19]
  Episodic normal/autonomic dysfunction

Loss of dipping status [18]

White coat HTN suspected

Masked HTN suspected
Nocturnal HTN
Symptomatic hypotension on therapy (patient may be
normotensive)
Unusual BP variability (may be associated with
increased risk)

Home/self-measured BP

Treatment: Nonpharmacologic [20]

Appropriate lifestyle modification [8] [29]

Treatment: Pharmacologic [11] [20]

Alpha-blockers [23]

Doxazosin
Prazosin
Terazosin

ACEIs [21]

Enalapril
Fosinopril
Lisinopril
Perindopril
Quinapril
Ramipril

ARBs [21]

Candesartan
Irbesartan
Losartan

Beta-Blockers [23]

> Atenolol
> Carvedilol
> Metoprolol
> Nebivolol
> Propranolol

CCBs

> Amlodipine
> Diltiazem
> Nifedipine
> Verapamil

Central beta-agonists [23]

> Clonidine
> Methyldopa

Direct renin inhibitors

> Aliskiren

Diuretics [21] [23]:

> Chlorothiazide
> Chlorthalidone
> Hydrochlorothiazide
> Indapamide

Guanethidine
Hydralazine

Treatment: Surgical/Invasive [12]

> Correction of secondary causes (e.g., aldosterone-secreting tumor resection, RAS angioplasty/stenting)
> Renal denervation [14]

Prevention

Adult screening (JNC 7): every 1–2 years depending on BP/other CV risk factors

Diet

Calorie control appropriate for weight management
Decreased Na
Increased K

Notes

[1] Severe hypertension crises requiring hospitalization/ emergency care include:

AMI
Aortic Dissection
Eclampsia
HF
Hypertensive encephalopathy
Intracranial hemorrhage
Post-CABG
Post-vascular surgery
Severe catecholamine excess, incl:
Clonidine withdrawal
Pheochromocytoma
Tyramine-MAOI interaction
Intoxication, including:

Cocaine
Phencyclidine
Phenylpropanolamine

Subarachnoid hemorrhage
Thrombotic stroke
Unstable angina

[2] Many in this list cause secondary HTN
[3] Often have coexisting CAD

[4] Renal damage secondary to increased intra-arterial pressures

[5] Does not include signs and symptoms of comorbid conditions/target organ damage

[6] Occult forms may be suspected in treatment-resistant HTN

[7] Basic tests for renal function, DM screen, and dyslipidemia screen indicated in all HTN patients; specific work-up for secondary causes reserved for high clinical suspicion or patients with resistant HTN

[8] Meticulous attention to:

Alcohol consumption (daily for males and 1/2 quantities for females)

2 mixed drinks; or
2 12 oz cans beer; or
2 4-oz glasses wine

CVD risk factors
Dietary sodium intake: no more than 2400 mg/day
Dyslipidemia
Regular aerobic exercise: 30 min most days of week
Tobacco cessation
Weight: maintain normal body weight (BMI 18.5–24.9 kg/m^2)

[9] Diagnostic ambulatory BP monitoring

[10] CXR and echo most often useful

[11] First-line treatment should comprise ACEI/ARB, thiazide, or CCB in non-blacks; avoid ACEI/ARB as first line therapy in black population

[12] Renal artery denervation for resistant HTN currently under investigation

[13] Includes bevacizumab, sorafenib, sunitinib, cisplatin, interferon-alpha

[14] Investigational

[15] Pseudohypertension: diagnose with Osler's maneuver: inflate cuff to 30 mmHg above palpable systolic pressure; try to "roll" brachial/radial artery under fingertips; healthy arteries should not be empty/not palpable; hard tube-like structure suggests pseudohypertension

[16] White coat HTN:

> Prevalence: 10–20 %
>
> Increased risk for overt Systemic Arterial Hypertension/ CVD
>
> Lifestyle modifications/regular follow-up recommended when diagnosed

[17] Masked HTN: 10–40 % of patients with HTN; associated with increased risk of sustained HTN/CV death

[18] Loss of dipping status: BP decreases <10 % at night compared to daytime BP

[19] Early AM BP surge: systolic BP 55 mmHg difference between sleep and early-hour awakening

[20] Target BP goals:

> AHA/ACC: All: <140/90 mmHg
>
> ESC: All: <140 mmHg (sys only)
>
> JNC 8 panel:
>
> > Patients <60 year of age: <140/90 mmHg
> > Patients >60 year of age: <150/90 mmHg
>
> Kidney disease improving global outcomes (KDIGO):
>
> > Patients with CKD: 130/80 mmHg
> > Patients with CKD/excreting >30 mg urine albumin/24 h: <130/80 mmHg

[21] JNC 8 panel members report: start treatment on thiazide diuretic except patients with DM or CKD for whom ACEI or ARB in combination with drug from another class is recommended; however some experts/British National Institute (NICE) recommend that chlorthalidone or indapamide should be used rather than hydrochlorothiazide as first-line drug for HTN

[22] JNC 7: compelling indications for specific drug classes:

> CKD:
>
> > ACEI
> > ARB

DM:

> ACEI
> ARB
> B-Blocker
> CCB
> Diuretic

HF:

> ACEI
> Aldosterone antagonist
> ARB
> Beta-blocker
> Diuretic

High CAD risk:

> ACEI
> ARB
> Beta-blocker
> CCB
> Diuretic

Post-AMI:

> ACEI
> Aldosterone antagonist
> B-Blocker

Recurrent stroke prevention

> ACEI
> Diuretic

[22] Increased ST2 correlates with presence of concentric LVH in patients with Systemic Arterial Hypertension
[23] Anti-sympathetic/adrenergic activity by drug treatment lowers BP but little/no evidence that this improves outcomes
[24] List comprises acute/chronic causes of BP elevation
[25] May be more common in African-Americans
[26] Higher visit-to-visit variability of systolic BP associated with increased risk for CVD and mortality, but unproven if treatment warranted

[27] Patient characteristics of resistant HTN in USA:

Black race
CKD
DM
Excessive dietary salt ingestion
Female sex
High baseline BP
LVH
Obesity
Older age
Residence in southeastern United States

[28] Medications that interfere with HTN treatment include:

Alcohol
Cyclosporine
Erythropoietin
Herbal compounds, including:

Ephedra
Ma huang

Natural licorice
Nonnarcotic analgesics

Nonsteroidal antiinflammatory agents, including aspirin
Selective COX-2 inhibitors

Oral contraceptives
Stimulants

Amphetamines
Dexmethylphenidate
Dextroamphetamine
Methamphetamines
Methylphenidate
Modafinil

Sympathomimetic agents

   Cocaine
   Decongestants
   Diet pills

[29] Lifestyle changes: **2013 ESH/ESC Guidelines for the management of arterial hypertension**

"5.1 Lifestyle changes

Appropriate lifestyle changes are the cornerstone for the prevention of hypertension. They are also important for its treatment, although they should never delay the initiation of drug therapy in patients at a high level of risk. Clinical studies show that the BP-lowering effects of targeted lifestyle modifications can be equivalent to drug monotherapy, although the major drawback is the low level of adherence over time—which requires special action to be overcome. Appropriate lifestyle changes may safely and effectively delay or prevent hypertension in non-hypertensive subjects, delay or prevent medical therapy in grade I hypertensive patients and contribute to BP reduction in hypertensive individuals already on medical therapy, allowing reduction of the number and doses of antihypertensive agents. Beside the BP-lowering effect, lifestyle changes contribute to the control of other CV risk factors and clinical conditions.

The recommended lifestyle measures that have been shown to be capable of reducing BP are: (i) salt restriction, (ii) moderation of alcohol consumption, (iii) high consumption of vegetables and fruits and low-fat and other types of diet, (iv) weight reduction and maintenance and (v) regular physical exercise. In addition, insistence on cessation of smoking is mandatory in order to improve CV risk, and because cigarette smoking has an acute pressor effect that may raise daytime ambulatory BP."

Guidelines

AHA/ACC/ASH scientific statement: treatment of hypertension in patients with coronary artery disease

Hypertension. 2015;65:1372–407. http://hyper.ahajournals.org/content/65/6/1372.full.

2013 ESH/ESC guidelines for the management of arterial hypertension

Eur Heart J.2014;34:2159–219. http://www.escardio.org/guidelines-surveys/esc-guidelines/Pages/arterial-hypertension.aspx.

JNC 7: Seventh Report of the Joint National Committee on Prevention, Detection, Evaluation, and Treatment of High Blood Pressure

Hypertension. 2003;42:1206–52. http://hyper.ahajournals.org/content/42/6/1206.long.

NICE: hypertension in adults: diagnosis and management. 2011

http://www.nice.org.uk/guidance/cg127/chapter/1-recommendations#choosing-antihypertensive-drug-treatment-2.

Patient Information

Medlineplus

ENGLISH
    http://www.nlm.nih.gov/medlineplus/highbloodpressure.html.
ESPANOL
    http://www.nlm.nih.gov/medlineplus/spanish/ency/article/000468.htm.

Mayo Clinic

http://www.mayoclinic.org/diseases-conditions/high-blood-pressure/basics/definition/con-20019580.

Genetics Home Reference

http://ghr.nlm.nih.gov/glossary=hypertension.

CDC

http://www.cdc.gov/bloodpressure/.

CDC: Reducing Sodium in Children's Diet

http://www.cdc.gov/vitalsigns/children-sodium/index.html.

Texas Heart Institute

http://www.texasheart.org/HIC/Topics/Cond/hbp.cfm.

Professional Information

AHA scientific statement: BP goals.
Hypertension. 2014;63:878–85. http://hyper.ahajournals.org/content/
    63/4/878.
AHA SC8IENTIFIC statement: resistant hypertension.
Hypertension. 2008;51:1403–19. https://c.ymcdn.com/sites/www.nyschp.
    org/resource/resmgr/Files/Resistant-Hypertension-2008-.pdf.

Review

Ann Intern Med. 2014;161(11):ITC1. http://annals.org/article.aspx?a
    rticleid=1984496&resultClick=24.

Review: Dietary Sodium

J Am Coll Cardiol. 2015;65:1042–50. http://content.onlinejacc.org/
    article.aspx?articleID=2194893.

Review: Drug Therapy

Eur Heart J. 2014;35:501–7. http://eurheartj.oxfordjournals.org/
    content/35/9/557.

Review: JNC 8/Future Recommendations

J Am Heart Assoc. 2015;4:e002315. http://jaha.ahajournals.org/content/4/12/e002315.full.

Review: Preeclampsia/Pregnancy Related HTN

Hypertension.   2016;67:238–42.   http://hyper.ahajournals.org/content/67/2/238.extract?etoc.

Review: Randomized RX Trials

Circulation Res. 2015;116:1058–73. http://circres.ahajournals.org/content/116/6/1058.full.

Review: Resistant HTN/CKD

Lancet.   2015;386:1588–98.   http://www.sciencedirect.com/science/article/pii/S0140673615004183.

Review: Resistant HTN

JAMA.   2014;311:2216–24.   http://jama.jamanetwork.com/article.aspx?articleid=1877189.

ACE Inhibitor Angioedema

Am J Med. 2015;128:120–5. http://www.sciencedirect.com/science/article/pii/S0002934314005919.

African Americans: Counseling

Circulation. 2014;129:2044–51. http://circ.ahajournals.org/content/129/20/2044.full.

Ambulatory BP Monitoring

Am J Med. 2015;128:14–20. http://www.sciencedirect.com/science/article/pii/S0002934314006597.

Ambulatory BP Monitoring

Circulation Res. 2015; 116:1034–45. http://circres.ahajournals.org/content/116/6/1034.full.

American Style Football

Circulation Cardio Qual Out. 2013;6:716–23. http://circoutcomes.ahajournals.org/content/6/6/716.full.

Aortic Stenosis: Treatment of HTN

Circulation.   2013;128:1349–53.   http://circ.ahajournals.org/content/128/12/1349.full.

Aortic Stiffness/Fibrosis

Hypertension.   2016;67:461–8.   http://hyper.ahajournals.org/content/67/2/461.abstract?etoc.

ARBS: Neuroprotection

Am J Hypertens. 2015;28:289–99. http://ajh.oxfordjournals.org/content/28/3/289.full?etoc.

Arterial Structural Changes

Circulation Res. 2015;116:1007–21. http://circres.ahajournals.org/content/116/6/1007.full.

Beta-Blockers: Central Systolic Pressure

Hypertension.   2016;67:316–24.   http://hyper.ahajournals.org/content/67/2/316.abstract?etoc.

CAD: BP Targets

Heart. 2013;99:601–13. http://heart.bmj.com/content/99/9/601.abstract.

CAD: Treatment-Resistant HTN

Am J Med. 2014;127:71–81. http://www.sciencedirect.com/science/article/pii/S0002934313007651.

Caffeine

Hypertension. 2015;65:691–6. http://hyper.ahajournals.org/content/65/3/691.abstract?etoc.

Cardiorespiratory Fitness

J Am Coll Cardiol. 2014;64:1245–53. http://content.onlinejacc.org/article.aspx?articleID=1905460.

Central Aortic Pressure: Effect of Antihypetensives

Am J Hypertens. 2016;29:448–57. http://ajh.oxfordjournals.org/content/29/4/448.abstract?etoc.

CKD: Resistant HTN

J Am Coll Cardiol. 2013;61:2461–7. http://content.onlinejacc.org/article.aspx?articleID=1696815.

CKD: Resistant HTN/Risk Stratification

J Am Coll Cardiol. 2013;61:2468–70. http://content.onlinejacc.org/article.aspx?articleID=1696808.

Children/Adolescents

N Engl J Med. 2014;370:2316–25. http://www.nejm.org/doi/full/10.1056/NEJMcp1001120.

Cognitive Changes: Racial Disparity

Am J Hypertens. 2016;29:185–93. http://ajh.oxfordjournals.org/content/29/2/185.abstract?etoc.

Cognitive Changes: Women

Am J Hypertens. 2016;29:202–16. http://ajh.oxfordjournals.org/content/29/2/202.abstract?etoc.

Cognitive Impairment: Progression with Excess BP Lowering

JAMA Intern Med. Online 2 Mar 2015. http://archinte.jamanetwork.com/article.aspx?articleID=2173093&utm-source=Silverchair%20Information%20Systems&utm-medium=email&utm-campaign=ArchivesofInternalMedicine%3AOnlineFirst03%2F02%2F2015.

Community-Wide HTN Intervention

Circ Cardiovasc Qual Out. 2014;7:828–34. http://circoutcomes.ahajournals.org/content/7/6/828.full.

CPAP

JAMA.   2013;310:2407–15.   http://jama.jamanetwork.com/article.aspx?articleid=1788459.

Diabetes Mellitus: New Onset/Mortality

Eur Heart J. 2016;37:968–74. http://eurheartj.oxfordjournals.org/content/37/12/968.abstract?etoc.

Diabetes Mellitus

JAMA.   2015;313:603–15.   http://jama.jamanetwork.com/article.aspx?articleid=2108887.

Diabetes Mellitus

Heart. 2013;99:577–85. http://heart.bmj.com/content/99/8/577.extract.

Dietary Effects on Blood Pressure

Hypertension.   2016;67:733–9.   http://hyper.ahajournals.org/content/67/4/733.abstract?etoc.

Dietary Sodium

Circulation Res. 2015;116:1046–57. http://circres.ahajournals.org/content/116/6/1046.full.

Dietary Sodium and Potassium

Mayo Clin Proc. 2013;88:987–95. http://www.sciencedirect.com/science/article/pii/S0025619613004631.

Dietary Sodium: Long-Term Effects on CVD Outcomes

BMJ. 2007;334:885–8. http://www.bmj.com/content/334/7599/885.

Dipping: Nocturnal

Expert Rev Cardiovasc Ther. 2010;8:781–92. http://informahealth-care.com/doi/abs/10.1586/erc.10.29.

Echo: Recommendations of ACE/EACVI

Eur Heart J Cardiovasc Imaging. 2015;16:577–605. http://ehjcimag-ing.oxfordjournals.org/content/16/6/577.full? .

Exercise: Benefits/Risks

Am J Hypertens. 2015;28:429–39. http://ajh.oxfordjournals.org/con-tent/28/4/429.abstract?etoc.

Garlic

Am J Hypertens. 2015;28:414–23. http://ajh.oxfordjournals.org/con-tent/28/3/414.abstract?etoc.

Genetics

Circulation Res.2015;116:937–59. http://circres.ahajournals.org/con-tent/116/6/937.full.

Home BP Monitoring

J Nurse Pract. 2014;10:607–10. http://www.sciencedirect.com/sci-ence/article/pii/S1555415514004127.

Home-Clinic BP Difference: Predictors

Am J Hypertens. 2016;29:614–25. http://ajh.oxfordjournals.org/content/29/5/614.full?etoc.

Hydrochlorothiazide Vs Chlorthalidone

Hypertension. 2004;43:4–9. http://hyper.ahajournals.org/content/43/1/4.full.

Hypertension Guidelines (Editorial)

J Clin Hypertens. 2014;16:251–4. http://onlinelibrary.wiley.com/doi/10.1111/jch.12306/full.

JNC8 Panel Members Report

JAMA. 2014;311:507–20. http://jama.jamanetwork.com/article.aspx?articleid=1791497.

KDIGO: BP Goals

Kidney Int. 2012;[Suppl]:2. http://www.nature.com/kisup/journal/v2/n5/index.html.

Large Scale Program

JAMA. 2013;310:699–705. http://jama.jamanetwork.com/article.aspx?articleid=1730511.

Metabolic Syndrome

J Am Coll Cardiol. 2013;61:12–9. http://content.onlinejacc.org/article.aspx?articleID=1555196.

Misconceptions about Treatment

Am J Med. 2015;128:450–5. http://www.sciencedirect.com/science/article/pii/S0002934314011383.

Morning BP Surge

Circulation. 2003;107:1401–6. http://circ.ahajournals.org/content/107/10/1401.full.

Morning BP Surge: White Population

Hypertension. 2014;64:943–50. http://hyper.ahajournals.org/content/64/5/943.full.

Obesity

Circulation Res. 2015;116:991–1006. http://circres.ahajournals.org/content/116/6/991.full.

Obesity: Role of Aldosterone

Am J Hypertens. 2016;29:415–23. http://ajh.oxfordjournals.org/content/29/4/415.abstract?etoc.

Osler Maneuver

Am J Med. 1986;80:906–10. http://www.sciencedirect.com/science/article/pii/0002934386906364.

Pregnancy

Circulation. 2014;129:1254–61. http://circ.ahajournals.org/content/129/11/1254.full.

Pregnancy

N Engl J Med. 2015;372:407–17. http://www.nejm.org/doi/full/10.1056/NEJMoa1404595?query=TOC.

Pregnancy: Future Risk

Circulation. 2013;127:681–90. http://circ.ahajournals.org/content/127/6/681.full.

Pregnancy/Preeclampsia: Future Risk

J Am Coll Cardiol. 2014;63:1815–22. http://content.onlinejacc.org/article.aspx?articleID=1841463.

Prehypertension: CAD Risk in Asians

J Am Heart Assoc. 2015;4:e001519. http://jaha.ahajournals.org/content/4/2/e001519.full.

RAAS

Circulation Res. 2015;116:960–75. http://circres.ahajournals.org/content/116/6/960.full.

Renal Denervation

N Engl J Med. 2014;370:1393–401. http://www.nejm.org/doi/full/10.1056/NEJMoa1402670.

Renal Denervation

Eur Heart J. 2014;36:219–27. http://dx.doi.org/10.1093/eurheartj/ehu441.

Resistant HTN

Eur Heart J. 2015;36:2686–95. http://eurheartj.oxfordjournals.org/
content/36/40/2686.

Resistant HTN

Int J Hypertens. 2011;598694. http://www.ncbi.nlm.nih.gov/pmc/arti-
cles/PMC3014709/.

Resistant HTN: Atherothrombosis

Eur Heart J. 2013;34:1204–14. http://eurheartj.oxfordjournals.org/
content/34/16/1204.

Resting Heart Rate/Incident HTN

Am J Hypertens. 2016;29:251–7. http://ajh.oxfordjournals.org/con-
tent/29/2/251.abstract?etoc.

Screening: USPSTF

Ann Intern Med. 2007;147:783–6. http://annals.org/article.
aspx?articleid=737820.

Secondary HTN: Screening

Eur Heart J. 2014;35:1245–54. http://eurheartj.oxfordjournals.org/
content/35/19/1245.

Self-monitoring/Self-titration

JAMA. 2014;312:799–808. http://jama.jamanetwork.com/article.
aspx?articleid=1899205.

Sex/Ethnicity: Incidence/Outcomes

Heart. 2013;99:715–21. http://heart.bmj.com/content/99/10/715.full.

Sympathetic Nervous System

Circulation Res. 2015;116:976–90. http://circres.ahajournals.org/content/116/6/976.full.

Sympathetic Overactivity

Indian Heart J. 2014;66:686–90. http://www.sciencedirect.com/science/article/pii/S0019483214007202.

ST2

J Clin Hypertension. 2013;15:899–904. http://onlinelibrary.wiley.com/doi/10.1111/jch.12205/full.

Systolic BP and Risk

JAMA Intern Med. 2014;174:1252–61. http://archinte.jamanetwork.com/article.aspx?articleid=1881014.

Treatment: Cost Effectiveness

N Engl J Med. 2015;372:447–55. http://www.nejm.org/doi/full/10.1056/NEJMsa1406751?query=TOC.

Treatment: Outcomes (Value Trial)

Eur Heart J. 2016;37:955–64. http://eurheartj.oxfordjournals.org/content/37/12/955.abstract?etoc.

Treatment: Sodium Reduction/Weight Loss

JAMA.   1998;279:839–46.   http://jama.jamanetwork.com/article.
aspx?articleid=187347.

Treatment: Systolic BP/Outcomes

Am J Med. 2013;126:501–08. http://www.sciencedirect.com/science/
article/pii/S0002934313000363.

Visceral Adiposity

J Am Coll Cardiol. 2014;64:997–1002. http://content.onlinejacc.org/
article.aspx?articleID=1900739.

Visit to Visit Variability

Ann Intern Med. 2015;163:329–38. http://annals.org/article.aspx?
articleID=2398909.

White Coat/Masked HTN

Hypertension.   2009;54:226–32.   http://hyper.ahajournals.org/con-
tent/54/2/226.full.

Updates and More

https://clinicalguidecvd.com/htn

Chapter 54
Inappropriate Sinus Tachycardia

ICD-10 Code

R00.0 (TACHYCARDIA UNSPECIFIED)

Alternate Names/Abbreviation

IST

Description/Etiology

Resting daytime HR >100 bpm and 24-h average HR >90 BPM not explainable by physiologic demands or conditions associated with increased HR

Cause unknown

Comorbid Conditions

ANXIETY/ANXIETY DISORDER

V.E. Friedewald, *Clinical Guide to Cardiovascular Disease*, 765
DOI 10.1007/978-1-4471-7293-2_54,
© Springer-Verlag London 2016

Demography

Females > males
More common in young adults

Pathophysiology

Form of dysautonomia, or intrinsic sinus node abnormality, or both, with no unified mechanism

Signs/Symptoms

BREATHING – DIFF (DYSPNEA)
CHEST – PALPITATIONS
CONSCIOUSNESS – LOSS, SUDDEN (SYNCOPE)
DIZZY/LIGHTHEADED/PRESYNCOPE
FATIGUE
HEART, RATE – RAPID (TACHYCARDIA) [2]
HEART, RATE, VAR – DECR [1]
MOOD – ANXIOUS

Differentiation

Ablation for Supraventricular Tachycardia
Acute Pulmonary Embolism
AMI
Anemia
Anxiety
Aortic Regurgitation
Dehydration
Drugs/substances including:

Alcohol
Anticholinergics
Beta-blocker withdrawal

Caffeine
Catecholamines
Cocaine
Tobacco

Duchenne Muscular Dystrophy
Exercise-Induced
Fever
Hyperthyroidism
Hypoglycemia
Mitral Regurgitation
Myocardial Ischemia
Pain
Pericarditis
Pneumothorax
Postural Orthostatic Tachycardia

Complications

Tachycardia-induced Cardiomyopathy [3]

Laboratory

NS; useful to R/O other causes of tachycardia, such as:

Hyperthyroidism
Hypoglycemia

ECG

RATE – INCREASED (SINUS TACHYCARDIA) [4]

Imaging

NS
R/O OTHER CAUSES OF TACHYCARDIA

Other Tests

24-h Ambulatory ECG
Tilt-table testing [5]

Treatment: Nonpharmacologic

Eliminate dietary stimulants, e.g., caffeine, alcohol
Psychiatric/psychologic consultation/support

Treatment: Pharmacologic

Benzodiazepines [6]
Beta-blockers [6]
Ivabradine

Treatment: Surgical/Invasive

Radiofrequency Ablation [7]
Surgical ablation [7]

Prevention

Avoid stimulants

Notes

[1] Often not present
[2] Rapid acceleration with exercise and slow return to base-line post-exercise
[3] Probably rare
[4] P wave morphology same during slow and fast rates

[5] For Postural Orthostatic Tachycardia

[6] Beta-blockers alone sometimes ineffective but may be more effective when taken in combination with a benzodiazepine

[7] Limited efficacy

Guidelines

2015 ACC/AHA/HRS Guideline for the Management of Adult Patients with Supraventricular Tachycardia

J Am Coll Cardiol. 2016;67:e27–115. http://content.onlinejacc.org/article.aspx?articleID=2443667.

Patient Information

Cardiac Health

http://www.cardiachealth.org/inappropriate-sinus-tachycardia-ist.

Professional Information

Review

J Am Coll Cardiol. 2013;61:793–801. http://content.onlinejacc.org/article.aspx?articleid=1486711&resultClick=3.

Review

Europace. 2005;7:104–12. http://europace.oxfordjournals.org/content/7/2/104.full.

Autoantibodies

Heart Rhythm. 2011;8:1788–95. http://www.heartrhythmjournal.com/article/S1547-5271(11)00787-9/abstract#SEC8.

RF Ablation

Circulation.   1995;92:2919–28.   http://circ.ahajournals.org/content/92/10/2919.full.

Ivabradine

J Am Coll Cardiol. 2012;60:1330–2. http://content.onlinejacc.org/article.aspx?articleid = 1358180.

Ivabradine: Efficacy

J Am Coll Cardiol. 2012;60:1323–9. http://content.onlinejacc.org/article.aspx?articleid = 1358179.

Sympathetic Tone

J Am Heart Assoc. 2014;3:e000700. http://jaha.ahajournals.org/content/3/2/e000700.full.

Updates and More

https://clinicalguidecvd.com/ist

Chapter 55
Infective Endocarditis (Subacute Bacterial Endocarditis/SBE)

ICD-10 Code

133.0

Alternate Names/Abbreviation

IE
SBE
SUBACUTE BACTERIAL ENDOCARDITIS

Description/Etiology

Bacterial/fungal infection of valve/endocardium/intracardiac foreign material due to (most common):

Streptococcus and Staphylococcus (80 % of cases) [1]
Enterococcus [2]
Hacek organisms [3]
Candida and other fungi [4]
Culture-negative [5]

Associated with increased cancer risk
See Duke Criteria for diagnosis [19]

V.E. Friedewald, *Clinical Guide to Cardiovascular Disease*,
DOI 10.1007/978-1-4471-7293-2_55,
© Springer-Verlag London 2016

Comorbid Conditions

ACUTE MYOCARDIAL INFARCTION [9]
BACTERIAL MENINGITIS [23]
CANCER
CARDIAC SURGERY
CARDIOMYOPATHY – HYPERTROPHIC
COLON POLYP
COLONOSCOPY [ESP WITH POLYP REMOVAL]
COLORECTAL ADENOCARCINOMA
COLOSTOMY
CONGENITAL HEART DISEASE [7] [8]
DENTAL INFECTION
DENTAL PROCEDURE
DIABETES MELLITUS
DIABETIC FOOT ULCER
ESOPHAGEAL VARICES
ESOPHAGUS ULCER
GASTRIC ANTRAL/FUNDUS ATROPHY
GASTROSTOMY
HIV [6]
IMMUNE DEFICIENCY
INSECT BITE
INTRACARDIAC DEVICES
INTRAVENOUS DRUG USE/ABUSE [6]
LOWER GI ANGIODYSPLASIA
MITRAL VALVE PROLAPSE [25]
NONRHEUMATIC VALVE DISEASE
OPERATIVE SITE INFECTION
PENETRATING CARDIAC FOREIGN BODY
PERIODONTITIS
PROSTHETIC VALVE
PRURIGO
RHEUMATIC VALVE DISEASE
SIGMOID DIVERTICULOSIS
SKIN WOUND
SKIN/SOFT TISSUE INFECTION
VENOUS LEG ULCER
VENOUS LINE – CENTRAL
VENOUS LINE – PERIPHERAL

Demography

Per underlying condition
Increased incidence in USA since 2007

Incubation

Varies with infecting agent

Signs/Symptoms

ABDOMEN, LUQ – TENDER [13]
CHEST, ANT, STERNUM – PAIN/TENDERNESS [14] [15]
CHILLS
COUGH [15]
EXTREM, HANDS/FEET – HEMORRHAGES, SUBUNGUAL (SPLINTER)
EXTREM, HANDS/FEET – NODULES, TENDER (OSLER NODES)
EXTREM, LONG BONES – PAIN/TENDERNESS [14] [15]
EYES, CONJUNCTIVAE – PETECHIAE
EYES, RETINA – WHITE SPOT AND HEMORRHAGE (ROTH SPOT)
EYES, VISION – DECR/LOSS
FATIGUE
FEVER [10] [11]
HEART – FRICTION RUB, PERICARD [15]
HEART – MURMUR, REGURG [12]
JOINTS – PAIN (ARTHRALGIA)
SKIN – PETECHIAE/ECCHYMOSES/PURPURA
SKIN, FEET/SOLES – MACULES, RED (JANEWAY LESION)
SPLEEN – TENDER [12]
SPLEEN, SIZE – INCR (SPLENOMEGALY)
URINE – BLOOD (HEMATURIA) [15]
VOICE – HOARSE (LARYNGITIS) [15]

Differentiation

All causes of unexplained fever lasting >72 h

Complications [26]

ACUTE VALVE REGURGITATION
ANNULAR ABSCESS
BLEEDING
CARDIAC FISTULA
CARDIAC PERFORATION
CEREBRAL ABSCESS
CEREBRAL MYCOTIC ANEURYSM
CORONARY ARTERY EMBOLUS
HF
INFECTIVE PERICARDITIS
MYOCARDIAL ABSCESS
PROSTHETIC   VALVE   SEPARATION   FORM
    ANNULUS
PROSTHETIC VALVE OBSTRUCTION
RENAL INFARCTION
SPLENIC ABSCESS
STROKE
SYSTEMIC ARTERIAL EMBOLUS [27]

Laboratory [19]

BLOOD, CULTURE – POS [5] [19]
BLOOD, ESR – INCR
BLOOD, HGB/HCT – DECR (ANEMIA)
BLOOD, LYMPHOCYTES – INCR (LYMPHOCYTOSIS)
BLOOD,   PLATELETS   –   DECR
    (THROMBOCYTOPENIA) [15]
BLOOD, RHEUMATOID FACTOR – POS
BLOOD, TROPONIN – INCR [WITH MYOCARD
    EXTENSION]
BLOOD, WBC – INCR (LEUKOCYTOSIS)
URINE, PROTEIN – INCR (PROTEINURIA)

ECG [16]

N/NS ABN
NS/VAR PER COMORBIDITY(S) [ESP VALVULAR
    HD/INTRACARD DEVICES]

Imaging [19] [21] [26] [29]

AV, FLOW – REGURG [NEW]
CARD ABSCESS
CARD MASS – OSCILLATING [20]
CARD VALVE, NATIVE – MASS [VEGETATION]
CARDIAC VALVE, PROS – DEHISCENCE
CARDIAC VALVE, PROS – MASS [VEGETATION]
MV, FLOW – REGURG [NEW]

Other Tests

NS

Treatment: Nonpharmacologic

Refer to guidelines for current recommendations

Treatment: Pharmacologic

Antibiotics [17]
Anticoagulation (controversial)
Refer to guidelines for current recommendations

Treatment: Surgical/Invasive [24] [26] [28]

Case-by-case basis for treatment of infection and sequelae of
valve leaflet and paravalvular tissue destruction [18] [24]

Prevention

IE prophylaxis [22]

Course

Mortality 40 % at 1 year; 15–20 % in-hospital
Increased long-term risks include:

All-cause mortality
AMI
HF
Stroke
Sudden death
Ventricular arrhythmias

Notes

[1] 80 % of TV infections are Staph Aureus; increased incidence due to Streptococcus since 2007
[2] Usually after GU/GI procedure; patients with malignancy
[3] Hemophilus, Actinobacillus, Cardiobacterium, Eikenella, Kingella species; cause large vegetations, large vessel embolism, HF
[4] Especially prosthetic valve IE
[5] 10 % negative due to prior antibiotic use; Candida; Aspergillus; slow growing organisms, eg, Coxiella Burnetii (Q Fever), Bartonella; Libman-Sacks (Systemic Lupus Erythematosus)
[6] Injection drug use or long-term indwelling central catheter
[7] Atrial Septal Defect uncommon cause except Atrioventricular type
[8] Most often with high pressure gradients
[9] At site of infarction or complicating ventricular aneurysm
[10] May be absent, especially with advanced age, prior antibiotic use, CNS hemorrhage, HF, renal failure
[11] Fever duration >72 h plus any murmur should raise suspicion of IE

[12] Changing or worsening of pre-existing murmur not diagnostic

[13] Splenic origin; acute stage

[14] Especially with severe anemia

[15] Uncommon/rare; when present initially in native left valve endocarditis, an early risk indicator of increased mortality

[16] Monitor for complications of heart block and dysrhythmias associated with septal abscess or Myocarditis

[17] Specific agents guided by causative organisms and susceptibility profiles; refer to current guidelines for detailed recommendations

[18] With heart valve team approach involving cardiologists, surgeons, infectious disease specialists

[19] Duke Criteria (Modified) for Infective Endocarditis (from Circulation 2015;132:1435–1486)

Major criteria

Blood culture positive for IE

Typical microorganisms consistent with IE from two separate blood cultures: Viridans streptococci, *Streptococcus bovis*, HACEK group, *Staphylococcus aureus*; or community-acquired enterococci in the absence of a primary focus, or microorganisms consistent with IE from persistently positive blood cultures defined as follows: at least two positive cultures of blood samples drawn >12 h apart or all 3 or a majority of ≥4 separate cultures of blood (with first and last sample drawn at least 1 h apart)

Single positive blood culture for *Coxiella burnetii* or anti–phase 1 IgG antibody titer ≥1:800

Evidence of endocardial involvement

Echocardiogram positive for IE (TEE recommended for patients with prosthetic valves, rated at least possible IE by clinical criteria, or complicated IE [paravalvular abscess]; TTE as first test in other patients) defined as follows: oscillating intracardiac mass on valve or supporting structures, in the path of regurgitant jets, or on implanted material in the absence of an alternative anatomic explanation; abscess; or new partial dehiscence of prosthetic valve or new valvular regurgitation (worsening or changing or pre-existing murmur not sufficient)

Minor criteria

Predisposition, predisposing heart condition, or IDU

Fever, temperature >38 °C

Vascular phenomena, major arterial emboli, septic pulmonary infarcts, mycotic aneurysm, intracranial hemorrhage, conjunctival hemorrhages, and Janeway lesions

Immunological phenomena: glomerulonephritis, Osler nodes, Roth spots, and rheumatoid factor

Microbiological evidence: positive blood culture but does not meet a major criterion as noted above (excludes single positive cultures for coagulase-negative staphylococci and organisms that do not cause endocarditis) or serological evidence of active infection with organism consistent with IE

---

[20] On valve, supporting structure, in path of regurgitant jet, implanted material

[21] TTE/TEE highly useful for all listed findings; CT indicated when echo insufficient

[22] Refer to guidelines

[23] Uncommon comorbidity, with mortality >60 %

[24] Surgical adverse outcomes correlate with:

> Increasing age
> Impaired LVEF (mod-severe)
> Prosthetic valve IE
> Staph aureus infection

[25] Infection on valve itself or in rare cases due to jet lesion in LA mural endocardium

[26] **Clinical and Echocardiographic Features That Suggest Potential Need for Surgical Intervention:** (from Circulation 2015;132:1435–1486)

> **Vegetation**
>
> > Persistent vegetation after systemic embolization
> > Anterior mitral leaflet vegetation, particularly with size >10 mm ≥1 Embolic events during first 2 weeks of antimicrobial therapy
> > Increase in vegetation size despite appropriate antimicrobial therapy

Valvular dysfunction

> Acute AR or MR with signs of ventricular failure
> HF unresponsive to medical therapy

Valve perforation or rupture

> Perivalvular extension
> Valvular dehiscence, rupture, or fistula
> New heart block
> Large abscess or extension of abscess despite appropriate antimicrobial therapy

[27] Systemic emboli:

> Occur in 22–25 % of cases of IE; rates can be higher if noninvasive imaging (including MRI/CT) routinely done to detect asymptomatic (silent) emboli
> Often involve major arterial beds, including brain, lungs, coronary arteries, spleen, bowel, extremities
> Up to 65 % of embolic events involve CNS, and >90 % of CNS emboli lodge in distribution of middle cerebral artery
> Highest incidence of embolic complications is seen with MV IE (more with anterior rather than posterior mitral leaflet involvement) and with IE caused by *S aureus*, *Candida*, and HACEK organisms.
> Emboli can occur before diagnosis, during treatment, or after treatment completion, although most emboli occur within first 2–4 weeks of antimicrobial therapy

[28] Valve surgery should be performed in most cases of fungal IE

[29] **Use of Echocardiography During Diagnosis and Treatment of Endocarditis** (from Circulation 2015;132:1435–1486)

Early

> Echocardiography as soon as possible (<12 h after initial evaluation)
> TEE preferred; obtain TTE views of any abnormal findings for later comparison

TTE if TEE is not immediately available

TTE may be sufficient in small children

Repeat echocardiography

TEE after positive TTE as soon as possible in patients at high risk for complications

TEE 3–5 days after initial TEE if suspicion exists without diagnosis of IE or with worrisome clinical course during early treatment of IE

Intraoperative/prepump

Identification of vegetations, mechanism of regurgitation, abscesses, fistulas, and pseudoaneurysms

Postpump

Confirmation of successful repair of abnormal findings

Assessment of residual valve dysfunction

Elevated afterload if necessary to avoid underestimating valve insufficiency or presence of residual abnormal flow

Completion of therapy

Establish new baseline for valve function and morphology and ventricular size and function

TTE usually adequate; TEE or review of intraoperative TEE may be needed for complex anatomy to establish new baseline

Guidelines

2014 AHA/ACC guideline for the management of patients with valvular heart disease

J Am Coll Cardiol. 2014;63:e57–185. http://content.onlinejacc.org/article.aspx?articleID=1838843.

2015 ESC guidelines for the management of infective endocarditis

Eur Heart J. 2015;36:3075–128. http://eurheartj.oxfordjournals.org/content/36/44/3075.

Patient Information

IMAGES

http://www.nlm.nih.gov/medlineplus/ency/imagepages/18142.htm.

Mayo Clinic

http://www.mayoclinic.org/diseases-conditions/endocarditis/basics/
definition/con-20022403.

AHA

http://www.heart.org/HEARTORG/Conditions/Congenital-
HeartDefects/TheImpactofCongenitalHeartDefects/Infective-
Endocarditis-UCM-307108-Article.jsp.

Merck

http://www.merckmanuals.com/home/heart-and-blood-vessel-disor-
ders/endocarditis/infective-endocarditis.

Cleveland Clinic

http://my.clevelandclinic.org/services/heart/disorders/heart-valve-
disease/endocarditis-protection.

Texas Heart Institute

http://www.texasheart.org/HIC/Topics/Cond/endocard.cfm.

Professional Information

AHA Scientific Statement: Adults

Circulation.   2015;132:1435–86.   http://circ.ahajournals.org/con-
tent/132/15/1435.full.

AHA Scientific Statement: Children

Circulation.   2015;132:1487–515.   http://circ.ahajournals.org/content/132/15/1487.full.

Early Description

Lancet.   1885.   http://www.sciencedirect.com/science/article/pii/S0140673602008279.

Review: Critical Questions

J Am Coll Cardiol. 2015;66:1068–76. http://content.onlinejacc.org/article.aspx?articleID=2430614.

Review

N Engl J Med. 2013;368:1425–33. http://www.nejm.org/doi/full/10.1056/NEJMcp1206782.

Review

Arch Intern Med. 2009;169463–73. http://archinte.jamanetwork.com/article.aspx?articleid=414841.

Review: Congenital Heart Disease

Circulation.   2013;128:1412–19.   http://circ.ahajournals.org/content/128/13/1412.full.

Review: Transaortic Valve IE

J Infect. 2015;70:565–76. http://www.sciencedirect.com/science/article/pii/S0163445314003843.

Cancer Risk

Am J Med. 2013;126:58–67. http://www.sciencedirect.com/science/article/pii/S0002934312007905.

Duke Criteria for Diagnosis

Clin Infect Dis. 2000;30:633–8. http://cid.oxfordjournals.org/content/30/4/633.full.

Enterococcus Faecalis Endocarditis

Circulation. 2013;127:1810–7. http://circ.ahajournals.org/content/127/17/1810.full.

Entry Portals

J Am Coll Cardiol. 2016;67:151–8. http://content.onlinejacc.org/article.aspx?articleID=2480639.

Epidemiology

J Am Coll Cardiol. 2012;59:1977–8. http://content.onlinejacc.org/article.aspx?articleid=1203852.

Epidemiology

PLoS One. 2013;8:e82665. http://journals.plos.org/plosone/article?id=10.1371/journal.pone.0082665.

IE with Bacterial Meningitis

Circulation. 2013;127:2056–62. http://circ.ahajournals.org/content/127/20/2056.full.

Imaging

Eur Heart J. 2014;35:624–32. http://eurheartj.oxfordjournals.org/content/35/10/624.

Imaging: Echo

Heart. 2004;90:614–7. http://www.ncbi.nlm.nih.gov/pmc/articles/PMC1768290/.

Imaging: CT

J Am Coll Cardiol. 2009;53:436–44. http://content.onlinejacc.org/article.aspx?articleid=1139382.

Imaging: 3D Echo

Circulation Card Imaging. 2014;7:149–54. http://circimaging.ahajournals.org/content/7/1/149.full?sid=aeab4f82-993f-45e1-ab08-efbec6dfe9ee.

Intracardiac Electronic Devices

Eur Heart J. 2015;36:2484–90. http://eurheartj.oxfordjournals.org/content/36/37/2484.

Implantable Cardiac Devices

JAMA. 2012;307:1727–35. http://jama.jamanetwork.com/article.aspx?articleid=1148195.

LA Mural Endocarditis Secondary to Jet Lesion

Circulation. 2015;131:1529–30. http://circ.ahajournals.org/content/131/17/1529.full.

Management

Lancet. 2012;379:965–75. http://www.ncbi.nlm.nih.gov/pubmed/2231 7840?dopt=Abstract.

Neurologic Complications

Circulation.   2013;127:2272–84.   http://circ.ahajournals.org/content/127/23/2272.full?sid=87d99194-91b1-4b54-ae6a-80b6c 2cdedf9.

Outcomes: Long-Term

Circulation.   2014;130:1684–91.   http://circ.ahajournals.org/content/130/19/1684.full.

Persistent Positive Blood Cultures: Prognosis

Eur Heart J. 2013;34:1749–54. http://eurheartj.oxfordjournals.org/content/34/23/1749.

Relapse Versus Reinfection

Clin Infect Dis. 2005;41:406–9. http://cid.oxfordjournals.org/content/41/3/406.abstract?ijkey=d759f594ada1e239672a304801ff9e0 5f4cd9c55&keytype2=tf-ipsecsha.

Roth Spots

Engl J Med. 2014;370:e38. http://www.nejm.org/doi/full/10.1056/ NEJMicm1312093.

Septic Shock

Eur Heart J. 2013;34:1999–2006. http://eurheartj.oxfordjournals.org/content/34/26/1999.

Surgery: Outcomes/Prognostic Factors

Eur J Cardiothorac Surg. 2015;47:826–32. http://ejcts.oxfordjournals. org/content/47/5/826.abstract.

Surgery: Early

N Engl J Med. 2012;366:2466–73. http://www.nejm.org/doi/ full/10.1056/NEJMoa1112843#t=articleDiscussion.

Surgery: Indications, Risks, Outcomes

Circulation. 2015;131:131–40. http://circ.ahajournals.org/content/131/2/131.abstract?etoc.

Surgery: Long-Term Outcomes

Eur Heart J. 2014;35:1195–204. http://eurheartj.oxfordjournals.org/ content/35/18/1195.

Surgery: Clinical Features/Outcomes

QJM. 2015;108:219–29. http://qjmed.oxfordjournals.org/content/108/3/219.abstract?etoc.

Thrombocytopenia: Risk Marker for INCR Mortality

An J Cardiol. 2015;115:950–5. http://www.ajconline.org/article/ S0002-9149(15)00056-9/abstract.

Trends in USA: Hospitalizations/Outcomes

J Am Coll Cardiol. 2013;62:2217–26. http://content.onlinejacc.org/ article.aspx?articleID=1732398.

Trends in USA: Incidence, Microbiology, Valve Replacement

J Am Coll Cardiol. 2015;65:2070–6. http://content.onlinejacc.org/article.aspx?articleID=2290815.

Updates and More

https://clinicalguidecvd.com/ie

Chapter 56
Leopard Syndrome

ICD-10 Code

Q87.1

Alternate Names/Abbreviation

Leopard: acronym for Lentigines, ECG-changes, ocular changes (Hypertelorism), Pulmonary Stenosis, anomalies in sex organs, growth retardation, deafness

CARDIOCUTANEOUS SYNDROME
LENTIGINOSIS PROFUSE
MOYNAHAN SYNDROME
MULTIPLE LENTIGINES SYNDROME
PROGRESSIVE CARDIOMYOPATHIC
LENTIGINOSIS

Description/Etiology

Autosomal dominant inherited condition affecting many areas of body, especially

Skin: brown spots (Lentigines) resembling freckles and Cafe Au Lait spots

V.E. Friedewald, *Clinical Guide to Cardiovascular Disease*, 789
DOI 10.1007/978-1-4471-7293-2_56,
© Springer-Verlag London 2016

Heart:

> Conduction system
> LVH
> PS

Facial structures
Genitalia
Stature: short
> Hearing (loss)

High penetrance and variable expression
Closely resembles Noonan Syndrome, especially in childhood [2]

Comorbid Conditions

ATRIAL FIBRILLATION
CARDIOMYOPATHY – HYPERTROPHIC
CELIAC DISEASE
PREEXCITATION SYNDROMES
PULMONARY STENOSIS

Pathophysiology

Cardiac structural: primarily Hypertrophic Cardiomyopathy and Pulmonary Valve Stenosis

Signs/Symptoms [3] [4]

BACK, CURV – LAT (SCOLIOSIS)
BACK, CURV – POST (KYPHOSIS)
BODY, GROWTH – DECR
BODY, HT – DECR
BREATHING – DIFF (DYSPNEA)
CHEST – PAIN, EFFORT (ANGINA PECTORIS)
CHEST – PALPITATIONS

CHEST, SHAPE – BARREL
CONSCIOUSNESS – LOSS, SUDDEN (SYNCOPE)
EARS, HEARING – LOSS (DEAFNESS) [8]
EARS, POSITION – LOW SET
EYES, LIDS – DROOPED (PTOSIS)
EYES, MOTION – JERKY (NYSTAGMUS)
EYES, SEPARATION – WIDE (HYPERTELORISM)
FACE, BROWS – PROTRUSION (FRONTAL
   BOSSING)
FACE, SHAPE – TRIANGULAR
FATIGUE
FERTILITY – DECR
GENITALS, TESTICLES, DESCENT – DELAYED/
   ABSENT (CRYPTORCHIDISM)
HEART, LSB, LOWER – THRILL, SYS
HEART, LSB, MID – MURMUR, SYS
HEART, LV, APEX – MURMUR, DIAS
HEART, LV, APEX – MURMUR, SYS
HEART, LV, APEX, IMP – FORCEFUL/SUSTAINED
HEART, LV, APEX, IMP – FORCEFUL/SUSTAINED
HEART, LV, APEX, IMP – DISPLACED, LAT
HEART, LV, APEX, IMP – DOUBLE
HEART, LV, APEX, IMP – TRIPLE
HEART, S2, SPLIT – REVERSED (PARADOXICAL)
HEART, S3 LV
JOINTS, MOVEMENT, RANGE – INCR
   (HYPERMOBILITY)
LIPS – THICK
MENTATION,
   LEARNING, DEVELOPMENT – DECR
NECK, POST, SKIN FOLDS – EXCESS
PENIS, OPENING – UNDERSIDE (HYPOSPADIAS)
PUBERTY, ONSET – DELAYED
SEIZURES
SKIN – LENTIGINES [1]
SKIN – SPOTS, HYPERPIGMENTED
   (CAFE – AU-LAIT) [9]
STERNUM, CURV – ANT (PECTUS CARINATUM)
STERNUM, CURV – POST (PECTUS EXCAVATUM)

Differentiation

Cardiac: other causes of LVOT obstruction

Complications

AF
Arterial dissection
HF
Sudden Death

Laboratory

NS

ECG

AV COND – 3RD DEGREE BLOCK
DYSRHYTHMIAS – ATRIAL (PACS/OTHERS)
DYSRHYTHMIAS – VENTRICULAR (PVCS/
OTHERS)
P WAVE, MORPH – VAR/ABN
Q WAVE – ABN
QRS – LVH PATTERN
QRS – RBBB/RBBB PATTERN
QRS – RVH PATTERN
QRS – S1S2S3 PATTERN
QRS, AXIS – L
QT/QTC INTERVAL – LONG
RATE – DECREASED (SINUS BRADYCARDIA)

Imaging [7]

ART, CORONARY, SIZE – INCR/ANEURYSM
AV, FLOW – REGURG

AV, LEAFLETS, MORPH – ABN
IVS, THICKNESS – INCR (SEPTAL HYPERTROPHY)
LA, CHAMBER, SIZE – INCR
LV, DIAS – DYSF
LV, MYOCARD, WALL THICKNESS – INCR
  (HYPERTROPHY) [5]
LV, OUTFLOW – OBS
LV, WALL THICKNESS, SEG – INCR [6]
MV, LEAFLETS – PROLAPSE
MV, LEAFLETS, MORPH – ABN
MV, MOTION SYS – ANT
PV, LEAFLETS, MORPH – ABN

Genomics

BRAF
PTPN11 [?]
RAF1

Other Tests

Ambulatory ECG monitoring
Cardiac Catheterization
EEG
Skin biopsy

Treatment: Nonpharmacologic

NS

Treatment: Pharmacologic

Variable according to associated abnormalities

Treatment: Surgical/Invasive

Septal ablation for LVOT obstruction
Variable according to associated abnormalities

Course

Highly variable; cardiac prognosis related to presence of
LVH

Notes

[1] Brown spots, more common on face, neck, upper body;
unaffected by sunlight; cardiac abnormalities may precede their appearance
[2] Differs   from   Noonan: deafness,   Hypertrophic
Cardiomyopathy, Lentigines more common in Leopard
[3] Highly variable, even within same family
[4] Cardiac signs/symptoms listed are due to LVOT obstruction caused by HCM; signs/symptoms of PS not listed
[5] LVH may be concentric or nonconcentric
[6] Isolated to cardiac apex reported in a few cases
[7] Great variability among reported cases; asymmetric and
concentric LVH most common abnormalities; other rare
findings sometimes found and not listed include:

Aortic Stenosis – Subvalvular
AV canal defect
LV dilatation
LV noncompaction
Multiple VSDs
LV apical aneurysm
RV moderator band

[8] Sensorineural; may be present at birth or develop later
[9] May precede Lentigines appearance

Guidelines

2014 ESC guidelines on diagnosis and management of hypertrophic cardiomyopathy
Eur Heart J. 2014;35:2733–79. http://eurheartj.oxfordjournals.org/content/35/39/2733.

Patient Information

Images

http://www.nlm.nih.gov/medlineplus/ency/imagepages/2927.htm.

Medlineplus

ENGLISH
  http://www.nlm.nih.gov/medlineplus/ency/article/001473.htm.
ESPANOL
  http://www.nlm.nih.gov/medlineplus/spanish/ency/article/001473.htm.

Nord

https://rarediseases.org/rare-diseases/leopard-syndrome/.

Genetics Home Reference

http://ghr.nlm.nih.gov/condition/multiple-lentigines-syndrome.

Professional Information

Review

Rev Esp Cardiol. 2013;66:350–6. http://www.revespcardiol.org/en/leopard-syndrome-a-variant-of/articulo/90198894/.

Arterial Dissection

N Engl J Med. 1995;332:576–9. http://www.nejm.org/doi/full/10.1056/NEJM199503023320905.

Cardiovascular Manifestations

Am J Cardiol. 2007;100:736–41. http://www.sciencedirect.com/science/article/pii/S000291490700968X.

Case Series

J Med Genet. 2004;41:5 e68. http://jmg.bmj.com/content/41/5/e68.full.

Images

Circulation. 2009;119:1328–9. http://circ.ahajournals.org/content/119/9.toc.

Images

Eur Heart J. 2007;28:3066. http://eurheartj.oxfordjournals.org/content/28/24/3066.full?sid=33a157c3-039c-4fd6-9021-f9f559b9c3c5.

Imaging: MRI

Eur Heart J. 2006;27:1407. http://eurheartj.oxfordjournals.org/content/27/12/1407.full?sid=33a157c3-039c-4fd6-9021-f9f559b9c3c5.

Updates and More

https://clinicalguidecvd.com/leopard

Chapter 57
Long QT Syndrome: Acquired (LQTS)

ICD-10 Code

I45.81

Alternate Names/Abbreviation

LQTS

Description/Etiology

Acquired long QT syndrome is manifest by ECG QT interval prolongation and Torsades de Pointes ventricular tachycardia triggered by drugs, electrolyte abnormalities, and other factors (see PREDISPOSING/COMORBID CONDITIONS)

In some persons QTc interval remains prolonged after elimination of triggers, suggesting an underlying genetic substrate as a causative factor

Predisposing/Comorbid Conditions

ANTIINFECTIVE DRUGS [2]
ATRIOVENTRICULAR HEART BLOCK

V.E. Friedewald, *Clinical Guide to Cardiovascular Disease*,
DOI 10.1007/978-1-4471-7293-2_57,
© Springer-Verlag London 2016

AUTONOMIC NEUROPATHY
CANCER CHEMOTHERAPY DRUGS [12]
CARDIOMYOPATHY – TAKOTSUBO
CARDIOVASCULAR DRUGS [1]
CENTRAL NERVOUS SYSTEM DRUGS [3]
CEREBRAL HEMORRHAGE
COCAINE
HIV
HYPOCALCEMIA
HYPOKALEMIA
HYPOMAGNESEMIA
HYPOTHERMIA
HYPOTHYROIDISM
LEFT VENTRICULAR HYPERTROPHY [4]
LONG QT SYNDROME – CONGENITAL
MYOCARDIAL FIBROSIS [4]
MYOCARDIAL ISCHEMIA [4]
NONALCOHOLIC FATTY LIVER DISEASE
ORGANOPHOSPHATES
PHEOCHROMOCYTOMA
POST-ACUTE MYOCARDIAL INFARCTION
PROPRIONIC ACIDEMIA [14]
PROTEIN-SPARING FASTING
SINUS NODE DYSFUNCTION
STROKE
SUBARACHNOID HEMORRHAGE

Demography

Variable per cause

Pathophysiology

Electrophysiological changes include:

Slowed outward repolarizing K currents
Enhanced inward calcium currents
Slowed inactivation of inward sodium currents

Signs/Symptoms

CONSCIOUSNESS – LOSS, SUDDEN (SYNCOPE)
DIZZY/LIGHTHEADED/PRESYNCOPE

Differentiation

Congenital Long QT Syndrome [15]
Other conditions causing ECG QTc interval prolongation

Complications

Polymorphic VT [5]
SCD

Laboratory

NS [6]

ECG

JT INTERVAL – LONG [13]
QT/QTc INTERVAL – LONG
T WAVE – ALTERNANS [7]
U WAVE – ALTERNANS
U WAVE – PROMINENT

Imaging

NS/VAR WITH COMORBID

Genomics

[15]

Other Tests

Ambulatory ECG monitoring

Treatment: Nonpharmacologic

Correct underlying cause

Treatment: Pharmacologic

Torsades: IV MGSO4 bolus followed by continuous infusion
Torsades: IV K [8]
Torsades: Mexiletine
Isoproterenol [11]
Long-term: beta-blocker

Treatment: Surgical/Invasive

Temporary pacing [9] [10]
Permanent pacing [10]
ICD
Left thoracic sympathectomy

Prevention

Avoid/DC causative agent

Course

Variable according to underlying condition

Notes

[1] Includes but not limited to:

Amiodarone
Azimilide
Bepridil
Disopyramide
Ibutilide
Quinidine
Phenylephrine
Procainamide

[2] Includes but not limited to:

Amantadine
Chloroquine
Erythromycin
Grepafloxacin
Moxifloxacin
Pentamidine
Trimethoprim-sulfamethoxazole

[3] Includes but not limited to:

Arsenic trioxide
Astemizole
Cisapride
Haloperidol
Itraconazole
Ketanserin
Ketoconazole
Papaverine
Phenothiazine
Probucol
Tacrolimus
Tricyclic antidepressants

[4] Promote drug-induced LQTS

[5] Torsades de Pointes; occurs after prolonged QTc interval in preceding sinus beats; usually short-lived and resolves spontaneously but may deteriorate to VF and SCD

[6] Eg, abnormal electrolytes

[7] Beat-to-beat variation in T wave amplitude; associated with marked increased risk of cardiac arrest

[8] Adjunct to IV MGSO4

[9] Prevent short-term recurrence of torsades

[10] Especially effective if precipitated by sinus pause/bradycardia

[11] Contraindicated for Congenital Long QT Syndrome

[12] Includes but not limited to:

> Arsenic Trioxide
> Dasatinib
> Lapatinib
> Nilotinib
> Vorinostat

[13] JT interval measure may be more accurate than QT in presence of prolonged QRS

[14] Propionic Acidemia: rare metabolic disorder due to propionyl-CoA carboxylase deficiency; affected persons have QT prolongation associated with VT/syncope

[15] Up to one-third of persons with Acquired LQTS may carry Congenital LQTS mutations, most often KCNH2

Guidelines

2013 ESC guidelines on cardiac pacing and cardiac resynchronization therapy

Eur Heart J. 2013:34;2318. http://www.escardio.org/guidelines-surveys/esc-guidelines/Pages/cardiac-pacing-and-cardiac-resynchronisation-therapy.aspx.

Patient Information

NIH

http://www.nhlbi.nih.gov/health/health-topics/topics/qt/.

Genetics Home Reference

http://ghr.nlm.nih.gov/glossary=longqtsyndrome.

ESPANOL
   http://es.heart.org/dheart/HEARTORG/Conditions/Answers-
   by-Heart-Fact-Sheets-Multi-language-Information-UCM-
   314158-Article.jsp.

Mayo Clinic

http://www.mayoclinic.org/diseases-conditions/long-qt-syndrome/
   basics/symptoms/con-20025388.

Cleveland Clinic

http://my.clevelandclinic.org/services/heart/disorders/arrhythmia/
   long-qt-syndrome.

Seattle Childrens

http://www.seattlechildrens.org/medical-conditions/heart-blood-
   conditions/long-qt-syndrome-symptoms/.

Texas Heart Institute

http://www.texasheart.org/HIC/Topics/Cond/longqts.cfm.

Professional Information

Arizona Health Foundation QT Drug List

http://crediblemeds.org/everyone/composite-list-all-qtdrugs/?rf=All.

Review: Drug-Induced QT Prolongation/ Torsades

J Am Coll Cardiol. 2016;67:1639–50. http://content.onlinejacc.org/article.aspx?articleID=2506371.

Atrial Fibrillation

J Am Coll Cardiol. 2008;51:836–42. http://content.onlinejacc.org/article.aspx?articleid=1138744.

Diagnostic Challenges

J Am Coll Cardiol. 2010;55:1962–4. http://content.onlinejacc.org/article.aspx?articleid=1142778#bib15.

Drug-Induced: Children

J Am Coll Cardiol. 2014;63:2272–9. http://content.onlinejacc.org/article.aspx?articleID=1851430.

Genetics

Eur Heart J. 2016;37:1456–64. http://eurheartj.oxfordjournals.org/content/37/18/1456.abstract?etoc.

JT Interval in Presence of Long QRS

Am J Cardiol. 2015;116:74–8. http://www.ajconline.org/article/S0002-9149(15)01044-9/abstract.

Mexiletine: Torsades

J Am Coll Cardiol EP. 2015;1:315–22. http://electrophysiology.onlinejacc.org/article.aspx?articleid=2411173&resultClick=24.

Nonalcoholic Fatty Liver DIS

J Am Heart Assoc. 2015;4:e001820. http://jaha.ahajournals.org/content/4/7/e001820.full.

Proprionic Acidemia

Heart Rhythm 2016: Feb (on line). http://www.heartrhythmjournal.com/article/S1547-5271(16)00137-5/abstract.

T Wave Alternans

Am J Med. 2015;128:480–3. http://www.sciencedirect.com/science/article/pii/S0002934315000741.

Updates and More

https://clinicalguidecvd.com/acqlqts

Chapter 58
Long QT Syndrome: Congenital

ICD-10 Code

I45.81

Alternate Names/Abbreviation

LQTS
ANDERSEN (ANDERSEN-TAWIL) SYNDROME
JERVELL-LANGE-NIELSEN (JLN) SYNDROME
ROMANO-WARD SYNDROME
TIMOTHY SYNDROME

Description/Etiology

Inherited ion channel disease (except LQT4) mainly manifest by life-threatening arrhythmias triggered by sudden increase in sympathetic activity, mediated by left-sided cardiac sympathetic nerves

Many affected persons also have hearing loss, seizures independent of ventricular dysrhythmias, and other neurodevelopmental anomalies

V.E. Friedewald, *Clinical Guide to Cardiovascular Disease*,
DOI 10.1007/978-1-4471-7293-2_58,
© Springer-Verlag London 2016

Etiology: genetic mutations affecting transmembrane Na or K ion channel proteins, comprising several Subtypes:

LQT1
LQT2
LQT3
LQT4
LQT5
LQT6
LQT7 [Andersen-Tawil Syndrome] [7]
LQT8 [Timothy Syndrome] [8]
LQT9
LQT10
LQT12
LQT13

Frequency:

LQT1–2: 90 % of cases
LQT3: 5 % of cases
LQT4 +: extremely rare

Predisposing/Comorbid Conditions

ATRIAL FIBRILLATION [12]
FAMILY HX: SUDDEN DEATH
SEIZURES [2]
SENSORINEURAL HEARING LOSS [1]

Demography

About 85 % inherited from 1 parent; remainder sporadic
Family history of SCD
Males at greater risk (especially LQT1) for arrhythmic event/SCD before puberty
Females have greater risk (especially LQT2) during pre-puberty, postmenopause, postpartum

Pathophysiology

Abnormal K and Na channel and channel-related proteins cause positive overcharge of myocytes and heterogeneous prolongation of repolarization in myocardial layers and regions

Signs/Symptoms

CHEST – PALPITATIONS
CONSCIOUSNESS – LOSS, SUDDEN (SYNCOPE) [14]
DIZZY/LIGHTHEADED/PRESYNCOPE
EARS, HEARING – LOSS (DEAFNESS) [1]
HEART, RATE – SLOW (BRADYCARDIA) [13]
SEIZURES

Differentiation

Acquired Long QT Syndrome
ARVD
Brugada Syndrome
Hypertrophc cardiomyopathy
Other causes of seizures
Other causes of sensorineural hearing loss
Other causes of ventricular dysrhythmias

Complications [24]

Polymorphic VT [5] [14]
SCD [14]

Laboratory

NS

ECG [3]

AV COND – 2ND DEGREE BLOCK, MOBITZ I (WENCKEBACH)
DYSRHYTHMIAS – ATRIAL (PACS/OTHERS) [12]
DYSRHYTHMIAS – VENTRICULAR (PVCS/OTHERS) [4]
JT INTERVAL – LONG [23]
QRS, AMP – VAR, RHYTHMIC
QT/QTC INTERVAL – LONG [19]
RATE – DECREASED (SINUS BRADYCARDIA) [12]
T WAVE – ALTERNANS [21]
T WAVE – NOTCHED [17]
T WAVE – POLYPHASIC [12]
T WAVE – TALL/PEAKED [15]
T WAVE – WIDE [18]
T WAVE, AMP – DECR/FLAT [16]
U WAVE – ALTERNANS
U WAVE – PROMINENT

Imaging

NS/VAR WITH COMORBID

Genomics [6] [24]

ACNK2
AKAP9
CACNA1C
CAV3
KCNE1
KCNE2
KCNH2
KCNJ2
KCNJ5

KCNQ1 [?]
SCN4B
SCN5A
SNTA1

Other Tests

Ambulatory 24 h ECG monitoring
Exercise test: QTc prolongation in patients with LQTS
Epinephrine infusion: QTc prolongation in patients with
    LQTS

Treatment: Nonpharmacologic

Avoid/caution in competitive sports [22]
Stress reduction (avoidance of alarm clocks, noise, etc.)
AED immediately available, e.g., at home

Treatment: Pharmacologic

Torsades: IV MGSO4 bolus followed by cont infusion
Torsades: IV K [9]
LQT1 and LQT2 (long-term): Beta-blockers [11]
LQT3 (long-term): Flecainide, Mexiletine [20]
LQT3 with KPQ mutation (short-term): IV Ranolazine
    [20]

Treatment: Surgical/Invasive

Temporary pacing [10]
Permament pacing [10]
ICD
Left thoracic sympathectomy

Notes

[1] Due to absent functional KCNQ1-KCNE1 pores in cochlea; occurs only in JLN Syndrome

[2] Independent of dysrhythmias

[3] T wave morphology, ST-T, repolarization pattern differ according to genotype

[4] Especially multifocal PVCs and Torsades de Pointes

[5] Torsades de Pointes; occurs after prolonged QTc in preceding sinus beats; usually short-lived and resolves spontaneously but may deteriorate to VF and SCD

[6] Mutations of KCNQ1, KCNH2, and SCN5A comprise most cases; all LQTS not yet genotyped

[7] Long QTc plus K-sensitive periodic paralysis, ventricular dysrhythmias, dysmorphic features

[8] Long QTc plus bradycardia, AV Block, other congenital cardiac defects and multiple other organ systems; longevity usually short with mean age of death at 2.5 years

[9] Adjunct to IV MGSO4

[10] Especially effective if precipitated by sinus pause/bradycardia

[11] Main efficacy in LQT1 and LQT2; decreased risk for cardiac event by >60 %; syncope occurring while on beta-blocker appears to convey no greater protection than on no drug treatment; efficacy may vary for preventing events in high-risk patients

[12] Especially LQT5, with AF and intense sinus bradycardia common

[13] May worsen with beta-blockers

[14] May be precipitated by:

Awakening from sleep (especially LQT3)
Emotions
Exercise (especially LQT1), particularly while swimming/diving
Stress
Sudden noise (especially LQT2)

[15] Especially LQT3

[16] Especially LQT2

[17] Especially LQT2

[18] Especially LQT1

[19] When >500 msc: highly likely to be LQTS

[20] Limited data but may be efficacious with decreased QTc interval and major reduction of life-threatening arrhythmic events in LQT3 patients

[21] T wave alternans associated with marked increasedly risk of cardiac arrest

[22] Outcome studies lacking; however, limited data show that in treatment-compliant persons, no adverse events occur in association with sports participation

[23] JT interval measure may be more accurate than QT in presence of prolonged QRS

[24] Family members should have genomic testing as asymptomatic carriers have 10× increased risk of cardiac events

Guidelines

HRS/EHRA/APHRS expert consensus statement on the diagnosis and management of patients with inherited primary arrhythmia syndromes

Heart Rhythm. 2013;10:1932–63. http://www.sciencedirect.com/science/article/pii/S1547527113005523.

Patient Information

NIH

http://www.nhlbi.nih.gov/health/health-topics/topics/qt/.

Genetics Home Reference

http://ghr.nlm.nih.gov/glossary=longqtsyndrome.

ESPANOL
http://es.heart.org/dheart/HEARTORG/Conditions/Answers-by-Heart-Fact-Sheets-Multi-language-Information-UCM-314158-Article.jsp.

Mayo Clinic

http://www.mayoclinic.org/diseases-conditions/long-qt-syndrome/basics/symptoms/con-20025388.

Cleveland Clinic

http://my.clevelandclinic.org/services/heart/disorders/arrhythmia/long-qt-syndrome.

Seattle Childrens

http://www.seattlechildrens.org/medical-conditions/heart-blood-conditions/long-qt-syndrome-symptoms/.

Texas Heart Institute

http://www.texasheart.org/HIC/Topics/Cond/longqts.cfm.

Professional Information

AHA Scientific Statement: Genomics

Circulation Cardiovasc Genetics. 2015;8:216–42. http://circgenetics.ahajournals.org/content/8/1/216.

Arizona Health Foundation QT Drug List

http://crediblemeds.org/everyone/composite-list-all-qtdrugs/?rf=All.

Review

Circulation. 2014;129:1524–9. http://circ.ahajournals.org/content/129/14/1524.full.

Review

Eur Heart J. 2013;34:3109–16. http://eurheartj.oxfordjournals.org/content/34/40/3109.

Review

J Am Coll Cardiol. 2008;51:2291–300. http://content.onlinejacc.org/article.aspx?articleid=1138983.

Review: Genetics of Sudden Cardiac Death

Circulation Res. 2015;116:1919–36. http://circres.ahajournals.org/content/116/12/1919.full.

Genetics Home Reference: Andersen-Tawil Syndrome

http://ghr.nlm.nih.gov/condition/andersen-tawil-syndrome.

Genetics Home Reference: Jervell and Lange-Nielsen Syndrome

http://ghr.nlm.nih.gov/condition/jervell-and-lange-nielsen-syndrome.

Genetics Home Reference: Romano Ward Syndrome

http://ghr.nlm.nih.gov/condition/romano-ward-syndrome.

Genetics Home Reference: Timothy Syndrome

http://ghr.nlm.nih.gov/condition/timothy-syndrome.

Arrhythmia: Mechanism

J Am Coll Cardiol. 1999;33:1415–23. http://content.onlinejacc.org/article.aspx?articleid=1125732.

Beta-Blockers: Differing Efficacy

J Am Coll Cardiol. 2014;64:1352–8. http://content.onlinejacc.org/article.aspx?articleID=1909594.

ECG Imaging: Electrophysiologic Substrate

Circulation. 2014;130:1936–43. http://circ.ahajournals.org/content/130/22/1936.full.

EPILEPSY

JACCCEP. 2016. doi:10.1016/j.jacep.2015.10.010. http://electrophysiology.onlinejacc.org/article.aspx?articleid=2482972.

Epinephrine Test

Circulation. 2006;113:1385–92. http://circ.ahajournals.org/content/113/11/1385.full.

Exercise Test

Circulation. 2003;107:838–44. http://circ.ahajournals.org/content/107/6/838.full.

Genotype-Specific ECG Patterns

J Electrocardiol. 2006;39(4 Suppl):S101–6. http://www.ncbi.nlm.nih.gov/pubmed/16963070.

JT Interval in Presence of Long QRS

Am J Cardiol. 2015;116:74–78. http://www.ajconline.org/article/S0002-9149(15)01044-9/abstract.

Longitudinal Family Study

Circulation. 1991;84:1136–44. http://www.ncbi.nlm.nih.gov/pubmed/1884444.

Mask with Many Faces

J Am Coll Cardiol. 2008;51:930–2. http://content.onlinejacc.org/article.aspx?articleid=1138772.

Mexiletine

J Am Coll Cardiol. 2016;67:1053–8. http://content.onlinejacc.org/article.aspx?articleID=2498347.

QT Clock

Heart Rhythm. 2016;13:190–8. http://www.heartrhythmjournal.com/article/S1547-5271(15)01127-3/abstract.

QT Interval and Incident Cardiovascular Events

J Am Coll Cardiol. 2014;64:2111–9. http://content.onlinejacc.org/article.aspx?articleID=1934902.

Risk Stratification

N Engl J Med. 2003;348:1866–74. http://www.nejm.org/doi/full/10.1056/NEJMoa022147.

Sports Participation Study in Treatment-Compliant Patients

JACCCEP. 2015;1:62–70. http://electrophysiology.onlinejacc.org/article.aspx?articleID=2277233.

(Editorial)

JACCCEP. 2015;1(1):71–3. http://electrophysiology.onlinejacc.org/article.aspx?articleID=2277236.

T Wave Alternans

Am J Med. 2015;128:480–3. http://www.sciencedirect.com/science/article/pii/S0002934315000741.

Ventricular Arrhythmias in Channelopathies: Management

Circulation Arrhythmia Electrophysiol. 2015;8:221–31. http://circep.ahajournals.org/content/8/1/221.extract?etoc.

Updates and More

https://clinicalguidecvd.com/conlqts

Chapter 59
Lower Exremity Artery Disease

ICD-10 Code

I74.3

Alternate Names/Abbreviation

LEAD
ARTERIOSCLEROSIS OBLITERANS
LERICHE SYNDROME [8]
LOWER EXTREMITY ARTERY DISEASE
PERIPHERAL ARTERIAL DISEASE (PAD)

Description/Etiology

A form of peripheral artery disease involving obstruction of arterial blood flow to pelvic organs/structures and lower extremities

Atherosclerosis most common cause but nonatherosclerotic forms exist, including:

Adventitial cysts
Aneurysmal disease
Congenital abnormalities
Entrapment syndromes

V.E. Friedewald, *Clinical Guide to Cardiovascular Disease*,
DOI 10.1007/978-1-4471-7293-2_59,
© Springer-Verlag London 2016

Fibromuscular Dysplasia
Inflammatory disease
Thromboembolic disease
Trauma

Underdiagnosed due to: [19]

High prevalence of asymptomatic patients with LEAD
Wide range of presenting leg symptoms

Predispoisng/Comorbid Conditions

ADVENTITIAL CYSTS
ATHEROSCLEROSIS IN OTHER CV AREAS [1]
DIABETES MELLITUS
DYSLIPIDEMIA
ENTRAPMENT SYNDROME
GOUT
HYPERCHOLESTEROLEMIA – FAMILIAL
HYPERHOMOCYSTEINEMIA
HYPERTENSION – SYSTEMIC ARTERIAL
INFLAMMATION
THROMBOEMBOLISM
TOBACCO USE
TRAUMA

Demography (Atherosclerotic Forms)

Age usually 70+ years except:

Age <50 years with DM and one or more other atherosclerotic risk factors
Age 50–69 years with history of tobacco use and DM

Pathophysiology

Mechanisms of functional impairment and decline in
LEAD poorly understood

Calf muscles in patients with LEAD show:

Apoptosis
Atrophy
Increased connective tissue
Loss of type II muscle fibers

Signs/Symptoms [10]

ARTERIAL PULSE, DORSALIS PEDIS – DECR/
    ABSENT [9]
ARTERIAL PULSE, FEMORAL – DECR/ABSENT
ARTERIAL PULSE, ILIAC – DECR/ABSENT
ARTERIAL PULSE, POPLITEAL – DECR/ABSENT
ARTERIAL PULSE, POST TIBILAL – DECR/
    ABSENT [9]
ARTERY, FEMORAL – BRUIT
ARTERY, ILIAC – BRUIT
ARTERY, POPLITEAL – BRUIT
EARS, BILAT, EARLOBE CREASE, DIAGONAL
EXTREM, BUTTOCK – PAIN, REST [5]
EXTREM, BUTTOCK – PAIN, WALKING
    (CLAUDICATION) [2] [4] [6]
EXTREM, CALF – PAIN, REST [5]
EXTREM, CALF – PAIN, WALKING
    (CLAUDICATION) [2] [3] [6]
EXTREM, FOOT, ARCH – PAIN, REST [5]
EXTREM, FOOT, ARCH – PAIN, WALKING
    (CLAUDICATION) [2] [6]
EXTREM, HIP – PAIN, REST [5]
EXTREM, HIP – PAIN, WALKING (INTERMITTENT
    CLAUDICATION) [4] [6]
EXTREM, THIGH – PAIN, REST [5] [8]
EXTREM, THIGH – PAIN, WALKING
    (INTERMITTENT CLAUDICATION) [2] [4] [6] [8]
EXTREM, UNILAT, TEMP – DECR
SEX, FUNCTION – DECR/ABSENT (IMPOTENCE) [8]
VEINS, FILLING TIME – INCR

Differentiation

Arthritis
Baker cyst
Chronic Exertional Compartment Syndrome [7]
DVT
Nerve root compression
Spinal Stenosis
Thromboangiitis Obliterans

Complications

Gangrene
Nonhealing skin ulcers

Laboratory [15]

BLOOD, BUN – INCR [18]
BLOOD, CHOLESTEROL, LDL (LDL-C) – INCR
BLOOD, CHOLESTEROL, TOTAL – INCR
BLOOD, ST2 – INCR [16]
BLOOD, TGS – INCR
BLOOD, TRIGLYCERIDES – INCR
BLOOD, TROPONIN – INCR [11]

ECG

NS/VAR PER COMORBIDITY(S) [ESP CAD]
N/NS ABN [12]

Imaging [13]

NS

Genomics [17]

NS

Other Tests

[13]

Treatment: Nonpharmacologic [14]

Exercise
Atherosclerosis risk factor modification

Treatment: Pharmacologic [14]

Atherosclerosis risk factor modification
Antiplatelet Rx
Phosphodiesterase inhibitor
Pentoxifylline
Vasodilator
Prostaglandins
Statins

Treatment: Surgical/Invasive [14]

Revascularization

Endovascular/stent
Surgical

Prevention

Atherosclerosis risk factor modification
Statins

Course

Highly variable; long-term outcomes usually determined by atherosclerosis in other arterial beds, especially coronary and cerebrovascular

Notes

[1] Careful evaluation for cerebrovascular, coronary, renal artery, and aortic disease important
[2] Relieved by rest within minutes
[3] Typically superficial femoral obstruction
[4] Typically aorto-iliac obstruction
[5] Typically nocturnal, with limb elevated, relieved by placing limb into dependent position
[6] May also be described as cramp, ache, numbness
[7] Exercise-induced muscle pain and swelling, usually in athletes
[8] Leriche Syndrome: aorto-iliac obstruction causing buttock/thigh claudication, impotence (due to decreased flow in pudendal artery), decreased/absent femoral artery pulses; less often: sciatica, paraplegia, renal Infarction
[9] Dorsalis pedis (8 %) and posterior tibial (3 %) arteries congenitally absent in many persons, but <1 % of individuals have congenital absence of both
[10] Significant arterial obstruction can be present in absence of any symptoms; clinical features of other common comorbid conditions, e.g., Carotid Stenosis, CAD, AAA, not listed here, but should be searched for in patients with LEAD
[11] Increased cardiac troponin associated with increased frequency of amputations/mortality
[12] ECG manifestations of CAD often present
[13] See current Guidelines for diagnostic details
[14] See current Guidelines for treatment details
[15] Serum lipids, CRP, other atherosclerosis risk factors often abnormal

[16] ST2 increase: correlates with increased mortality in DM/critical limb ischemia

[17] Genetics of LEAD not established, although associations have been strongly suggested in ongoing investigations

[18] Increased BUN may be independent risk factor for critical limb ischemia

[19] In primary care settings, 30–60 % of patients with LEAD have no exertional leg symptoms and up to 50 % have exertional leg symptoms atypical for classic intermittent claudication

Guidelines

Management of patients with peripheral artery disease (Compilation of 2005 and 2011 ACCF/AHA Guideline Recommendations)

J Am Coll Cardiol. 2013;61:1555–70. http://content.onlinejacc.org/article.aspx?articleid=1659662.

ESC guidelines on the diagnosis and treatment of peripheral artery diseases

Eur Heart J. 2011;32:2851–906. http://eurheartj.oxfordjournals.org/content/ehj/32/22/2851.full.pdf.

Patient Information

Images

http://www.nlm.nih.gov/medlineplus/ency/imagepages/18077.htm.

http://www.mayoclinic.org/diseases-conditions/peripheral-artery-disease/multimedia/intermittent-claudication/img-20008123.

Medlineplus

ENGLISH
http://www.nlm.nih.gov/medlineplus/ency/article/000170.htm.
ESPANOL
http://www.nlm.nih.gov/medlineplus/spanish/ency/article/000170.htm.

Mayo Clinic

http://www.mayoclinic.org/diseases-conditions/peripheral-artery-disease/basics/definition/con-20028731.

AHA

http://www.heart.org/HEARTORG/Conditions/More/Peripheral ArteryDisease/About-Peripheral-Artery-Disease-PAD-UCM-301301-Article.jsp.

Cleveland Clinic

http://my.clevelandclinic.org/services/heart/disorders/pad.

ADA

http://www.diabetes.org/living-with-diabetes/complications/heart-disease/peripheral-arterial-disease.html?referrer=https://www.google.com/" style="text-decoration:none;" target="_blank"> https://www.google.com/" style="text-decoration:none;" target="_blank">http://www.diabetes.org/living-with-diabetes/complications/heart-disease/peripheral-arterial-disease.html?referrer=https://www.google.com/.

Merck

http://www.merckmanuals.com/home/heart-and-blood-vessel-disorders/peripheral-arterial-disease/overview-of-peripheral-arterial-disease.

CDC: PAD Fact Sheet

http://www.cdc.gov/dhdsp/data-statistics/fact-sheets/fs-pad.htm.

Professional Information

Review

J Am Coll Cardiol. 2016;67:1338–57. http://content.onlinejacc.org/article.aspx?articleID=2502814.

Review

Circulation.   2013;128:2241–50.   http://circ.ahajournals.org/content/128/20/2241.full.

Review

J Am Acad Phys Assist. 2012;25:52–6. http://journals.lww.com/jaapa/Fulltext/2012/09000/Medical-and-surgical-management-of-peripheral.9.aspx.

Review

N Engl J Med. 2007;356:1241–50. http://www.nejm.org/doi/full/10.1056/NEJMcp064483.

Review

Circulation. 1996;94:3026–49. http://circ.ahajournals.org/content/94/11/3026.full.

Review of Literature

Br Med Bull. 2012;104:21–39. http://bmb.oxfordjournals.org/content/104/1/21.

Atrial Fibrillation/Stroke Risk

J Am Heart Assoc. 2014;3:e001270. http://jaha.ahajournals.org/content/3/6/e001270.long.

Angiogenic/Cell RX

Circ Res. 2015;116:1561–78. http://circres.ahajournals.org/content/116/9/1561.full.

Antithrombotic RX

Rev Vasc Med. 2014;2:37–42. http://www.sciencedirect.com/science/article/pii/S2212021113000490.

Bun: Risk Factor for Critical Limb Ischemia

Med. 2015;94:e948. http://journals.lww.com/md-journal/Fulltext/2015/06030/Elevated-Blood-Urea-Nitrogen-is-Associated-With.11.aspx.

Coronary Kartery Disease

Circulation. 2004;109:3136–44. http://circ.ahajournals.org/content/109/25/3136.full.

Diabetes Mellitus

J Am Coll Cardiol. 2006;47:921–9. http://www.sciencedirect.com/science/article/pii/S0735109705028627.

Early Diagnosis in Smokers

J Nurse Pract. 2014;10:611–5. http://www.sciencedirect.com/science/article/pii/S1555415514004620.

Endovascular Treatment

Circ Res. 2015;116:1599–613. http://circres.ahajournals.org/content/116/9/1599.full.

Epidemiology

Circ Res. 2015;116:1509–26. http://circres.ahajournals.org/content/116/9/1509.full.

Exercise/Medical/Stent Revasc Comparison (Aorto-Iliac Obstruction)

J Am Coll Cardiol. 2015;65:999–1009. http://content.onlinejacc.org/article.aspx?articleID=2194897.

Foot Infection

J Nurse Pract. 2008;4:208–15. http://www.sciencedirect.com/science/article/pii/S1555415508000196.

Genetics

Circ Res. 2015;116:1551–60. http://circres.ahajournals.org/content/116/9/1551.full.

Gout: Increased Risk

Ann Rheum Dis. 2015;74:642–7. http://ard.bmj.com/content/74/4/642.full.

Hypertension: Treatment

Prog Cardiovasc Dis. 2008;50:238–63. http://www.sciencedirect.com/science/article/pii/S0033062007000758.

Leriche Syndrome

Int J Geron. 2013;7:239–40. http://www.sciencedirect.com/science/
article/pii/S1873959813000914.

Leriche Syndrome

Am J Med. 2014;127:291–4. http://www.sciencedirect.com/science/
article/pii/S0002934314000722.

Lower Extremity Manifestations

Cir Res. 2015;116:1540–50. http://circres.ahajournals.org/content/
116/9/1540.full.

Mediterranean Diet: Decreased Risk

JAMA. 2014;311:415–7. http://jama.jamanetwork.com/article.aspx?a
rticleid=1817779#jld130034r2.

Morbidity/In-Hospital Outcomes

Eur Heart J. 2013;34:2706–14. http://eurheartj.oxfordjournals.org/
content/34/34/2706.abstract.

Nonatheromatous Lesions

Arteriosclerosis Thromb Vas Biol. 2015;35:439–47. http://atvb.
ahajournals.org/content/35/2/439.abstract?etoc.

Pathogenesis of Clinical Manifestations

Circ Res. 2015;116:1527–39. http://circres.ahajournals.org/content/
116/9/1527.full.

PAR-1 Inhibition: Vorapaxor

Circulation. 2013;127:1522–9. http://circ.ahajournals.org/content/127/14/1522.full.

PAR-1 Inhibition: Vorapaxor

N Engl J Med. 2012;366:1404–13. http://www.nejm.org/doi/full/10.1056/NEJMoa1200933.

Pharmacologic Treatment

Circ Res. 2015;116:1579–98. http://circres.ahajournals.org/content/116/9/1579.full.

Revascularization: Below Knee Balloon Angioplasty

Circulation. 2013;128:615–21. http://circ.ahajournals.org/content/128/6/615.full.

Revascularization: Infrapopliteal

J Am Coll Cardiol. 2014;64:1568–76. http://content.onlinejacc.org/article.aspx?articleID=1911033.

Revascularization: Long-Term Outcomes

Circulation. 2013;127:1241–50. http://circ.ahajournals.org/content/127/11/1241.full.

Revascularization: Post-procedure Management

Circulation. 2013;128:749–57. http://circ.ahajournals.org/content/128/7/749.full.

Revascularization Compared to Noninvasive Therapy: 1 YR Follow-Up

Circulation. 2014;130:939–47. http://circ.ahajournals.org/content/130/12/939.full.

Revascularization: Surgery

Circ Res. 2015;116:1614–28. http://circres.ahajournals.org/content/116/9/1614.full.

ST2 Increase: Predictor of Mortality in DM/Critical Limb Ischemia

Arterioscler Thromb Vasc Biol. 2012;32:e149–60. http://atvb.ahajournals.org/content/32/12/e149.full.

Statins

Eur Heart J. 2014;35:2864–72. http://eurheartj.oxfordjournals.org/content/35/41/2864.

Stents: Femoropopliteal

J Am Coll Cardiol. 2013;62:1320–7. http://content.onlinejacc.org/article.aspx?articleID=1710964.

Tobacco Smoke: Second-Hand

Heart.   2013;99:1342–5.   http://heart.bmj.com/content/99/18/1342.
abstract.

Tobacco Use

Rev Cardiovasc Med. 2004;5:189–93. http://www.ncbi.nlm.nih.gov/
pubmed/15580157.

Tobacco Use

Heart.   2014;100:414–23.   http://heart.bmj.com/content/100/5/414.
abstract.

Troponin T: Mortality/Amputation Rates

J Am Coll Cardiol. 2014;63:1529–38. http://content.onlinejacc.org/
article.aspx?articleID=1700991.

Updates and More

https://clinicalguidecvd.com/lead

Chapter 60
Marfan Syndrome

ICD-10 Code

Q87.40 Unspecified
Q87.41 CV manifestations
Q87.410 Aortic Dilation
Q87.418 Other CV manifestations
Q87.42 Ocular manifestations
Q87.43 Skeletal manifestation

Description/Etiology

Inherited connective disorder (usually dominant inheritance) involving mainly cardiovascular, skeletal, ocular tissues

Usually caused by mutations in FBN1 gene, which encodes matrix protein Fibrillin 1

Ghent diagnostic criteria [35]:

In the absence of family history:

1. Aortic Root Dilatation Z score ≥ 2 and Ectopia Lentis = Marfan syndrome [28].

V.E. Friedewald, *Clinical Guide to Cardiovascular Disease*,
DOI 10.1007/978-1-4471-7293-2_60,
© Springer-Verlag London 2016

2. Aortic Root Dilatation Z score ≥ 2 and FBN1 = Marfan syndrome [29]
3. Aortic Root Dilatation Z score ≥ 2 and Systemic Score ≥ 7pts = Marfan syndrome [30]
4. Ectopia lentis and FBN1 with known Aortic Root Dilatation = Marfan syndrome [31]

In the presence of family history:

1. Ectopia lentis and Family History of Marfan syndrome (as defined above) = Marfan syndrome [32]
2. A systemic score ≥ 7 points and Family History of Marfan syndrome (as defined above) = Marfan syndrome [33]
3. Aortic Root Dilatation Z score (≥ 2 above 20 years old, ≥ 3 below 20 years old) + Family History of Marfan syndrome (as defined above) = Marfan syndrome [34].

Predisposing/Comorbid Conditions

BICUSPID AORTIC VALVE
CARDIOMYOPATHY – DILATED
COARCTATION OF AORTA
DILATATION: ABDOMINAL AORTA
DILATATION: ASCENDING AORTA
DILATATION: DESCENDING THORACIC AORTA
DILATATION: MAIN PULMONARY ARTERY
ECTOPIA LENTIS [26]
FAMILY HX: SUDDEN DEATH
FH: MARFAN
LUMBOSACRAL DURAL ECTASIA
MITRAL ANNULUS CALCIFICATION
MITRAL VALVE PROLAPSE
RESTRICTIVE LUNG DISEASE
SCOLIOSIS
SPONTANEOUS PNEUMOTHORAX
STRIAE ATROPHICA

Demography

Global
Gender equal
More common in amateur and professional basketball and
volleyball athletes

Pathophysiology [13]

FBN1 mutation causes:

Decreased amount of functional Fibrillin-1 available to
form microfibrils
Decreased tissue elastin content (eg, aortic wall)
Excess release of growth factors
Tissue overgrowth/instability

Cardiovascular morphologic changes include:

Aortic root/descending thoracic aorta dilatation
Mitral valve prolapse
Sinuses of Valsalva dilatation (begins in utero)
Thickened AV valves with regurgitation

Signs/Symptoms

BACK – PAIN [17]
BACK, CURV – LAT (SCOLIOSIS) [5]
BODY, HT – INCR [20]
EXTREM – LONG [2]
EXTREM, ELBOW, EXTENSION – DECR/ABSENT [1]
EXTREM, FEET – FLAT (PES PLANUS)
EXTREM, FEET, ARCH – HIGH (PES CAVUS) **[6]**
EXTREM,   FINGERS   –   CONTRACTURES
(CAMPTODACTYLY)
EXTREM, FINGERS – LONG (ARACHNODACTYLY)
[3] [4]

EYES – GLAUCOMA
EYES, CORNEA – FLAT
EYES, GLOBE, AXIAL LENGTH – INCR
EYES, IRIS – HYPOPLASTIC
EYES, LENS – DISLOCATION (ECTOPIA LENTIS) [26]
EYES, LENS – OPACITY (CATARACT)
EYES, PALPEBRAL FISS – DOWN-SLANTING
EYES, PUPILS – MIOSIS, INCR [7]
EYES, RETINA – DETACHED
EYES, VISION – MYOPIA
FACE, CHEEKS – FLAT
FACE, CHIN – SMALL (MICROGNATHIA)
FACE, JAW – DISPLACED, POST (RETROGNATHISM)
HEAD, SKULL – LONG/NARROW (DOLICHOCEPHALY)
HEART, LSB, LOWER – CLICK, SYS [8]
HEART, LSB, LOWER – MURMUR, SYS [8]
HEART, LSB, MID – MURMUR, DIAS [10]
HEART, LV, APEX – CLICK(S), SYS [9]
HEART, LV, APEX – MURMUR, SYS [9]
HEART, RSB, UPPER – MURMUR, DIAS [10]
JOINTS, MOVEMENT, RANGE – INCR (HYPERMOBILITY)
MOUTH, PALATE – HIGH/ARCHED
MOUTH, TEETH – CROWDING
SKIN, GEN – STRIAE ATROPHICA [16]
STERNUM, CURV – ANT (PECTUS CARINATUM)
STERNUM, CURV – POST (PECTUS EXCAVATUM)

Differentiation

Aneurysms-Osteoarthritis Syndrome
Ascending Aortic Aneurysm Syndrome
Bicommissural Aortic Valve Syndrome
Cutis Laxa

Ehlers-Danlos Syndrome
Familial Ectopic Lentis
Familial Mitral Valve Prolapse Syndrome
Familial Thoracic Aortic Aneurysm Syndrome
Homocystinuria
Loeys-Dietz Syndrome
MASS phenotype [18]

Complications [13]

AMI [12]
Aortic Aneurysm
Aortic Dissection [21]
Coronary Aneurysm
Dilated Cardiomyopathy [23]
Dysrhythmias – atrial [19]
Dysrhythmias – ventricular
HF
Mitral Regurgitation
Pulmonary Hypertension
Restrictive lung disease [15]
Spontaneous Pneumothorax [14]
Stroke [11]
Sudden Athletic-Related Death
Sudden Infant Death

Laboratory

GENETIC TESTING

ECG

NS/VAR PER COMORBIDITY(S) [ESP CARDIAC
ABN]

Imaging [22]

AORTA, ASCEND, SIZE – INCR
AORTA, ROOT, SIZE – INCR [25]
AV, FLOW – REGURG
LV, DIAS – DYSF [23]
LV, SYS – DYSF [23]
MV, ANNULUS – CALCIUM
MV, LEAFLETS – PROLAPSE
TV, LEAFLET, MOTION – PROLAPSE

Genomics

FBN1

Other Tests

Contrast aortography

Treatment: Nonpharmacologic

Avoidance/caution in contact/competitive sports
Avoidance/caution in isometric exercise

Treatment: Pharmacologic

ARBs [27]
Beta-blockers [24]

Treatment: Surgical/Invasive

Elective: aortic root repair with/without AV replacement

Course

Variable according to pathology

Notes

[1] <170°
[2] Arm span to height ratio >1.05
[3] Walker-Murdoch/wrist sign: full overlap of thumb over 5th finger when wrapped over contralateral wrist
[4] Steinberg/thumb sign: distal thumb phalanx fully extends beyond ulnar border of hand when fully extended across palm
[5] >20°
[6] Occurs less often than pes planus
[7] Due to ciliary muscle hypoplasia
[8] TV prolapse/regurgitation
[9] MV prolapse/regurgitation
[10] AR secondary to aortic root dilatation
[11] Involvement of carotid arteries
[12] Involvement of coronary arteries
[13] Pertaining to CV system only
[14] Due to widening of distal lung airspaces
[15] Due to sternum deformities/scoliosis
[16] Occur in areas not subject to stretch, such as anterior shoulder, low back
[17] Due to dural ectasia; usually not symptomatic
[18] MASS: mitral, aortic, skin, skeletal features in persons without true Marfan
[19] Especially AF
[20] Due to long bone overgrowth (dolichostenomelia)
[21] Main risk factors are family history of Aortic Dissection and increased maximal aortic dimension by echo
[22] Echo/Doppler may be used serially for monitoring, especially for aortic root size
[23] LV dysfunction independent of valve regurgitation may occur in some persons

[24] To reduce proximal aortic sheer stress

[25] Echo measures internal aortic diameter; MRI and CT measure external diameter, which is 0.2-0.4 larger than echo measures

[26] Ectopia lentis: affects 60 % of Marfan patients; other causes include:

Familial Ectopia Lentis
Homocystinuria
Weill-Marchesani Syndrome

Brachydactyly
Joint stiffness
Other eye abnormalities
Short stature

[27] Decreases aortic dilatation rates (losartan)

[28] *** Presence of aortic root dilatation (Z-score ≥ 2 when standardized to age and body size) or dissection and ectopia lentis allows unequivocal diagnosis of Marfan syndrome, regardless of presence or absence of systemic features except where these are indicative of Shprintzen Goldberg syndrome, Loeys-Dietz syndrome, or vascular Ehlers Danlos syndrome

[29] *** Presence of aortic root dilatation ($Z \geq 2$) or dissection and identification of a bona fide FBN1 mutation are sufficient to establish the diagnosis, even when ectopia lentis is absent.

[30] *** Where aortic root dilatation ($Z \geq 2$) or dissection is present, but ectopia lentis is absent and the FBN1 status is either unknown or negative, a Marfan syndrome diagnosis is confirmed by the presence of sufficient systemic findings (≥ 7 points, according to a scoring system) confirms the diagnosis. However, features suggestive of Shprintzen Goldberg syndrome, Loeys-Dietz syndrome, or vascular Ehlers Danlos syndrome must be excluded and appropriate alternative genetic testing (TGFBR1/2,

SMAD3, TGFB2, TGFB3, collagen biochemistry, COL3A1, and other relevant genetic testing when indicated and available upon the discovery of other genes) should be performed.

[31] *** In the presence of ectopia lentis, but absence of aortic root dilatation/dissection, the identification of an FBN1 mutation previously associated with aortic disease is required before making the diagnosis of Marfan syndrome

[32] *** The presence of ectopia lentis and a family history of Marfan syndrome (as defined in 1–4 above) is sufficient for a diagnosis of Marfan syndrome

[33] *** A systemic score of greater than or equal to 7 points and a family history of Marfan syndrome (as defined in 1–4 above) is sufficient for a diagnosis of Marfan syndrome. However, features suggestive of Shprintzen Goldberg syndrome, Loeys-Dietz syndrome, or vascular Ehlers Danlos syndrome must be excluded and appropriate alternative genetic testing (TGFBR1/2, SMAD3, TGFB2, TGFB3 collagen biochemistry, COL3A1, and other relevant genetic testing when indicated and available upon the discovery of other genes) should be performed

[34] *** The presence of aortic root dilatation (Z≥2 above 20 year old, ≥ 3 below 20 year old) and a family history of Marfan syndrome (as defined in 1–4 above) is sufficient for a diagnosis of Marfan syndrome. However, features suggestive of Shprintzen Goldberg syndrome, Loeys-Dietz syndrome, or vascular Ehlers Danlos syndrome must be excluded and appropriate alternative genetic testing (TGFBR1/2, SMAD3, TGFB2, TGFB3, collagen biochemistry, COL3A1, and other relevant genetic testing when indicated and available upon the discovery of other genes) should be performed

[35] *** From: The Marfan Foundation https://www.marfan.org/dx/rules

Guidelines

2010   ACCF/AHA/AATS/ACR/ASA/SCA/SCAI/SIR/STS/SVM Guidelines for the Diagnosis and Management of Patients with Thoracic Aortic Disease

Circulation.   2010:121;1544–79.   http://circ.ahajournals.org/content/121/13/e266.full.pdf.

2014 ESC Guidelines on the diagnosis and treatment of aortic diseases

Eur Heart J. doi:10.1093/eurheartj/ehu281. https://www.nvvc.nl/media/richtlijn/187/2014_ESC_Guidelines_on_Diagnosis_and_Treatment_of_Aortic_Disease.pdf.

Patient Information

Genetics Home Reference

http://ghr.nlm.nih.gov/condition/marfan-syndrome.

Medlineplus

http://www.nlm.nih.gov/medlineplus/marfansyndrome.html.
http://www.nlm.nih.gov/medlineplus/ency/imagepages/9611.htm.

Marfan Foundation

http://www.marfan.org/.

Mayo Clinic

http://www.mayoclinic.org/diseases-conditions/marfan-syndrome/basics/definition/con-20025944.

Espanol

http://www.nlm.nih.gov/medlineplus/spanish/marfansyndrome.html.

Professional Information

Review

J Nurse Pract. 2014;10:594–602. http://www.sciencedirect.com/science/article/pii/S1555415514004140.

Review

Lancet. 2005;366:1965–76. http://www.sciencedirect.com/science/article/pii/S0140673605677896.

Aortic Type A Dissection/Marfan: Surgery

Circulation. 2014;129:1381–6. http://circ.ahajournals.org/content/129/13/1381.full.

Aortic Root Dissection Prevention: Atenolol Versus Losartan

N Engl J Med. 2014;371:2061–71. http://www.nejm.org/doi/full/10.1056/NEJMoa1404731.

Aortic Dilatation/Bicuspid Aortic Valve

Heart. 2014;100:126–34. http://heart.bmj.com/content/100/2/126.full.

Coronary Aneurysm

Circulation.   2014;129:1791–2.   http://circ.ahajournals.org/content/129/17/1791.full.

Cardiovascular Involvement: Natural History/Followup

J Am Coll Cardiol. 1989;14:422–8. http://www.sciencedirect.com/science/article/pii/0735109789901976.

Familial Thoracic Aorta Aneurysms

Curr Opin Cardiol. 2014;29:492–8. http://www.ncbi.nlm.nih.gov/pubmed/25290696.

Ghent Nosology for Marfan Syndrome (Revised)

J Med Genet. 2010;47:476–85. http://jmg.bmj.com/content/47/7/476.abstract.

Losartan Versus Atenolol: Aortic Dilatation

Eur Heart J. 2016;37:978–85. http://eurheartj.oxfordjournals.org/content/37/12/978.abstract?etoc.

Losartan: Decreased Aortic Dilatation Rates

Eur Heart J. 2013;34:3491–500. http://eurheartj.oxfordjournals.org/content/34/45/3491.

Mitral Valve Prolapse

Echocardiography. 2009;26:357–64. http://www.ncbi.nlm.nih.gov/pubmed/19054044?dopt=Abstract.

Pregnancy

Int J Cardiol. 2009;136;156–61. http://www.sciencedirect.com/science/article/pii/S0167527308006177.

Pulmonary Artery Aneurysm

Circulation. 2015;131:310–6. http://circ.ahajournals.org/content/131/3/310.extract.

Pulmonary Artery Aneurysm/Dissection

J Am Coll Cardiol. 2013;61:685. http://content.onlinejacc.org/article.aspx?articleID=1567630.

Surgery: Aortic Root Aneurysm

J Thorac Cardiovasc Surg. 2003;125:789–96. http://www.sciencedirect.com/science/article/pii/S0022522302733047.

Surgery: Bentall/Valve-Sparing Aortic Root Procedures

Ann Thor Surg. 2008;85:2003–11. http://www.sciencedirect.com/science/article/pii/S000349750800163X.

Updates and More

https://clinicalguidecvd.com/marfan

Chapter 61
Mitral Regurgitation: Acute

Management Keys

Diagnosis of presence and determination of etiology are urgent in order to initiate appropriate interventional therapy, which may be lifesaving

ICD-10 Code

I34.0

Alternate Names/Abbreviation

ACUTE MR

Description/Etiology

Acute compromise of MV apparatus due to many causes, including:

Chordal rupture [13]
Infective Endocarditis
Papillary muscle rupture [12]
Papillary muscle dysfunction [1]
Prosthetic valve dysfunction

V.E. Friedewald, *Clinical Guide to Cardiovascular Disease*,
DOI 10.1007/978-1-4471-7293-2_61,
© Springer-Verlag London 2016

Predisposing/Comorbid Conditions

CORONARY ARTERY DISEASE
MYXOMATOUS MV
RHEUMATIC VALVE DISEASE

Demography

Per etiology

Pathophysiology

Sudden increase in LA/LV blood volume without corresponding LA/LV dilatation, causing:

Decreased LV stoke volume
Rapid increase in pulmonary venous pressure/acute pulmonary edema
Systemic Hypotension

Signs/Symptoms

BREATH SOUNDS – CRACKLES (RALES)
BREATHING – DIFF (DYSPNEA)
BREATHING – RAPID (TACHYPNEA)
EXTREM, HANDS/FEET, COLOR – BLUE (ACROCYANOSIS) [5]
FATIGUE
FEVER [6]
HEART, LV, APEX – MURMUR, DIAS [2, 3]
HEART, LV, APEX – MURMUR, SYS [4]
HEART, LV, APEX, IMP – FORCEFUL/SUSTAINED [8]
HEART, RATE – RAPID (TACHYCARDIA)
HEART, S3 LV [2]

HYPOTENSION   (BLOOD   PRESSURE   –
  DECREASED/LOW)
NECK, JVP, V WAVE – INCR/LARGE
SKIN, TEMP – DECR [5]

Differentiation

HF
Non-cardiac pulmonary edema
Other causes of circulatory collapse
Pneumonia

Complications

Acute pulmonary edema
Dysrhythmias
HF
SHOCK

Laboratory

BLOOD, NT-PROBNP – INCR
BLOOD, WBC – INCR (LEUKOCYTOSIS) [6]

ECG [7]

DYSRHYTHMIAS – ATRIAL (PACS/OTHERS)
DYSRHYTHMIAS – VENTRICULAR (PVCS/
  OTHERS)
RATE – INCREASED (SINUS TACHYCARDIA)
ST-T WAVE – ABN, NS

Imaging

CARD SIZE MAY BE N [10]
LV, WALL MOTION – INCR/HYPERDYNAMIC
MV, FLOW – REGURG
MV, LEAFLET MORPH – ABN
MV, LEAFLET, MOTION – ABN
PUL – EDEMA [9]

Other Tests

Coronary angiography if ischemic etiology possible

Treatment: Nonpharmacologic

O_2

Treatment: Pharmacologic

Antibiotics [6]
Inotropes [11]
Vasodilators [11]

Treatment: Surgical/Invasive

Intraaortic balloon counterpulsation
MV repair
MV replacement

Prevention

Variable per etiology

Course

Variable per etiology

Notes

[1] Due to acute Myocarditis or acute myocardial ischemia causing papillary muscle displacement
[2] May be only auscultatory findings
[3] Early diastole
[4] May be best heard at cardiac base; may be soft/absent or not holosystolic; may radiate to neck, spine, top of head
[5] Peripheral vasoconstriction
[6] With Infective Endocarditis (bacterial)
[7] Often normal; ischemic changes signify acute coronary etiology of MR
[8] Often absent; if present, hyperdynamic LV in presence of normal cardiac size suggests acute MR
[9] Rarely, edema may be isolated to 1 segment if preferentially directed to a single pulmonary vein
[10] Unless prior chronic MR present
[11] To stabilize prior to surgery only
[12] STEMI, usually inferior AMI
[13] May occur with degenerative MV disease

Guidelines

2014 AHA/ACC Guideline for the Management of Patients with Valvular Heart Disease
J Am Coll Cardiol. 2014;63:e57–e185. http://www.content.onlinejacc.org/article.aspx?articleID=1838843.
Guidelines on the management of valvular heart disease (version 2012)
Eur Heart J. 2012;33:2469–75. http://www.escardio.org/guidelines-surveys/esc-guidelines/Pages/valvular-heart-disease.aspx.

Patient Information

Images

http://www.nlm.nih.gov/medlineplus/ency/imagepages/1056.htm.
http://www.nlm.nih.gov/medlineplus/ency/imagepages/1097.htm.

Medlineplus

ENGLISH
http://www.nlm.nih.gov/medlineplus/ency/article/ 000176.htm.
ESPANOL.
http://www.nlm.nih.gov/medlineplus/spanish/ency/ article/000176.htm.

Cleveland Clinic

http://www.clevelandclinicmeded.com/medicalpubs/disease management/cardiology/mitral-valve-disease/#s0065.

Mayo Clinic

http://www.mayoclinic.org/diseases-conditions/mitral-valve-regurgitation/basics/definition/con-20022644.

AHA

http://www.heart.org/HEARTORG/Conditions/More/ HeartValveProblemsandDisease/Problem-Mitral-Valve-Regurgitation-UCM-450612-Article.jsp.

Merck

http://www.merckmanuals.com/home/heart-and-blood-vessel-disorders/heart-valve-disorders/mitral-regurgitation.

Professional Information

Review: Basic Mechanisms

Can J Cardiol. 2014;30:971–81. http://www.sciencedirect.com/science/article/pii/S0828282X14004280.

AMI: Shock Trial

J Am Coll Cardiol. 2000;36:1104–9. http://www.sciencedirect.com/science/article/pii/S0735109700008469.

AMI: Outcomes

Ann Intern Med. 1992;117:18–24. http://www.annals.org/article.aspx?articleid=705627&resultClick=3.

Diagnosis and Treatment

J Heart Valve Dis. 1993;2:512–22. http://www.ncbi.nlm.nih.gov/pubmed/8269160.

PAP Muscle Rupture (Case Report)

Circulation. 2013;127:e586-8. http://www.circ.ahajournals.org/content/127/18/e586.full.

Post-valvotomy Acute MR

Catheter Cardiovasc Interv. 2013;81:603–8. http://www.onlinelibrary.wiley.com/doi/10.1002/ccd.24417/abstract.

Vasodilator Therapy

Am J Cardiol. 1979;43:773–7. http://www.ajconline.org/article/0002-9149(79)90077-8/abstract.

Updates and More

https://clinicalguidecvd.com/amr

Chapter 62
Mitral Regurgitation: Chronic

ICD-10 Code

I34.1

Alternate Names/Abbreviation

MR
MITRAL INSUFFICIENCY

Description/Etiology

50 % of LV stroke volume diverted to regurgitant flow into LA due to primary or secondary abnormalities of structure/function of mitral apparatus, including:

MV leaflets [1]
MV annulus [2]
Chordae tendineae [3]
Papillary muscles [4]

Stages (secondary form):

A. At risk

Normal valve leaflets/chords/annulus with CAD or cardiomyopathy

V.E. Friedewald, *Clinical Guide to Cardiovascular Disease*, 857
DOI 10.1007/978-1-4471-7293-2_62,
© Springer-Verlag London 2016

B. Progressive

Abnormal regional wall motion with mild MV leaflet tethering

Annular dilatation with mild loss of central leaflet coaptation

C. Asymptomatic severe

Abnormal regional wall motion/LV dilatation with severe MV leaflet tethering

Annular dilatation with severe loss of central leaflet coaptation

D. Symptomatic severe

Abnormal regional wall motion/LV dilatation with severe MV leaflet tethering

Annular dilatation with severe loss of central leaflet coaptation

Most common cause: degenerative MV disease

Comorbid Conditions

ANTIPHOSPHOLIPID SYNDROME
AORTIC REGURGITATION – CHRONIC
ATRIAL FIBRILLATION
CARCINOID HEART DISEASE
CARDIAC AMYLOIDOSIS
CARDIAC SARCOIDOSIS
CARDIOMYOPATHY – DILATED
CARDIOMYOPATHY – HYPERTROPHIC
CARDIOMYOPATHY – RESTRICTIVE
CARDIOMYOPATHY – TAKOTSUBO
DRUGS: ERGOTAMINES
DRUGS: METHYSERGIDE
DRUGS: PERGOLIDE
ENDOMYOCARDIAL FIBROSIS
GIANT CELL MYOCARDITIS
HEART FAILURE
INFECTIVE ENDOCARDITIS

KAWASAKI DISEASE
MARFAN SYNDROME
MITRAL ANNULUS CALCIFICATION
MITRAL VALVE PROLAPSE [INCL BARLOW]
MYOCARDITIS
MYXOMA – LEFT ATRIUM
RADIATION
RHEUMATIC FEVER [See Appendix A]
RHEUMATOID ARTHRITIS
STABLE ISCHEMIC HEART DISEASE
SYSTEMIC LUPUS ERYTHEMATOSUS
VON WILLEBRAND SYNDROME [ACQUIRED]

Demography

Variable according to etiology
Prevalence: 10 % in persons > age 75 years

Pathophysiology

Abnormal reverse blood flow from LV to LA and resultant LV and LA dilatation and LV compensatory changes to maintain cardiac output

Cardiac function in patients with primary MV abnormalities tends to deteriorate with time as volume overload progresses and effective valve orifice area increases

Both RV systolic dysfunction (due to LV remodeling/abnormal septal function/increased PA pressure) and LV dysfunction contribute to abnormal hemodynamics

Degenerative MV disease consists of myxomatous degeneration of MV leaflets with:

Elongated/redundant chordal apparatus

Prolapse of leaflets into LA causing leaflet edge malcoaptation/subsequent regurgitation

Rupture of chordal structures (sometimes), especially in older males, causing further increase in MR severity due to unsupported leaflet segments

Signs/Symptoms [5]

ARTERIAL PULSE, AMP – DECR/ABS
ARTERIAL PULSE, FALL – RAPID
ARTERIAL PULSE, RISE – RAPID
BREATHING – DIFF (DYSPNEA)
CHEST, ANT, L – BULGE
FATIGUE
HEART, LV, APEX – MURMUR, DIAS
HEART, LV, APEX – MURMUR, SYS [12, 16]
HEART, LV, APEX, IMP – FORCEFUL/SUSTAINED
HEART, LV, APEX, IMP – DIFFUSE
HEART, P2, INTENSITY – INCR
HEART, S2, SPLIT – WIDE [SEVERE; EARLY AV
    CLOSURE]
HEART, S3 LV [12]
SKIN, TEMP – DECR
SWEATING – INCR (DIAPHORESIS/
    HYPERHIDROSIS)

Differentiation (of MR Systolic Murmur)

AS – Valvular
HCM (with LVOT obstruction)
TR
VSD

Complications

AF/Flutter (30 % 10-year incidence)
Bleeding [14]
Other dysrhythmias
HF
IE
Peripheral emboli
Pulmonary edema
SCD [6]

Laboratory

BLOOD, NT-PROBNP – INCR [13]
BLOOD, ST2 – INCR [17]

ECG

P WAVE, DUR – INCR
QRS – LBBB/LBBB PATTERN
QRS – LVH PATTERN

Imaging [7] [15]

CARDIOMEGALY
LUNGS, INTERSTITIUM – EDEMA/INFILTRATES
LA, CHAMBER, SIZE – INCR
LV, CHAMBER, SIZE – INCR
LV, WALL MOTION – INCR/HYPERDYNAMIC
MV, FLOW – REGURG
MV, LEAFLET MORPH – ABN [11]
MV, LEAFLETS, MOTION – ABN [11]

Other Tests

Exercise Doppler [8]
Cardiac catheterization [9]

Treatment: Nonpharmacologic

NS

Treatment: Pharmacologic

Asymptomatic: NS
AF: rate control and anticoagulation

Primary versus secondary considerations [19] [20]
Aldosterone antagonists
ACEIs
ARBs
Beta-blockers

Treatment: Surgical/Invasive [10]

MV repair
   Surgical
   Transcatheter [18]
MV replacement with mitral apparatus preservation
MV replacement with mitral apparatus removal

Course

Primary MR asymptomatic 5 year rates:

Death from any cause: 22 %
HF: 14 %
New AF: 14 %

Primary MR predictors of poor outcome include:

Age
AF
Decreased LVEF
Increased LV end-systolic volume
LA dilatation
MR severity
PAH

Notes

[1] Eg, myxomatous degeneration, rheumatic heart disease, congenital deformity, radiation
[2] Eg, annular calcification, myxomatous degeneration, connective tissue disease

[3] Eg, Rheumatic Carditis, radiation, IE, drugs

[4] Eg, ischemia, DCM, HCM

[5] Patients with mild-moderate MR often are asymptomatic for many years; symptoms of dyspnea/exercise intolerance develop slowly as compensatory mechanisms are overwhelmed by volume overload and irreversible LV dysfunction occurs

[6] May occur in asymptomatic patients

[7] Echo: Principle means of investigation for severity, mechanisms, reparability, consequences, RV function, PA pressure; high degree of operator skill required

[8] To assess patients with severe MR who are asymptomatic for exercise tolerance and effects of exercise on PA pressure and MR severity

[9] When noninvasive testing is unsatisfactory or incongruent with clinical findings or when surgery is contemplated

[10] In patients with primary MR, surgical intervention with repair/replacement indicated with severe MR and symptoms or LV dysfunction (EF <60 % or end systolic diameter >40 mm); surgical repair is preferred treatment for primary MR and is associated with better outcomes than MV replacement; see guidelines for detailed current specific recommendations

[11] According to etiology

[12] Primary MR: increased intensity/long duration of MR murmur and presence of S3 suggest significant MR; in secondary MR, murmur intensity often soft/unrelated to severity

[13] Blood BNP/Pro-BNP level increases/changes may be outcome predictors

[14] Due to acquired von Willebrand syndrome and reversible with MV surgery

[15] CMRI may be superior to echo for quantifying MR

[16] Usually blowing quality; harsh/musical suggests ruptured chordae tendineae/MVP

[17] Increased ST2 correlates with higher level of LVEF and lower LVEDD post-MV repair

[18] Early data: significant MR treated with transcatheter repair results in significant clinical improvements at 12 months

[19] Primary MR: pharmacologic treatment does not alter natural history of severe primary MR; for symptomatic patients with severe primary MR, diuretics and afterload reduction help relieve signs/symptoms of HF, but intervention is ultimate treatment; see guidelines for detailed current specific recommendations

[20] Secondary MR: first-line treatment consists of guideline-directed medical therapy for LV dysfunction, including ACEIs, ARBs, beta-blockers, and aldosterone antagonists; see guidelines for detailed current specific recommendations

Appendix A: World Heart Federation Echo Criteria for Diagnosis of Rheumatic Fever

Individuals Age <20 Years

Definite RHD (either A, B, C, or D):

A. Pathological MR and at least two morphological features of RHD of the MV

B. MS mean gradient = 4 mmHg*

C. Pathological AR and at least two morphological features of RHD of the AV‡

D. Borderline disease of both the AV and MV§

Borderline RHD (either A, B, or C):

A. At least two morphological features of RHD of the MV without pathological MR or MS

B. Pathological MR

C. Pathological AR

Normal echocardiographic findings (all of A, B, C, and D):

A. MR that does not meet all four Doppler echocardiographic criteria (physiological MR)
B. AR that does not meet all four Doppler echocardiographic criteria (physiological AR)
C. An isolated morphological feature of RHD of the MV (for example, valvular thickening) without any associated pathological stenosis or regurgitation
D. Morphological feature of RHD of the AV (for example, valvular thickening) without any associated pathological stenosis or regurgitation

Individuals Age 20+ Years

Definite RHD (either A, B, C, or D):

A. Pathological MR and at least two morphological features of RHD of the MV
B. MS mean gradient =4 mmHg*
C. Pathological AR and at least two morphological features of RHD of the AV, only in individuals aged <35 years‡
D. Pathological AR and at least two morphological features of RHD of the MV

*Congenital MV anomalies must be excluded. Furthermore, inflow obstruction due to nonrheumatic mitral annular calcification must be excluded in adults. ‡Bicuspid AV, dilated aortic root, and hypertension must be excluded. §Combined AR and MR in high prevalence regions and in the absence of congenital heart disease is regarded as rheumatic. Abbreviations: AR, aortic regurgitation; AV, aortic valve; MR, mitral regurgitation; MS, mitral stenosis; MV, mitral valve; RHD, rheumatic heart disease; WHF, World Heart Federation.

Guidelines

2014 AHA/ACC Guideline for the Management of Patients with Valvular Heart Disease

J Am Coll Cardiol. 2014;63:e57–e185. http://content.onlinejacc.org/article.aspx?articleID=1838843.

Guidelines on the management of valvular heart disease (version 2012)

Eur Heart J.2012;33:2469–75. http://www.escardio.org/guidelines-surveys/esc-guidelines/Pages/valvular-heart-disease.aspx.

The American Association for Thoracic Surgery Consensus Guidelines: Ischemic mitral valve regurgitation

J Thor Card Surg. 2016;151:940–56. http://www.sciencedirect.com/science/article/pii/S0022522316000453.

Surgical and interventional management of mitral valve regurgitation: a position statement from the European Society of Cardiology Working Groups on Cardiovascular Surgery and Valvular Heart Disease

Eur Heart J. 2016;37:133–9. http://eurheartj.oxfordjournals.org/content/37/2/133.

Patient Information

Images

http://www.nlm.nih.gov/medlineplus/ency/imagepages/1056.htm.
http://www.nlm.nih.gov/medlineplus/ency/imagepages/1097.htm.

Medlineplus

ENGLISH
http://www.nlm.nih.gov/medlineplus/ency/article/000176.htm.

ESPANOL.
http://www.nlm.nih.gov/medlineplus/spanish/ency/article/000176.htm.

Cleveland Clinic

http://www.clevelandclinicmeded.com/medicalpubs/disease
management/cardiology/mitral-valve-disease/#s0065.

Mayo Clinic

http://www.mayoclinic.org/diseases-conditions/mitral-valve-
regurgitation/basics/definition/con-20022644.

AHA

http://www.heart.org/HEARTORG/Conditions/More/HeartValve
ProblemsandDisease/Problem-Mitral-Valve-Regurgitation-
UCM-450612-Article.jsp.

Merck

http://www.merckmanuals.com/home/heart-and-blood-vessel-
disorders/heart-valve-disorders/mitral-regurgitation.

Professional Information

Review

Lancet.   2016;387:1324–34.   http://www.sciencedirect.com/science/
article/pii/S0140673616005584.

Review: Ischemic MR

Eur Heart J. 2010;31:2996–3005. http://eurheartj.oxfordjournals.org/
content/31/24/2996.

Review: Rheumatic Heart Disease

Lancet. 2016;387:1335–46. http://www.sciencedirect.com/science/article/pii/S014067361600547X.

Acquired Von Willebrand Syndrome

J Thromb Haemost. 2014;12:1966–74. http://onlinelibrary.wiley.com/doi/10.1111/jth.12734/abstract;jsessionid=9163877EC098A19CBBBB67A067BBAA8D.f03t02.

Annular Calcification (Image)

N Engl J Med. 2015;372:e23. http://www.nejm.org/doi/full/10.1056/NEJMicm1404772

Aortic Valve Replacement: Preop/Outcomes

Circulation. 2013;128:2776–84. http://circ.ahajournals.org/content/128/25/2776.full.

Asymptomatic MR: Treatment

J Am Coll Cardiol. 2014;63:2398–407. http://content.onlinejacc.org/article.aspx?articleID=1851448.

Diagnosing Severity

J Am Coll Cardiol. 2014;64:2792–801. http://content.onlinejacc.org/article.aspx?articleID=2085767.

Functional MR: Leaflet Remodeling

Eur Heart J Cardiovasc Imaging. 2015;16:290–9. http://ehjcimaging.oxfordjournals.org/content/16/3/290.full?etoc.

Imaging: Giant LA

J Am Coll Cardiol. 2013;62:e9. http://content.onlinejacc.org/article.aspx?articleID=1692247.

Schemic MR: Repair During CABG

N Engl J Med. 2014;371:2178–88. http://www.nejm.org/doi/full/10.1056/NEJMoa1410490?query=cardiology.

Ischemic MR: Repair Versus Replacement

N Engl J Med. 2014;370:23–32. http://www.nejm.org/doi/full/10.1056/NEJMoa1312808.

MR/Flail Leaflet: Effect of Age on Outcomes

Eur Heart J. 2013;34:2600–9. http://eurheartj.oxfordjournals.org/content/34/33/2600.abstract.

Post-NSTEMI: Long-Term Follow-Up

Heart. 2013;99:1502–8. http://heart.bmj.com/content/99/20/1502.abstract.

Percutaneous MV Repair

J Am Coll Cardiol. 2014;63:2057–68. http://content.onlinejacc.org/article.aspx?articleID=1838310.

Post-traumatic Stress Disorder

Am J Med. 2013;126:916–24. http://www.sciencedirect.com/science/article/pii/S0002934313004932.

Quantification

Circulation. 2012;126:2005–17. http://circ.ahajournals.org/content/126/16/2005.full.

Quantification by Echo

Eur J Echocardiogr. 2010;11:307–32. http://ehjcimaging.oxfordjournals.org/content/11/4/307.

Quantification: MRI Vs ECHO

J Am Coll Cardiol. 2015;65:1078–88. http://content.onlinejacc.org/article.aspx?articleID=2199424.

RV Systolic Dysfunction

Circulation. 2013;127:1597–608. http://circ.ahajournals.org/content/127/15/1597.full.

ST2 Increase Clinical Correlates

Thorac Cardiovasc Surg. 2014;62:47–51. http://www.scopus.com/record/display.url?eid=2-s2.0-84895059363&origin=inward&txGid=49E4F72486868669DB4D6A7B011E2689.Vdktg6RVtMfaQJ4pNTCQ%3a1.

Surgical Approaches

J Am Coll Cardiol. 2012;60:1315–22. http://content.onlinejacc.org/article.aspx?articleid=1355817.

Transcatheter Repair: Review

J Am Coll Cardiol. 2014;64:2688–700. http://content.onlinejacc.org/article.aspx?articleID=2042954.

Transcatheter Repair: Cardioband Feasibility

Eur Heart J. 2016;37:817–25. http://eurheartj.oxfordjournals.org/content/37/10/817.full.

Transcatheter Repair: Mitraclip Comparison with Surgery (Everest)

J Am Coll Cardiol. 2015;66:2844–54. http://content.onlinejacc.org/article.aspx?articleID=2476627.

Transcatheter Repair: MitraClip Safety/Efficacy

Heart. 2014;100:473–8. http://heart.bmj.com/content/100/6/473.abstract.

Transcatheter Repair: Multisociety Overview

J Am Coll Cardiol. 2014;63:840–52. http://content.onlinejacc.org/article.aspx?articleID=1785971.

Transcatheter Repair

Circulation. 2014;130:1712–22. http://circ.ahajournals.org/content/130/19/1712.full.

Traumatic Papillary Muscle Dysfunction

Eur Heart J. 1988;9:1030–3. http://eurheartj.oxfordjournals.org/content/9/9/1030.

WHF Echo Criteria for Rheumatic Heart Disease

Nature Reviews Cardiology. 2012;9:297–309. http://www.nature.com/nrcardio/journal/v9/n5/box/nrcardio.2012.7-BX1.html.

Updates and More

https://clinicalguidecvd.com/cmr

Chapter 63
Mitral Stenosis: Acquired

Management Keys

Perform TTE to establish diagnosis, quantify hemodynamic severity, assess concomitant valvular lesions, and
demonstrate valve morphology to determine suitability
for mitral commissurotomy

Anticoagulate for AF (all types), prior systemic embolus,
LA thrombus

Control heart rate for AF with rapid ventricular response
and for normal sinus rhythm when symptoms occur
with effort

Perform percutaneous mitral balloon commissurotomy in
symptomatic patients with severe MS and favorable
valve morphology in absence of LA thrombus or
moderate-to-severe MR

Perform mitral valve surgery (repair, commissurotomy, or
valve replacement) in severely symptomatic patients with
severe MS who are not high risk for surgery and who are
not candidates for or who have failed previous percutaneous mitral balloon commissurotomy

ICD-10 Code

I05.0

V.E. Friedewald, *Clinical Guide to Cardiovascular Disease*, 873
DOI 10.1007/978-1-4471-7293-2_63,
© Springer-Verlag London 2016

Alternate Names/Abbreviation

MS

Description/Etiology [8]

Structural obstruction of blood flow through mitral valve, due to:

Annular calcification
Rheumatic Carditis [17]

Comorbid Conditions

AORTIC   REGURGITATION   –   CHRONIC [RHEUMATIC HEART DIS]
AORTIC STENOSIS – VALVULAR [RHEUMATIC HEART DIS]
CARCINOID HEART DISEASE [RARE]
HUNTERS SYNDROME
MITRAL ANNULUS CALCIFICATION
MITRAL   REGURGITATION   –   CHRONIC [RHEUMATIC HEART DIS]
RHEUMATIC FEVER [17]
TRICUSPID STENOSIS [RHEUMATIC HEART DIS]

Demography

F > M 2:1
More common in undeveloped countries [2]

Pathophysiology [12]

Morphology:

MV leaflet thickening
MV leaflet calcification

MV commissural fusion
MV chordal fusion

Transmitral pressure gradient causes increased LA and pulmonary pressures and LA dilatation
Concomitant MR usually present

Signs/Symptoms [3]

ABDOMEN – PAIN
ARTERIAL PULSE, AMP – DECR/ABS
BREATH SOUNDS – WHEEZES
BREATHING – DIFF (DYSPNEA)
BREATHING – DIFF, NOCTURNAL (DYSPNEA, NOCT)
BREATHING – DIFF, RECLINING FLAT (ORTHOPNEA)
BREATHING – RAPID (TACHYPNEA)
CHEST – PAIN
CHEST – PALPITATIONS
COUGH
EXTREM, LOWER, BILAT – EDEMA
FATIGUE
HEART, BASE – MURMUR, DIAS [10]
HEART, LSB, LOWER – IMP, SYS
HEART, LSB, LOWER – MURMUR, DIAS
HEART, LSB, MID – PERCUSSION, DULLNESS
HEART, LV, APEX – MURMUR, DIAS [11]
HEART, LV, APEX – OPENING SNAP, MITRAL
HEART, LV, APEX – THRILL, DIAS
HEART, P2 – PALPABLE
HEART, P2, INTENSITY – INCR
HEART, RATE – RAPID (TACHYCARDIA)
HEART, RSB – SOUND, SYS EJECTION
HEART, S1, INTENSITY – DECR/ABSENT
HEART, S1, INTENSITY – INCR
HYPOTENSION (BLOOD PRESSURE – DECREASED/LOW)

LIVER – ENLARGED (HEPATOMEGALY)
NECK, JVP – ELEV
NECK, JVP, A WAVE – INCR/LARGE (CANNON WAVE)
SKIN, CHEEKS, COLOR – PINK PURPLE (MALAR FACIES)
SKIN, COLOR – BLUE (CYANOSIS)
SPUTUM – BLOOD (HEMOPTYSIS)
VOICE – HOARSE (LARYNGITIS) [ORTNER-S SYNDROME] [9]

ECG

P WAVE, DUR – INCR, NOTCHED (P MITRALE)
QRS – RVH PATTERN
QRS, AXIS – R

Differentiation

ASD
Cor Triatriatum
Myxoma – Left Atrium
Papillary Fibroelastoma
TV stenosis

Complications

Acute pulmonary edema [5]
Acute Pulmonary Embolism [4]
AF [4]
Pulmonary Hypertension
Stroke – Ischemic
Systemic embolism [4]

Laboratory

NS

Imaging [17]

LA, CHAMBER, SIZE – INCR
LUNGS, INTERSTITIUM – EDEMA, CV ANGLE (KERLEY B LINES) [1]
LUNGS, INTERSTITIUM – EDEMA, HILA (KERLEY A LINES) [1]
LUNGS, INTERSTITIUM – EDEMA/INFILTRATES
MV, ANNULUS – CALCIUM
MV, LEAFLET, MOTION – ABN
MV, LEAFLETS – CALCIUM
MV, LEAFLETS – THICK
MV, LEAFLETS, MORPH – ABN
MV, LEAFLETS, MOTION – DECR
MV, LEAFLETS, MOTION – DOMED
MV, ORIFICE, AREA – DECR
MV, TRANSVALVE PRESS – GRADIENT
PA, MAIN,SIZE – INCR
PA. PRESS – INCR
RA, CHAMBER, SIZE – INCR
RV, CHAMBER, SIZE – INCR

Other Tests

Cardiac catheterization when noninvasive tests are unsatisfactory or discordant with clinical findings

Treatment: Nonpharmacologic

Dietary salt restriction (for pulmonary congestion)

Treatment: Pharmacologic

Anticoagulation for:

AF (paroxysmal, persistent, permanent)
LA thrombus
Prior systemic embolus

Diuretic for pulmonary congestion
Inhaled corticosteroid for bronchial hyperreactivity
Negative chronotropic agent for tachycardia [18]

Beta-blocker
CCB

Rheumatic Fever prophylaxis

Treatment: Surgical/Invasive [15]

Percutaneous mitral balloon valvotomy [6]
MV replacement [7]
Surgical commissurotomy

Prevention

Rheumatic fever prevention protocol

Course [12]

Time of Rheumatic Fever to initial symptoms: 20–40 years
Mean age of presentation (developed countries): 5-6th decade
After onset of limiting symptoms, untreated 10-year survival: 0–15 %

Notes

[1]   CXR: indicates severe MS

[2] In developed countries, many cases of MS are among immigrants

[3] Symptoms usually absent until valve area decreased to 1.5 cm^2 but other factors (e.g., sinus tachycardia, supraventricular tachycardia, AF, pregnancy, concomitant valve lesions, PAH, anemia) can cause earlier onset of symptoms or symptoms disproportionate to valve area

[4] Sometimes initial MS clinical manifestation

[5] Especially with sudden AF and rapid ventricular response rate

[6] Preferred over surgical commissurotomy, which remains procedure of choice in some developing countries

[7] For patients not candidates for commissurotomy, including:

Significant valve calcification/fibrosis
Subvalvular fusion of MV apparatus

[8] Other uncommon/rare causes of MS include:

Anorectic drugs
Carcinoid Syndrome
Mitral annulus calcification

[9] Due to large LA impingement on recurrent laryngeal nerve

[10] Graham-Steel murmur, due to either pulmonary regurgitation secondary to Pulmonary Hypertension or Rheumatic AR

[11] C-reactive protein may be increased as manifestation of ongoing rheumatic inflammation

[12] Disease progression highly variable between populations and among individuals; usually slow with average decrease in MV area of $0\cdot01$ cm^2 per year, but >1/3 of patients have no decline in valve area over several years

[14] Presenting symptom usually dyspnea precipitated by effort, pregnancy, stress, infection, AF with rapid ventricular response

[15] Data inadequate for evidence-based recommendation for mixed valve disease, which predominates with Rheumatic Heart Disease

[16] In selected patients with reduction in transmitral gradient/increased MV area from about 1–2 cm², early outcomes include rapid decrease in LA pressure, increased cardiac output, subsequent decrease in PA pressure

[17] **World Heart Federation echo criteria for diagnosis of Rheumatic Fever***

Individuals age <20 years:
Definite RHD (either A, B, C, or D):

A. Pathological MR and at least two morphological features of RHD of MV
B. MS mean gradient: 4 mmHg
C. Pathological AR and at least two morphological features of RHD of AV
D. Borderline disease of both AV and MV§

Borderline RHD (either A, B, or C):

A. At least two morphological features of RHD of MV without pathological MR or MS
B. Pathological MR
C. Pathological AR

Normal echocardiographic findings (all of A, B, C, and D):

A. MR that does not meet all four Doppler echocardiographic criteria (physiological MR)
B. AR that does not meet all four Doppler echocardiographic criteria (physiological AR)
C. An isolated morphological feature of RHD of MV (for example, valvular thickening) without any associated pathological stenosis or regurgitation
D. Morphological feature of RHD of AV (for example, valvular thickening) without any associated pathological stenosis or regurgitation

Individuals age >20 years:
Definite RHD (either A, B, C, or D):

A. Pathological MR and at least two morphological features of RHD of MV

B. MS mean gradient; 4 mmHg
C. Pathological AR and at least two morphological features of RHD of AV, only in individuals aged <35 years
D. Pathological AR and at least two morphological features of RHD of MV

*Congenital MV anomalies must be excluded; inflow obstruction due to nonrheumatic mitral annular calcification must be excluded in adults

[18] For patients with MS in normal sinus rhythm and symptoms associated with exercise

Guidelines

2014 AHA/ACC Guideline for the Management of Patients with Valvular Heart Disease
J Am Coll Cardiol. 2014;63:e57–e185. http://content.onlinejacc.org/article.aspx?articleID=1838843.
Guidelines on the management of valvular heart disease (version 2012)
Eur Heart J. 2012;33:2469–75. http://www.escardio.org/guidelines-surveys/esc-guidelines/Pages/valvular-heart-disease.aspx.

Patient Information

Images

http://www.nlm.nih.gov/medlineplus/ency/imagepages/18147.htm.

Medlineplus

ENGLISH
http://www.nlm.nih.gov/medlineplus/ency/article/000175.htm.
ESPANOL
http://www.nlm.nih.gov/medlineplus/spanish/ency/article/000175.htm.

Cleveland Clinic

http://www.clevelandclinicmeded.com/medicalpubs/
diseasemanagement/cardiology/mitral-valve-disease/.

Mayo Clinic

http://www.mayoclinic.org/diseases-conditions/mitral-valve-
stenosis/basics/definition/con-20022582.

AHA

http://www.heart.org/HEARTORG/Conditions/More/
HeartValveProblemsandDisease/Problem-Mitral-Valve-
Stenosis-UCM-450370-Article.jsp.

Merck

http://www.merckmanuals.com/home/heart-and-blood-vessel-
disorders/heart-valve-disorders/mitral-stenosis.

Texas Heart Institute

http://www.texasheart.org/HIC/Topics/Cond/vmitral.cfm.

Professional Information

Review: Mitral Commissurotomy
Heart. 2016;102:500–7. http://heart.bmj.com/content/102/7/500?etoc.

Review: Rheumatic Heart Disease

Lancet.   2016;387:1335–46.   http://www.sciencedirect.com/science/
article/pii/S014067361600547X.

Annular Calcification

J Am Coll Cardiol. 2015;66:1934–41. http://content.onlinejacc.org/
article.aspx?articleid=2461798#tab1.

Annular Calcification (Image)

N Engl J Med. 2015;372:e23. http://www.nejm.org/doi/full/10.1056/
NEJMicm1404772.

Balloon Mitral Valvuloplasty

Am J Med. 2014;127:1126.e1–1126.e12. http://www.sciencedirect.
com/science/article/pii/S000293431400401X.

Commissurotomy: Reintervention

Eur Heart J. 2013;34:1923–30. http://eurheartj.oxfordjournals.org/
content/34/25/1923.

Echo: 2D Versus 3D for MV Area

Heart.   2013;99:253–8.   http://heart.bmj.com/content/99/4/253.
abstract.

Hunter Syndrome

Circulation. 2013;128:1269–70. http://circ.ahajournals.org/content/
128/11/1269.full.

Mitral Commissurotomy for Restenosis After Previous Mitral Commissurotomy

Heart. 2013;99:1336–41. http://heart.bmj.com/content/99/18/1336.

Mitral Valvuloplasty Versus Surgical Treatment in MS with Severe TR

Circulation. 2007;116:I246–I250. http://circ.ahajournals.org/content/ 116/11_suppl/I-246.full.

Non-rheumatic MS

Eur   J   Echocardiogr   2009;10:103–105.   http://ehjcimaging. oxfordjournals.org/content/10/1/103.

Post-valvuloplasty Tricuspid Regurgitation

Heart. 2013;99:91–7. http://heart.bmj.com/content/99/2/91.abstract.

Rheumatic Heart Disease in Bangladesh

Indian Heart J. 2016;68:88–98. http://www.sciencedirect.com/science/ article/pii/S0019483215003181.

Systemic Embolism: Predictors

Ann   Intern   Med.   1998;128:885–9.   http://annals.org/article.aspx? articleid=711449.

Updates and More

https://clinicalguidecvd.com/mvs

Chapter 64
Mitral Valve Prolapse (Barlow/Parachute Mitral Valve Syndrome)

ICD-10 Code

I34.1

Alternate Names/Abbreviation

BARLOW SYNDROME
PARACHUTE MITRAL VALVE SYNDROME

Description/Etiology

The most common cause of chronic MR in developed countries; younger populations with MVP present with Barlow's disease; older populations present with fibro-elastic deficiency disease

Barlow's Disease:

Thickened/diffusely redundant myxomatous leaflet tissue with disrupted collagen and elastic layers
Prolapse of most mitral leaflet segments
Severe mitral annular enlargement
Elongated chordae
Patients usually present in young/middle-aged at time of surgery after long history of murmur or MR [15]

V.E. Friedewald, *Clinical Guide to Cardiovascular Disease*, 885
DOI 10.1007/978-1-4471-7293-2_64,
© Springer-Verlag London 2016

Fibroelastic deficiency:

> Decreased connective tissue deficient in collagen, elastin, proteoglycans
> Thin, smooth, translucent leaflets without excess tissue
> Moderate annulus dilatation
> Thin, slightly elongated chordae
> Patients often present at older age with chordal rupture and flail leaflet after a short clinical history

Familial [14] and nonfamilial forms

Secondary forms of MVP occurring in other known conditions listed in Predisposing/Comorbid Conditions

Predisposing/Comorbid Conditions

ANEURYSMS-OSTEOARTHRITIS SYNDROME
ATRIAL SEPTAL DEFECT – SECUNDUM
ATRIOVENTRICULAR   LEFT-SIDED   BYPASS TRACTS
CARDIOMYOPATHY – HYPERTROPHIC
EHLERS-DANLOS SYNDROME
HOMOCYSTINURIA
LOEYS-DIETZ SYNDROME
MARFAN SYNDROME
OPEN ANGLE GLAUCOMA [10]
OSTEOGENESIS IMPERFECTA
PRIMARY HYPOMASTIA
PSEUDOXANTHOMA ELASTICUM
VON   WILLEBRAND   DISEASE   [AND   OTHER COAGULOPATHIES]

Demography

2–3 % of general population (global: >176 million persons)
Often familial [14]

Pathophysiology

Morphology of Barlow's:

Expansion of middle spongiosa layer of MV due to proteoglycan accumulation

Structural alterations of collagen in all components of leaflets

Structurally abnormal chordae (composed of increased amounts of glycosaminoglycans) [13]

Systolic billowing of either or both MV leaflets into LA, with or without MR [3]

Signs/Symptoms [1]

CHEST – PAIN [2]
CHEST – PALPITATIONS
CHEST, STERNUM, CURV – POST (PECTUS EXCAVATUM)
CONSCIOUSNESS – LOSS, SUDDEN (SYNCOPE)
DIZZY/LIGHTHEADED/PRESYNCOPE
FATIGUE
HEART, LV, APEX – CLICK(S), SYS [5, 15]
HEART, LV, APEX – MURMUR, DIAS
HEART, LV, APEX – MURMUR, SYS [5, 15]
HEART, LV, APEX – SOUNDS, EARLY DIAS
HYPOTENSION   (BLOOD   PRESSURE   – DECREASED/LOW)
SPINE, THORACIC – STRAIGHT

Differentiation

Other causes of MR

Complications

Fibrin emboli [4]

Infective Endocarditis
Progressive MR
Ruptured chordae [13]
Stroke
Sudden Death

Laboratory

NS

ECG [6]

DYSRHY – PREEXCITATION
DYSRHYTHMIAS – ATRIAL (PACS/OTHERS)
DYSRHYTHMIAS – VENTRICULAR (PVCS/OTHERS)
Q WAVE – ABN
QT/QTC INTERVAL – LONG
ST-T WAVE – ABN, NS
T WAVE – INVER, ABN
U WAVE – PROMINENT

Imaging

MV, FLOW – REGURG
MV, LEAFLETS – THICK [ECHO: ≥5 MM]
MV, LEAFLETS, MOTION – PROLAPSE [ECHO: >2 MM
    ABOVE ANNULUS IN PARASTERNAL VIEW]

Genomics [14]

DCHS1

Other Tests

Ambulatory ECG monitoring [7]

Treatment: Nonpharmacologic

Reassurance of benign prognosis except in patients with severe forms
DC stimulants

Treatment: Pharmacologic

Endocarditis prophylaxis – patients with:

Definite MR
Thick leaflets
Elongated chordae
Dilated LA/LV

ASA [8]
Warfarin [8]
Beta-blockers [8]

Treatment: Surgical/Invasive

MV repair

Prevention

Infective Endocarditis prophylaxis for severe forms

Course

Benign in most cases, with no lifestyle restrictions, but may progress to significant MR over subsequent 1–2 decades in up to 1/4 of persons with mild MVP

Notes

[1] A variety of additional symptoms, many neuropsychiatric, such as panic disorder, have been described but are debated as part of a syndrome related to MVP

[2] Seldom resembles angina pectoris

[3] MR severity ranges from mild to severe

[4] May cause ophthalmic abnormalities such as visual field loss

[5] Timing highly variable under different conditions; occurs earlier (closer to S1) with decreased ventricular preload (Valsalva, upright position); occurs later with increased preload (squatting, handgrip)

[6] NS changes; may be normal

[7] Palpitations may be noted in absence of dysrhythmia

[8] No specific guideline recommendations available for medical therapy; drug Rx, if any, should be on case-by-case basis

[9] May be abnormal when secondary to predisposing congenital conditions

[10] MVP and open angle glaucoma may share same pathophysiologic basis involving proteoglycans and glycosaminoglycans

[11] May occur on MV leaflets/apparatus or in rare cases due to jet lesion in LA mural endocardium

[12] Especially in young females; correlates with fibrosis of papillary muscles and inferobasal LV wall, which is structural hallmark and correlates with ventricular arrhythmia origin, possibly due to myocardial stretch by prolapsing leaflet

[13] Chordal rupture: frequent pathological finding; may be secondary to mechanical weakening, combined with abnormal hemodynamic stresses arising from valve leaflet redundancy

[14] Inheritance: autosomal-dominant with variable penetrance influenced by age/sex; marked heterogeneity of clinical presentation including affected members within a family

[15] Classic auscultatory finding in MVP: dynamic, mid-late systolic click often associated with high-pitched, late systolic murmur; careful physical examination is highly sensitive for making MVP diagnosis, but specificity limited with echo as gold standard

Guidelines

2014 AHA/ACC Guideline for the Management of Patients with Valvular Heart Disease
J Am Coll Cardiol. 2014;63:e57–e185. http://content.onlinejacc.org/article.aspx?articleID=1838843.
Guidelines on the management of valvular heart disease (version 2012)
Eur Heart J. 2012;33:2469–75. http://www.escardio.org/guidelines-surveys/esc-guidelines/Pages/valvular-heart-disease.aspx.

Patient Information

Medlineplus

ENGLISH
http://www.nlm.nih.gov/medlineplus/mitralvalveprolapse.html.
ESPANOL
http://www.nlm.nih.gov/medlineplus/spanish/mitralvalveprolapse.html.

Genetics Home Reference

http://ghr.nlm.nih.gov/glossary=mitralvalveprolapse.

Mayo Clinic

http://www.mayoclinic.org/diseases-conditions/mitral-valve-prolapse/basics/definition/con-20024748.

Texas Heart Institute

http://www.texasheartinstitute.org/HIC/Topics/Cond/mvp.cfm.

AHA

http://www.heart.org/HEARTORG/Conditions/More/HeartValveProblemsandDisease/Problem-Mitral-Valve-Prolapse-UCM-450441-Article.jsp.

Cleveland Clinic

http://my.clevelandclinic.org/services/heart/disorders/mitral-valve-prolapse.

Harvard

http://www.health.harvard.edu/heart-health/mitral-valve-prolapse.

Professional Information

DCHS1 Mutation

Nature. 2015. doi:10.1038/nature14670. http://www.nature.com/nature/journal/vaop/ncurrent/full/nature14670.html?WT.ec-id=NATURE-20150813&spMailingID=49306476&spUserID=MTM4MTQzNTcyMTQxS0&spJobID=741956713&spReportId=NzQxOTU2NzEzS0.

Epidemiology/Pathophysiology

Circulation. 2014;129:2158–70. http://circ.ahajournals.org/content/129/21/2158.full.

Left Atrial Mural Endocarditis Secondary to MVP JET Lesion

Circulation. 2015;131:1529–30. http://circ.ahajournals.org/content/131/17/1529.full.

Mitral Valve Morphology

Circulation. 2013;127:832–41. http://circ.ahajournals.org/content/127/7/832.full.

MR/Flail Leaflet: Effect of Age on Outcomes

Eur Heart J. 2013;34:2600–09. http://eurheartj.oxfordjournals.org/content/34/33/2600.abstract.

Natural History

Circulation.   2002;106:1355–61.   http://circ.ahajournals.org/content/106/11/1355.full.pdf+html?sid=1a6c50a2-20e9-4419-a523-b5484f3dcee3.

Open Angle Glaucoma

Heart.2015;101:609–15.http://heart.bmj.com/content/101/8/609?etoc.

Sudden Cardiac Death

Heart Rhythm. 2016;13:498–503. http://www.heartrhythmjournal.com/article/S1547-5271(15)01196-0/abstract.

Sudden Cardiac Death

Circulation. 2015;132:556–66.http://circ.ahajournals.org/content/132/7/556.full.

VF/Sudden Cardiac Death

J Am Coll Cardiol. 2013;62:222–30. http://content.onlinejacc.org/article.aspx?articleID=1709682.

Updates and More

https://clinicalguidecvd.com/mvp

Chapter 65
Myocarditis

Management Keys

Evaluate for underlying/treatable cause

Monitor for possible progression to Dilated Cardiomyopathy and HF

Special vigilance (especially for dysrhythmias) when low voltage or LBBB present on ECG [7]

ICD-10 Code

I40.1

Alternate Names/Abbreviation

NS

Description/Etiology [22]

Cardiac inflammation due to a wide variety of causes (see PREDISPOSING/COMORBID CONDITIONS, below) other than those due to CAD

V.E. Friedewald, *Clinical Guide to Cardiovascular Disease*,
DOI 10.1007/978-1-4471-7293-2_65,
© Springer-Verlag London 2016

Clinical presentation varies, including: [3]

Acute chest pain
Acute dysrhythmias with

Palpitations
Syncope

Cardiogenic shock
New onset/worsening HF

Predisposing/Comorbid Conditions [1]

AUTOIMMUNE

CHURG-STRAUSS SYNDROME
DIABETES MELLITUS [TYPE 1]
HYPERTHYROIDISM
INFLAMMATORY BOWEL DISEASE
KAWASAKI DIS
MYASTHENIA GRAVIS
POLYMYOSITIS
RHEUMATOID ARTHRITIS
SARCOIDOSIS
SCLERODERMA
SYSTEMIC LUPUS ERYTHEMATOSUS
WEGENER GRANULOMATOSIS

DRUGS – ALLERGIC [23]

AMITRYPTYLINE
CEFACLOR
COLCHICINE
ISONIAZID
LIDOCAINE
LOOP/THIAZIDE DIURETICS
METHYL DOPA
PENICILLIN
PHENYLBUTAZONE
PHENYTOIN

SULFONAMIDES
TETRACYCLINE

DRUGS – TOXIC

AMPHETAMINES
ANTHRACYCLINES
CATECHOLAMINES
CLOZAPINE
COCAINE
CYCLOPHOSPHAMIDE
FLUOURACIL
HEMETINE
INTERLEUKIN 2
LITHIUM
TRASTUZUMAB

HEAVY METAL TOXICITY

COPPER TOXICITY
IRON TOXICITY
LEAD TOXICITY

IMMUNE-MEDIATED

SERUM SICKNESS
TETANUS TOXIOD
VACCINES

INFECTIONS – BACTERIAL

CHAGAS DISEASE
DIPHTHERIA   (CORYNEBACTERIUM
   DIPHTHERIA)
HEMOPHILUS INFLUENZA
LEGIONELLOSIS (LEGIONELLA)
LEPTOSPIROSIS
LYME DISEASE (BORRELIA BURGDORFERI)
MENINGOCOCCEMIA   (NEISSERIA
   MENINGITIDIS)
MYCOBACTERIUM TUBERCULOSIS
MYCOPLASMA PNEUMONIAE

Q FEVER
ROCKY   MOUNTAIN   SPOTTED   FEVER
(RICKETTSIA RICKETTSII)
SCRUBTYPHUS(RICKETTSIATSUTSUGAMUSHI)
SHIGELLOSIS (S BOYDII, S DYSENTERIAE, S
FLEXNERI, S SONNEI)
TYPHOID FEVER
TYPHUS – SCRUB
YERSINIOSIS (Y ENTEROCOLITICA)

INFECTIONS – VIRAL

ADENOVIRUS [MAINLY CHILDREN]
CHICKENPOX (VARICELLA)
COXSACKIE VIRUS A
COXSACKIE VIRUS B
CYTOMEGALOVIRUS   [MAINLY
IMMUNOCOMPROMISED PTS]
DENGUE FEVER
EBOLA VIRUS DISEASE
ECHOVIRUS
ENTEROVIRUS
HEMORRHAGIC   FEVER   WITH   RENAL
SYNDROME
HEPATITIS C
HERPES SIMPLEX
HIV
HUMAN HERPES VIRUS 6
INFECTIOUS MONONUCLEOSIS
INFLUENZA – SEASONAL
LASSA FEVER
LYMPHOCYTIC CHORIOMENINGITIS
MARBURG FEVER
MUMPS
PARVOVIRUS B19 INFECTION
POLIOMYELITIS- ACUTE

PSITTACOSIS
RABIES
RUBEOLA
SMALLPOX (VARIOLA)
WEST NILE FEVER

OTHERS

ALCOHOL USE/EXCESS
ARSINE POISONING
BEE STING
BERI BERI
CARBON MONOXIDE POISONING
CELIAC DISEASE
ELECTRIC SHOCK
HEART TRANSPLANT [REJECTION]
MALARIA
PHEOCHROMOCYTOMA
PHOSPHOROUS
RADIATION
SCORPION STING
SNAKE BITE
SODIUM AZIDE
SPIDER BITE
WASP STING
CARDIOMYOPATHY – PERIPARTUM
CARDIOMYOPATHY – TAKOTSUBO
GIANT CELL ARTERITIS
INFLUENZA – AVIANl
TRICHINELLOSIS

Demography

Varies with etiology
More common in males
All ages, especially young adults

Pathophysiology

Acute myocyte Injury due to various mechanisms including:

Autoimmune cell invasion of myocardium
Infectious pathogen entry/replication
Intracellular antigen exposure
Immune system activation
Myocyte ischemia/necrosis

Signs/Symptoms [8]

APPETITE – DECR (ANOREXIA) [INCL POOR FEEDING]
BREATHING – DIFF (DYSPNEA) [20]
BREATHING – RAPID (TACHYPNEA)
CHEST – PAIN [6, 11]
CHEST – PALPITATIONS
CONSCIOUSNESS – LOSS, SUDDEN (SYNCOPE)
COUGH
FATIGUE
FEVER [10]
HEART – FRICTION RUB, PERICARD
HEART, LV, APEX – MURMUR, SYS
HEART, RATE – RAPID (TACHYCARDIA) [WITH/WITHOUT FEVER]
HEART, RHYTHM – IRREG
HEART, S1, INTENSITY – DECR/ABSENT
HEART, S3 LV
JOINTS – PAIN (ARTHRALGIA) [10]
LIVER – ENLARGED (HEPATOMEGALY)
MENTATION – WEAKNESS (MALAISE)
MUSCLES – PAIN (MYALGIA) [10]
VOMITING (EMESIS)

Differentiation

AMI
Other causes of HF/LV dysfunction

Complications

Cardiogenic Shock
Dysrhythmias [7]
HF
SCD [7] [9]

Laboratory

BLOOD, TROPONIN – INCR [2]

ECG

T WAVE – INVER, ABN [4]
AV COND – 1ST DEGREE BLOCK
AV COND – 2ND DEGREE BLOCK
AV COND – 3RD DEGREE BLOCK
DYSRHYTHMIAS – ATRIAL (PACS/OTHERS)
DYSRHYTHMIAS – VENTRICULAR (PVCS/ OTHERS) [7]
PR SEGMENT – DEPRESSED
Q WAVE – ABN [6] [UNCOMMON]
QRS – LBBB/LBBB PATTERN [18]
QRS – LONG, NS
QRS, AXIS – L [7]
QT/QTC INTERVAL – LONG [7]
RATE – DECREASED (SINUS BRADYCARDIA)

ST SEGMENT – DEPR
ST SEGMENT – ELEV [5] [6]
ST-T WAVE – ABN, NS [4]
VOLTAGE, GEN – DECR [19]

Imaging

CARDIOMEGALY [12]
LUNGS – INFILTRATES
LV, INTRACAVITY – MASS [14]
LV, MYOCARD – LGE [21]
LV, SYS – DYSF [13]
MRI: INTRACELLULAR EDEMA; INTERSTITIAL
  EDEMA; HYPEREMIA; CAPILLARY LEAKAGE;
  MYOCARD FIBROSIS/NECROSIS
PERICARD – FLUID
PLEURA – FLUID
PUL, VASCULARITY – INCR

Other Tests

EMB

Treatment: Nonpharmacologic

SCD prevention: withdraw from competitive athletics and
  vigorous exertion for prescribed period

Treatment: Pharmacologic

Antiarrhythmic [17]
Antivirals [15]
HF protocol
Immunosuppressives [16]

Treatment: Surgical/Invasive

Mechanical circulatory support and card transplant
Pacemaker [17]

Prevention

Varies with etiology

Course

Varies with etiology
Viral Myocarditis: 19 % mortality in <5 years

Notes

[1] Partial list
[2] Cardiac troponins: limited value because:

Do not differentiate from myocardial ischemia
Normal value does not exclude Myocarditis
May be increased in many other conditions

[3] Consider this diagnosis in absence of other explanations of these manifestations, especially CAD
[4] T wave inversion usually occurs after complete normalization of ST-T wave changes in Myocarditis (usually occurs while ST segment elevation still present in AMI)
[5] May resemble AMI
[6] ST segment usually concave upward vs convex upward in myocardial ischemia/AMI
[7] Tachyarrhythmias associated with increased mortality in children
[8] Often asymptomatic; clinical manifestations highly variable
[9] Including young children
[10] Prodromal phase preceding by days-weeks in viral form

[11] Pericardial involvement

[12] Due to chamber enlargement/pericardial effusion

[13] LV dysfunction common; RV dysfunction uncommon

[14] Thrombus; occurs in up to 25 % of patients

[15] Limited effectiveness because viral infection usually precedes Myocarditis by weeks

[16] Eg, corticosteroids and cyclosporine for Giant Cell Myocarditis

[17] When specifically indicated for significant arrhythmias/high grade HB

[18] LBBB associated with worse outcome (up to 8x in children)

[19] Low voltage is risk factor for dysrhythmias; mechanism unknown

[20] Difficult breathing is most common complaint in children

[21] Presence of LGE may be best independent predictor of all-cause and cardiac mortality in biopsy-proven viral Myocarditis

[22] ACC/AHA Guideline Description***

Sec 5.6.1 Myocarditis

Inflammation of the heart may cause HF in about 10 % of cases of initially unexplained cardiomyopathy. A variety of infectious organisms, as well as toxins and medications, most often postviral in origin, may cause myocarditis. In addition, myocarditis is also seen as part of other systemic diseases such as systemic lupus erythematosus and other myocardial muscle diseases such as HIV cardiomyopathy and possibly peripartum cardiomyopathy. Presentation may be acute, with a distinct onset, severe hemodynamic compromise, and severe LV dysfunction as seen in acute fulminant myocarditis, or it may be subacute, with an indistinct onset and better-tolerated LV dysfunction. Prognosis varies, with spontaneous complete resolution (paradoxically most often seen with acute fulminant myocarditis) to the development of DCM despite immunosuppressive therapy. The role of immunosuppressive therapy is controversial.

Targeting such therapy to specific individuals based on the presence or absence of viral genome in myocardial biopsy samples may improve response to immunosuppressive therapy.

[23] ACC/AHA Guideline description***

Sec 5.7.1 Hypersensitivity Myocarditis

Hypersensitivity to a variety of agents may result in allergic reactions that involve the myocardium, characterized by peripheral eosinophilia and a perivascular infiltration of the myocardium by eosinophils, lymphocytes, and histiocytes. A variety of drugs, most commonly the sulfonamides, penicillins, methyldopa, and other agents such as amphotericin B, streptomycin, phenytoin, isoniazid, tetanus toxoid, hydrochlorothiazide, dobutamine, and chlorthalidone, have been reported to cause allergic hypersensitivity myocarditis. Most patients are not clinically ill but may die suddenly, presumably secondary to an arrhythmia.

***From 2013 ACCF/AHA Guideline for the Management of Heart Failure: A Report of the American College of Cardiology Foundation/American Heart Association Task Force on Practice Guidelines. J Am Coll Cardiol. 2013;62(16):e147–e239

Guidelines

2013 ACCF/AHA Guideline for the Management of Heart Failure
J Am Coll Cardiol. 2013;62:e147–e239. http://content.onlinejacc.org/article.aspx?articleid=1695825.
ESC Guidelines for the diagnosis and treatment of acute and chronic heart failure 2012
Eur Heart J. 2012;33:1787–1847. http://eurheartj.oxfordjournals.org/content/ehj/33/14/1787.full.pdf.
HFSA: Myocarditis: Current Treatment
J Card Fail. 2010;16:e176–e179. http://www.onlinejcf.com/article/S1071-9164(10)00231-9/fulltext.

Patient Information

Medlineplus

ENGLISH
  http://www.nlm.nih.gov/medlineplus/ency/article/000149.htm.
ESPANOL.
  http://www.nlm.nih.gov/medlineplus/spanish/ency/
  article/000149.htm.

Texas Heart Institute

http://www.texasheartinstitute.org/HIC/Topics/Cond/myocard.cfm.

Mayo Clinic

http://www.mayoclinic.org/diseases-conditions/myocarditis/basics/
  definition/con-20027303.

Myocarditis Foundation

http://www.myocarditisfoundation.org/about-myocarditis/.

Nord

https://rarediseases.org/rare-diseases/giant-cell-myocarditis/.

Cincinnati Childrens: Pediatric Myocarditis

http://www.cincinnatichildrens.org/health/m/myocarditis/.

Johns Hopkins

http://www.hopkinsmedicine.org/heart-vascular-institute/
  conditions-treatments/conditions/myocarditis.html.

Seattle Childrens

http://www.seattlechildrens.org/medical-conditions/heart-blood-conditions/myocarditis/.

Professional Information

History

Heart Vessels. 1985;1(Supplement):1–3. http://link.springer.com/article/10.1007%2FBF02072348.

ESC Position Statement

Eur Heart J. 2013;34:2636–48. http://eurheartj.oxfordjournals.org/content/34/33/2636.

Review

Lancet. 2012;379:738–47. http://www.sciencedirect.com/science/article/pii/S014067361160648X.

Review

Circulation. 2006;113:876–90. http://www.circ.ahajournals.org/content/113/6/876.full.

Review

Mayo Clin Proc. 2009;84:1001–9. http://www.ncbi.nlm.nih.gov/pmc/articles/PMC2770911/.

Review

Circulation. 2009;119:2615–24. http://circ.ahajournals.org/content/119/19/2615.full.

Review: Clinical Presentation/Diagnosis

Heart. 2015;101:1332–44. http://heart.bmj.com/content/101/16/1332. extract.

Review: Diagnosis/Treatment in Children

Circulation.   2014;129:115–28.   http://circ.ahajournals.org/content/129/1/115.extract.

Review: State of Art Update

J Am Coll Cardiol. 2012;59:779–92. http://content.onlinejacc.org/article.aspx?articleid=1201151&resultClick=3.

Autoimmunity

J Clin Invest. 2011;121:1561–73. http://www.jci.org/articles/view/44583.

Children: Clinical Presentation

Am J Emerg Med. 2009;27:942–7. http://www.sciencedirect.com/science/article/pii/S0735675708005573#.

Diagnosis of Myocarditis

J Am Coll Cardiol. 2016;67:1812–4. http://content.onlinejacc.org/article.aspx?articleID=2512991#tab1.

Endomyocardial Biopsy

Eur Heart J. 2007;28:3076–93. http://www.escardio.org/guidelines-surveys/esc-guidelines/Pages/endomyocardial-biopsy.aspx.

Gender/Age Characteristics

Heart. 2013;99:1681–4. http://heart.bmj.com/content/99/22/1681. abstract.

Giant Cell Arteritis (Case Report)

Circ Heart Fail. 2016;9:e002778. http://circheartfailure.ahajournals. org/content/9/2/e002778.full.

Imaging: CMR

J Am Coll Cardiol. 2016;67:1800–11. http://content.onlinejacc.org/ article.aspx?articleID=2512985#tab1.

LGE: Long-Term Predictor of Mortality in Viral Myocarditis

J Am Coll Cardiol. 2012;59:1604–15. http://content.onlinejacc.org/ article.aspx?articleID=1203136.

Pheochromocytoma

Circulation. 2014;129:1348–9. http://circ.ahajournals.org/content/ 129/12/1348.full.

Tachyarrhythmias and Increased Mortality in Children

Am   J   Cardiol.   2014;113:535–40.   http://www.sciencedirect.com/science/article/pii/S0002914913021516.

Tuberculous Myocarditis (Case Report)

Circulation.   2013;128:271–7.   http://circ.ahajournals.org/content/128/3/271.full.

Viral Myocarditis: Diagnosis

Arch Cardiovasc Dis. 2009;102:559–68. http://www.ncbi.nlm.nih.gov/pubmed/19664576?dopt=Abstract.

Updates and More

https://clinicalguidecvd.com/myocard

Chapter 66
Myxoma: Left Atrium

ICD-10 Code

D15.1

Description/Etiology

Most common primary benign cardiac tumor in adults;
75 % of all cardiac myxomas

Etiology either idiopathic or congenital as part of Carney
Complex [5]

Predisposing/Comorbid Conditions

BREAST FIBROADENOMA
CARDIAC TUMOR(S)
CARNEY COMPLEX [5]
DYSRHYTHMIAS – ATRIAL [13]

Demography

More common in females

All ages

Cardiac myxomas may be more common and present at
younger age in developing countries

V.E. Friedewald, *Clinical Guide to Cardiovascular Disease*,
DOI 10.1007/978-1-4471-7293-2_66,
© Springer-Verlag London 2016

Pathophysiology

Most often attached by stalk to region of fossa ovalis

Composition: gelatinous (myxoid); heterogeneous, often with areas of necrosis, cysts, hemorrhage

Flow obstruction/regurgitation at level of MV due to mobile, pedunculated tumor

Constitutional symptoms (e.g., fever) due to tumor secretion of IL-6

Metastatic embolization [16]

Signs/Symptoms [7] [12]

BEHAVIOR – BIZARRE/CHANGED

BODY, APPEARANCE – WASTING (CACHEXIA)

BREATH SOUNDS – CRACKLES (RALES) [MAY BE LOCAL]

BREATHING – DIFF (DYSPNEA)

BREATHING – DIFF, NOCTURNAL (DYSPNEA, NOCT)

CHEST – PAIN

CONSCIOUSNESS – LOSS, SUDDEN (SYNCOPE)

CONSCIOUSNESS – LOSS, SUDDEN, UPRIGHT (ORTHOSTATIC SYNCOPE)

COUGH

EXTREM – RAYNAUD PHENOMENON

EXTREM, DIGITS – CLUBBED

EXTREM, LOWER, BILAT – EDEMA

EYES, VISION – DECR/LOSS

FATIGUE

FEVER

HEART, LV, APEX – MURMUR, DIAS [2]

HEART, LV, APEX – MURMUR, SYS [2]

HEART, P2, INTENSITY – INCR [2]

HEART, S1, INTENSITY – INCR [2]

HEART, S1, SPLIT – WIDE [2]

HEART, S4 LV [2]

HEART, SOUND – EARLY DIAS [1] [2]
SKIN – LENTIGINES [CARNEY COMPLEX] [5]
SKIN – PETECHIAE/ECCHYMOSES/PURPURA
SKIN, COLOR – PALE (PALLOR)
SPUTUM – BLOOD (HEMOPTYSIS)
WEIGHT – LOSS

Differentiation

Acute Rheumatic Fever
Cerebrovascular Disease
Infective Endocarditis
Mitral Regurgitation
Mitral Stenosis
Myocarditis
Pulmonary disease
Pulmonary Hypertension
Vasculitis

Complications

Acute Mitral Regurgitation [8]
AMI
Acute Pulmonary Edema
Detach/Lodge at Aortic Bifurcation
Endocarditis
Extension Locally
Intracranial Arterial Aneurysm
LV dysfunction
Metastasis [16]
Peripheral emboli [4] [16]
Pulmonary Arterial Hypertension
Stroke
Sudden Death
Visceral infarction

Laboratory [12]

BLOOD, ESR – INCR
BLOOD, HGB/HCT – DECR (ANEMIA) [6]
BLOOD, IGG – INCR
BLOOD, IL-6 – INCR
BLOOD,   PLATELETS   –   DECR
(THROMBOCYTOPENIA)

ECG [10] [12]

DYSRHYTHMIAS – ATRIAL (PACS/OTHERS)
N/NS ABN
P WAVE, DUR – INCR
QRS – RBBB/RBBB PATTERN
QRS – RVH PATTERN
QRS, AXIS – R
RATE – INCREASED (SINUS TACHYCARDIA)

Imaging [9] [10] [12]

LA, CHAMBER, SIZE – INCR [MAY BE NORMAL
SIZE]
LA, INTRACAVITY – MASS [MAY BE CALCIFIED]
LGE, TUMOR [14]
MV, FLOW – REGURG
MV, LEAFLETS, MOTION – ABN [FLUTTERING]
PA, PRESS – INCR
PUL, VASCULARITY – INCR
RV, CHAMBER, SIZE – INCR [MAY BE NORMAL
SIZE]

Genomics

PRKAR1A

Other Tests

> Cardiac catheterization/coronary angiography – mainly for CAD

EMB

Treatment: Nonpharmacologic

NS

Treatment: Pharmacologic

NS

Treatment: Surgical/Invasive

> Surgical resection: usually curative

Course

> Recurrence after surgical resection [9]:
>
>> About 13 %;
>> Higher in Carney Complex
>> Rare after 4 years
>> Usually at same site
>
> Normal lifespan after complete resection

Notes

[1] "Tumor plop" low-pitch; caused by tumor prolapse across MV; diastolic murmur usually absent

[2] Auscultatory findings may vary with time/patient position

[3] May protrude through MV orifice

[4] Tumor particle or superimposed thrombus; occurs in up to 50 % of patients; most common sites are CNS, retina, coronary artery, extremities; embolic event may be initial clinical manifestation

[5] Carney Complex: autosomal dominant condition, including mammary myxoid fibroadenoma, skin pigmented lesions, endocrine disorders, testicular tumors, psammomatous melanotic schwannoma; 2/3 s have cardiac myxomas

[6] Hemolytic; associated with calcified tumor

[7] Occurrence of symptoms acutely with upright or other certain body positions should raise this diagnostic possibility

[8] Ruptured chordae tendineae due to "wrecking ball effect" of calcified tumor

[9] TEE especially valuable; MRI used when echo inadequate/further characterization needed; semi-annual follow-up echo for 4 years after surgical resection recommended for recurrence detection

[10] Often normal

[11] Adult benign cardiac tumors (frequency):

> Myxoma (45 %)
> Lipoma (20 %)
> Papillary Fibroelastoma (15 %)
> Hemangioma (5 %)
> Fibroma (3 %)
> Rhabdomyoma (1 %)
> Teratoma (<1 %)
> Others (10 %)

Pediatric benign cardiac tumors:

> Rhabdomyoma (45 %)
> Fibroma (15 %)
> Myxoma (15 %)
> Teratoma (15 %)
> Hemangioma (5 %)
> Others (5 %)

[12] Clinical manifestations highly variable and mainly determined by tumor location/size
[13] Especially Supraventricular Tachycardia, which may be initial manifestation
[14] For tumor vascularity
[16] Embolic tumor cells may remain viable at site of embolization, thereby becoming distant metastases or peripheral tumor masses

Guidelines

NS

Patient Information

Genetics Home Reference: Carney Complex

http://ghr.nlm.nih.gov/condition/carney-complex.

Images

http://www.nlm.nih.gov/medlineplus/ency/imagepages/18078.htm.

Medlineplus

ENGLISH

http://www.nlm.nih.gov/medlineplus/ency/article/007273.htm.

ESPANOL

http://www.nlm.nih.gov/medlineplus/spanish/ency/article/007273.htm.

Patient Journey

BMJ. 2013;347:f4430. http://www.bmj.com/content/347/bmj.f4430.

Pubmed

http://www.ncbi.nlm.nih.gov/pubmedhealth/PMH0004532/.

Merck

http://www.merckmanuals.com/home/heart-and-blood-vessel-disorders/heart-tumors/myxomas.

Professional Information

Carney Complex

J Cardiothorac Surg. 2011;6:25. doi: 10.1186/1749-8090-6-25. http://www.cardiothoracicsurgery.org/content/6/1/25.

Clinical Presentation

Medicine.   2001;80:159–72.   http://journals.lww.com/md-journal/Fulltext/2001/05000/Clinical-Presentation-of-Left-Atrial-Cardiac.2.aspx.

Carney Complex

http://ghr.nlm.nih.gov/condition/carney-complex.

Case Report from THIJ: Catastrophic Systemic Embolization

Tex Heart Inst J. 2014;41;64–6. http://www.thij.org/doi/full/10.14503/THIJ-12-2964?=.

Echo

J Am Soc Echocardiogr. 2011;24:618–24. http://www.sciencedirect.com/science/article/pii/S089473171100040X.

Endocarditis

Eur Heart J. 1992;13:1592–3. http://eurheartj.oxfordjournals.org/content/13/11/1592.3.

Familial Multicentric

Eur J Echocardiogr. 2005;6:148–50. http://ehjcimaging.oxfordjournals.org/content/6/2/148.long.

Giant LA Myxoma/Eye Embolism/Endocarditis: Case Report

J Am Coll Cardiol. 2014;63:2049. http://content.onlinejacc.org/article.aspx?articleID=1851444.

Image: Carney's Complex

J Am Coll Cardiol. 2010;55:1395. http://content.onlinejacc.org/article.aspx?articleid=1142663&resultClick=3.

Image: CT

N Engl J Med. 2008;358:728. http://www.nejm.org/doi/full/10.1056/NEJMicm0708551.

Image: Echo

N Engl J Med. 2009;361:e51. http://www.nejm.org/doi/full/10.1056/NEJMicm0807505.

Imaging Cardiac Tumors: MRI/CT

Clin Radiol. 2009;64:1214–30. http://www.ncbi.nlm.nih.gov/pubmed/19913133.

Left Atrial Rhabdomyosarcoma: Case Report

Circulation. 2014;129:e503–e505. http://circ.ahajournals.org/content/
129/21/e503.full.

Left Atrial Thrombus Mimicking Myxoma

Circulation. 2006;113:e456–e457. http://circ.ahajournals.org/content/
113/11/e456.full?sid=c1d4e4bc-f477-401a-9e82-fa4ac143d123.

Left Ventricular Dysfunction

Angiology. 2006;57:119–22. http://www.ncbi.nlm.nih.gov/pubmed/
16444467.

Survival After Resection

Circulation. 2008;118:S7–S15. http://circ.ahajournals.org/content/
118/14-suppl-1/S7.full.

Updates and More

https://clinicalguidecvd.com/lamyx

Chapter 67
Myxoma: Left Ventricle

ICD-10 Code

D15.1

Alternate Names/Abbreviation

NS

Description/Etiology

Rare LV intracardiac pedunculated or intramural tumor
Idiopathic or congenital etiology as part of Carney
   Complex [9]
Clinical features depend on tumor location

Predisposing/Comorbid Conditions

OTHER CARDIAC TUMOR(S)

V.E. Friedewald, *Clinical Guide to Cardiovascular Disease*,
DOI 10.1007/978-1-4471-7293-2_67,
© Springer-Verlag London 2016

Demography

Females 3:1
Cardiac myxomas may be more common and present at younger age in developing countries

Pathophysiology

Composition: gelatinous (myxoid); heterogeneous, often with areas of necrosis, cysts, hemorrhage
Depending on tumor location/mobility, hemodynamic effects primarily:

LVOT obstruction
MR

Signs/Symptoms [5] [9]

BREATHING – DIFF (DYSPNEA) [3]
CHEST – PAIN [4]
CHEST – PALPITATIONS
CONSCIOUSNESS – LOSS, SUDDEN (SYNCOPE) [3]
DIZZY/LIGHTHEADED/PRESYNCOPE [3]
EYES, VISION – DECR/LOSS
HEART – MURMURS, CHANGING
HEART, LSB, MID – MURMUR, SYS [6]
SPUTUM – BLOOD (HEMOPTYSIS)

Differentiation

Aortic Stenosis – Subaortic
Aortic Stenosis – Valvular
HF
Ventricular metastatic tumor
Ventricular septal Rhabdomyoma
Ventricular thrombus

Complications [2]

Conduction defects
Dysrhythmias
Stroke
Sudden Death
Systemic embolus [1]

Laboratory

NS

ECG [7]

N/NS ABN
QRS – LVH PATTERN

Imaging [8]

CARDIOMEGALY
LV, INTRACAVITY – MASS

Genomics

PRKAR1A

Other Tests

NS

Treatment: Nonpharmacologic

NS

Treatment: Pharmacologic

NS

Treatment: Surgical/Invasive

Tumor resection

Prevention

After resection monitor for tumor recurrence in LV/other cardiac chambers

Notes

[1] 2/3 s of patients; cerebral embolus most common
[2] May be initial presentation
[3] 50 % of patients; may be related to position
[4] May resemble angina pectoris; due to direct tumor obstruction or embolic obstruction of coronary artery
[5] Unlike atrial myxomas, constitutional symptoms uncommon
[6] Resembles AS
[7] May be normal
[8] Incidental finding of LV mass by imaging for another indication may be first manifestation
[9] Carney Complex: autosomal dominant condition, including mammary myxoid fibroadenoma, skin pigmented lesions, endocrine disorders, testicular tumors, psammomatous melanotic schwannoma; 2/3 s have cardiac myxomas

Guidelines

NS

Patient Information

Genetics Home Reference: Carney Complex

http://ghr.nlm.nih.gov/condition/carney-complex.

Images

http://www.nlm.nih.gov/medlineplus/ency/imagepages/18078.htm.

Medlineplus

ENGLISH
http://www.nlm.nih.gov/medlineplus/ency/article/007273.htm.

ESPANOL
http://www.nlm.nih.gov/medlineplus/spanish/ency/article/007273.
htm.

Patient Journey

BMJ. 2013;347:f4430. http://www.bmj.com/content/347/bmj.f4430.

Pubmed

http://www.ncbi.nlm.nih.gov/pubmedhealth/PMH0004532/.

Merck

http://www.merckmanuals.com/home/heart-and-blood-vessel-disor-
ders/heart-tumors/myxomas.

Professional Information

Carney Complex

J Cardiothorac Surg. 2011;6:25. doi: 10.1186/1749-8090-6-25. http://
www.cardiothoracicsurgery.org/content/6/1/25.

Case Report

Egyptian Heart J. 2014;66:375–7. http://www.sciencedirect.com/science/article/pii/S1110260814000386.

Case Report

Eur J Echocardiog. 2009;10:593–5. http://ehjcimaging.oxfordjournals.org/content/10/4/593.

Missed Metastatic

World J Cardiol. 2013;5:387–90. http://www.ncbi.nlm.nih.gov/pmc/articles/PMC3817281/.

Stroke Presentation (Case Report)

Egyptian Heart J. 2014;66:375–7. http://www.sciencedirect.com/science/article/pii/S1110260814000386.

Ventricular Metastatic Liposarcoma (Case Report)

Circulation. 2013;127:e443–e445. http://circ.ahajournals.org/content/127/6/e443.full.

Updates and More

https://clinicalguidecvd.com/lvmyx

Chapter 68
Myxoma: Right Atrium

ICD-10 Code

D15.1

Description/Etiology

Tumor usually attached to interatrial septum; may be very large, pedunculated, often calcified; may be biatrial with dumbbell shape with common stalk attached to fossa ovalis

Etiology: idiopathic or congenital as part of Carney Complex [10]

Predisposing/Comorbid Conditions

CARDIAC TUMOR(S)

Demography

All ages

Cardiac myxomas may be more common and present at younger age in developing countries

V.E. Friedewald, *Clinical Guide to Cardiovascular Disease*,
DOI 10.1007/978-1-4471-7293-2_68,
© Springer-Verlag London 2016

Pathophysiology

Composition: gelatinous (myxoid); heterogeneous, often with areas of necrosis, cysts, hemorrhage
Functional TV stenosis
R-L shunting in presence of patent foramen ovale may cause paradoxical (systemic) embolism

Signs/Symptoms

ABDOMEN – FLUID (ASCITES)
BODY, APPEARANCE – WASTING (CACHEXIA)
BREATHING – DIFF (DYSPNEA) [9]
CONSCIOUSNESS – LOSS, SUDDEN (SYNCOPE)
CONSCIOUSNESS – LOSS, SUDDEN, UPRIGHT (ORTHOSTATIC SYNCOPE)
EXTREM – RAYNAUD PHENOMENON
EXTREM, DIGITS – CLUBBED
EXTREM, LOWER, BILAT – EDEMA
FATIGUE
FEVER
HEART, LSB, LOWER – MURMUR, DIAS [3] [4] [6] [7]
HEART, LSB, LOWER – MURMUR, SHORT, EARLY, SYS [2] [4] [6] [7]
HEART, LSB, LOWER – MURMUR, SYS [HOLOSYS] [4] [5] [6] [7]
HEART, SOUND – EARLY SYS [1] [6]
JOINTS – PAIN (ARTHRALGIA)
LIVER – ENLARGED (HEPATOMEGALY)
MUSCLES – PAIN (MYALGIA)
NECK, JVP – ELEV
NECK, JVP, V WAVE – INCR/LARGE [5] [6]
SKIN, COLOR – BLUE (CYANOSIS) [8]
SKIN, COLOR – RED (ERYTHEMA)
WEIGHT – LOSS

Differentiation

Carcinoid Syndrome
Constrictive Pericarditis
Ebstein Anomaly
Pulmonary Arterial Hypertension
Pulmonary Embolism
Pulmonary Stenosis
Pulmonary Venous Hypertension
Rheumatic Valve Disease
Tricuspid Stenosis

Complications

Acute Pulmonary Embolism
LV Dysfunction
Paradoxical Systemic Embolism
RHF

Laboratory

BLOOD, ESR – INCR
BLOOD, HGB/HCT – DECR (ANEMIA)
BLOOD, IGG – INCR
BLOOD, IL-6 – INCR
BLOOD, PLATELETS – DECR
(THROMBOCYTOPENIA)

ECG

P WAVE – TALL/PEAKED
QRS – RBBB/RBBB PATTERN
QRS, AXIS – R

Imaging

RA, CHAMBER, SIZE – INCR
RA, INTRACAVITY – MASS [MAY BE CALCIFIED]
RV, CHAMBER, SIZE – INCR
TV, FLOW – REGURG

Genomics

PRKAR1A

Other Tests

Cardiac catheterization (caution: has risk of provoking pulmonary embolization)

Treatment: Nonpharmacologic

NS

Treatment: Pharmacologic

NS

Treatment: Surgical/Invasive

Tumor resection

Course

Recurrence after surgical resection:

About 13 %; probably lower in sporadic cases, higher in familial forms (eg, Carney Complex)

Usually at same site
Rare after 4 years

High incidence of perioperative arrhythmias but lower long term prevalence
Normal longevity usual after complete resection

Notes

[1] Due to expulsion of tumor from RV; may be associated with palpable tumor shock
[2] Caused by TR due to tumor holding open TV in early systole; precedes early systolic sound
[3] Long or only late diastole
[4] Accentuated by inspiration
[5] Large TR when TV damaged by tumor
[6] May change with position
[7] Murmurs may resemble friction rub
[8] With patent foramen ovale
[9] Most common first symptom
[10] Carney Complex: autosomal dominant condition, includes mammary myxoid fibroadenoma, skin pigmented lesions, endocrine disorders, testicular tumors, psammomatous melanotic schwannoma; 2/3 s have cardiac myxomas

Guidelines

NS

Patient Information

Genetics Home Reference: Carney Complex

http://ghr.nlm.nih.gov/condition/carney-complex.

Images

http://www.nlm.nih.gov/medlineplus/ency/imagepages/18078.htm.

Medlineplus

ENGLISH
http://www.nlm.nih.gov/medlineplus/ency/article/007273.htm.

ESPANOL
http://www.nlm.nih.gov/medlineplus/spanish/ency/article/007273.htm.

Patient Journey

BMJ. 2013;347:f4430. http://www.bmj.com/content/347/bmj.f4430.

Pubmed

http://www.ncbi.nlm.nih.gov/pubmedhealth/PMH0004532/.

Merck

http://www.merckmanuals.com/home/heart-and-blood-vessel-disorders/heart-tumors/myxomas.

Professional Information

Ascites/Extra-Cardiac Manifestations

Angiology. 2005;56:357–60. http://www.ncbi.nlm.nih.gov/pubmed/15889208.

Carney Complex

J Cardiothorac Surg. 2011;6:25. doi: 10.1186/1749-8090-6-25. http://www.cardiothoracicsurgery.org/content/6/1/25.

Images: Right Atrial Hemangioma

J Am Coll Cardiol. 2014;63:e41–e41. http://content.onlinejacc.org/article.aspx?articleID=1841608.

Left Ventricular Dysfunction

Heart Lung Circ. 2013;22:309–11. http://www.ncbi.nlm.nih.gov/pubmed/23098892.

Pulmonary Embolism

J Surg Case Rep. 2014. doi: 10.1093/jscr/rju115.. pii: rju115. http://jscr.oxfordjournals.org/content/2014/10/rju115.long.

Pulmonary Embolism

J Forensic Leg Med. 2008;15:454–6. http://www.ncbi.nlm.nih.gov/pubmed/18761314.

Updates and More

https://clinicalguidecvd.com/ramyx

Chapter 69
Myxoma: Right Ventricle

ICD-10 Code

D15.1

Description/Etiology

Usually attached to free wall or IVS
  Usually pedunculated, sometimes with long stalk
Tend to extend into RVOT tract and sometimes prolapse
  through PV during ventricular systole [1]
Etiology: idiopathic or congenital as part of Carney
  Complex [6]

Comorbid Conditions

Other cardiac tumors

Demography

All ages

V.E. Friedewald, *Clinical Guide to Cardiovascular Disease*,
DOI 10.1007/978-1-4471-7293-2_69,
© Springer-Verlag London 2016

Pathophysiology

Composition: gelatinous (myxoid); heterogeneous, often
with areas of necrosis, cysts, hemorrhage
Physiologic effects:

RVOT obstruction
Pulmonary regurgitation

Signs/Symptoms

BREATHING – DIFF (DYSPNEA)
CHEST – PAIN
CHEST – PALPITATIONS
CONSCIOUSNESS – LOSS, SUDDEN (SYNCOPE)
DIZZY/LIGHTHEADED/PRESYNCOPE
HEART, LSB, LOWER – MURMUR, DIAS [5]
HEART, LSB, MID – MURMUR, DIAS [4]
HEART, LSB, MID – MURMUR, SYS [2]
HEART, LSB, UPPER – MURMUR, DIAS [4]
HEART, LSB, UPPER – MURMUR, SYS [2]
HEART, LSB, UPPER – SOUND, DIAS
    [MID-DIASTOLE] [3]
HEART, LSB, UPPER – SOUND, EJECTION
HEART, LSB, UPPER – THRILL, SYS
NECK, JVP, A WAVE – INCR/LARGE
    (CANNON WAVE)

Differentiation

Pulmonary Artery Stenosis
Pulmonary Arterial Hypertension
Pulmonary Subvalvar Stenosis
Pulmonary Valve Stenosis

Complications

Pulmonary Embolism
RHF
Sudden death

Laboratory

NS

ECG

QRS – RVH PATTERN
QRS, AXIS – R

Imaging

CARDIOMEGALY [CXR: MILD; MAY BE N SIZE]
RV, CHAMBER, SIZE – INCR
RV, INTRACAVITY – MASS

Other Tests

Cardiac catheterization: determine RVOT gradient

Treatment: Nonpharmacologic

NS

Treatment: Pharmacologic

NS

Treatment: Surgical/Invasive

Tumor resection

Prevention

NS

Course

Post-tumor resection longevity approaches normal
Recurrence risk low (2–14 %)

Notes

[1] Consistent with high frequency of RVOT murmurs
[2] Intensity may be highly variable with time and body position but has inconsistent changes with inspiration
[3] "Tumor plop"
[4] Pulmonary regurgitation
[5] Flow across TV
[6] Carney Complex: autosomal dominant condition, including mammary myxoid fibroadenoma, skin pigmented lesions, endocrine disorders, testicular tumors, psammomatous melanotic schwannoma; 2/3 s have cardiac myxomas

Guidelines

NS

Patient Information

Genetics Home Reference: Carney Complex

http://ghr.nlm.nih.gov/condition/carney-complex.

Images

http://www.nlm.nih.gov/medlineplus/ency/imagepages/18078.htm.

Medlineplus

ENGLISH

http://www.nlm.nih.gov/medlineplus/ency/article/007273.htm.

ESPANOL

http://www.nlm.nih.gov/medlineplus/spanish/ency/article/007273.htm.

Patient Journey

BMJ. 2013;347:f4430. http://www.bmj.com/content/347/bmj.f4430.

Pubmed

http://www.ncbi.nlm.nih.gov/pubmedhealth/PMH0004532/.

Merck

http://www.merckmanuals.com/home/heart-and-blood-vessel-disorders/heart-tumors/myxomas.

Professional Information

Carney Complex

J Cardiothorac Surg. 2011;6:25. doi: 10.1186/1749-8090-6-25. http://www.cardiothoracicsurgery.org/content/6/1/25.

Case Report

Circulation. 2000;102:e14–e15. http://circ.ahajournals.org/content/102/2/e14.long.

Case Report

N Engl J Med. 2000;342:295. http://www.nejm.org/doi/full/10.1056/NEJM200001273420418.

Right Ventricular Hemangioma (Case Report)

J Am Coll Cardiol. 2013;61:2388. http://content.onlinejacc.org/article.aspx?articleID=1695217.

Right Ventricular Sarcoma (Case Report)

Eur Heart J. 2014;35:2509. http://eurheartj.oxfordjournals.org/content/35/37/2509.

Updates and More

https://clinicalguidecvd.com/rvmyx

Chapter 70
Nonsustained Ventricular Tachycardia (NSVT)

Management Keys

Post-acute coronary syndrome patients with NSVT should be investigated for evidence of ischemia (e.g., angina, ECG changes) and have evaluation of serum electrolytes, especially those taking diuretics or have had hypokalemia or hypomagnesemia

ICD-10 Code

I47.2

Alternate Names/Abbreviation

NSVT

Description/Etiology [1]

Ventricular tachycardia (≥3 consecutive beats arising below AV node, with wide QRS complex) that:

Does not lead to hemodynamic compromise
<30 s in duration
Rate >125/min

V.E. Friedewald, *Clinical Guide to Cardiovascular Disease*,
DOI 10.1007/978-1-4471-7293-2_70,
© Springer-Verlag London 2016

May occur secondary to structural heart disease or in idiopathic form in otherwise apparently normal heart [2]

Predisposing/Comorbid Conditions

ACUTE MYOCARDIAL INFARCTION [2]
ARRHYTHMOGENIC RIGHT VENTRICULAR
    DYSPLASIA/CARDIOMYOPATHY
ATHLETES [8]
BRUGADA SYNDROME
CABG
CARDIAC AMYLOIDOSIS
CARDIOMYOPATHY – DILATED
CARDIOMYOPATHY – HYPERTROPHIC
CARDIOMYOPATHY – RESTRICTIVE
CATECHOLAMINERGIC POLYMORPHIC
    VENTRICULAR TACHYCARDIA
CHAGAS DISEASE
EARLY REPOLARIZATION [3]
GIANT CELL MYOCARDITIS
HEART FAILURE
HYPERTENSION – SYSTEMIC ARTERIAL
LONG QT SYNDROME – CONGENITAL
OBSTRUCTIVE SLEEP APNEA [9]
VALVULAR HEART DISEASE

Demography

All populations; varies according to etiology

Pathophysiology

Idiopathic: most likely triggered by adrenergic stimulation
    (eg, exercise)
Usually arises in RV

Signs/Symptoms [4]

CHEST – PALPITATIONS
CONSCIOUSNESS – LOSS, SUDDEN (SYNCOPE)
DIZZY/LIGHTHEADED/PRESYNCOPE
HEART, RATE – RAPID (TACHYCARDIA)
HYPOTENSION (BLOOD PRESSURE –
    DECREASED/LOW)

Differentiation

ECG: Supraventricular Tachycardia with aberrant
    conduction
Other causes of syncope

Complications

Tachycardia-Induced Cardiomyopathy
SCD [7] [10]

Laboratory

NS

ECG

DYSRHYTHMIAS – VENTRICULAR (PVCS/OTHERS)
QRS – LBBB/LBBB PATTERN [USUAL] [5]
QRS – LONG, NS [5]

Imaging [6]

NS/VAR WITH COMORBID

Other Tests

Ambulatory ECG monitoring
EP testing

Treatment: Nonpharmacologic

Avoidance of proven triggers

Treatment: Pharmacologic

Beta-blockers
Other drug indications dictated by underlying etiology

Treatment: Surgical/Invasive

ICD
Other interventions dictated by underlying etiology (eg, CABG for CAD)

Prevention

NS

Course

Varies according to etiology
Exercise-induced occurrence in asymptomatic persons: unaffected

Notes

[1] No universal definition
[2] Common post-AMI (40-70 % of pts) in first 24 h
[3] QRS slurring/notching, most often in young male athletes
[4] In addition to findings due to underlying disease
[5] During VT
[6] For risk stratification and decision for ICD
[7] Uncommon in idiopathic form
[8] Considered benign when suppressed by exercise; may be suppressed during deconditioning and resume with conditioning; mechanism unknown
[9] Especially during sleep
[10] High risk features:

> Long duration (>7 beats)
> Increasing frequency
> Polymorphic appearance
> ECG changes/biomarker elevation
> Recurrent ischemia
> Low LVEF
> HF (Killip II-IV)
> Prior ventricular arrhythmia
> Occurrence more than 12–24 h after ACS
> BBB

Guidelines

2012 ACCF/AHA/HRS Focused Update Incorporated Into the ACCF/AHA/HRS 2008 Guidelines for Device-Based Therapy of Cardiac Rhythm Abnormalities

J Am Coll Cardiol. 2013;61:e6–e75. http://content.onlinejacc.org/article.aspx?articleid=1486116#tab1.

Patient Information

Medlineplus

ENGLISH

http://www.nlm.nih.gov/medlineplus/ency/article/000187.htm.

ESPANOL

http://www.nlm.nih.gov/medlineplus/spanish/ency/article/000187.htm.

Merck

http://www.merckmanuals.com/home/heart-and-blood-vessel-disorders/abnormal-heart-rhythms/ventricular-tachycardia.

AHA

http://www.heart.org/HEARTORG/Conditions/Arrhythmia/AboutArrhythmia/Tachycardia-Fast-Heart-Rate-UCM-302018-Article.jsp#.

Cleveland Clinic

http://my.clevelandclinic.org/services/heart/disorders/arrhythmia/Ventricular-Tachycardia.

Mayo Clinic

http://www.mayoclinic.org/diseases-conditions/ventricular-tachycardia/basics/definition/con-20036846.

Stanford

https://stanfordhealthcare.org/medical-conditions/blood-heart-circulation/ventricular-tachycardia.html.

Professional Information

Review

J Am Coll Cardiol. 2012;60:1993–2004. http://content.onlinejacc.org/
article.aspx?articleid=1378223.

Review

Eur Heart J. 2004;25:1093–9. http://eurheartj.oxfordjournals.org/
content/25/13/1093.long.

Acute Myocardial Infarction

Circulation. 1998;98:2030–6. http://circ.ahajournals.org/content/
98/19/2030.

ARVD

Circulation, 2010;122:1144–52. http://circ.ahajournals.org/content/
122/12/1144.abstract.

Cardiac Amyloidosis

Pacing Clin Electrophysiol. 2001;24:1228–33. http://onlinelibrary.
wiley.com/doi/10.1046/j.1460-9592.2001.01228.x/abstract

Chagas Disease

Pacing Clin Electrophysiol. 2011;34:54–62. http://onlinelibrary.wiley.
com/doi/10.1111/j.1540-8159.2010.02896.x/abstract.

Dilated Cardiomyopathy

Curr Cardiol Rep. 2005;7:368–75. http://www.ncbi.nlm.nih.gov/pubmed/16105493.

Exercise-Induced: Prognosis/Asymptomatic Persons

J Am Coll Cardiol. 2013;62:595–600. http://content.onlinejacc.org/article.aspx?articleID=1697402.

Giant Cell Myocarditis

N Engl J Med. 1997;336:1860–6. http://www.nejm.org/doi/full/10.1056/NEJM199706263362603.

Post-CABG

J Cardiovasc Electrophysiol. 2002;13:757–63. http://onlinelibrary.wiley.com/doi/10.1046/j.1540-8167.2002.00757.x/abstract.

Post-revascularization

J Cardiovasc Electrophysiol. 2002;13:342–6. http://onlinelibrary.wiley.com/doi/10.1046/j.1540-8167.2002.00342.x/abstract.

Updates and More

https://clinicalguidecvd.com/nsvt

Chapter 71
Obstructive Sleep Apnea

Management Keys

Consider this diagnosis in all pts with CVD/increased risk of CVD [1] [24]

ICD-10 Code

G47.33

Alternate Names/Abbreviation

OSA
SLEEP RELATED BREATHING DISORDER

Description/Etiology

Recurrent collapse of pharyngeal airway causing intermittent hypoxemia and CO_2 retention during sleep, disrupting normal autonomic and hemodynamic sleep responses; excess sympathetic drive may extend to waking hours, causing increased BP and increased HR [1]

V.E. Friedewald, *Clinical Guide to Cardiovascular Disease*,
DOI 10.1007/978-1-4471-7293-2_71,
© Springer-Verlag London 2016

Apnea: ≥10 s pause in respiration associated with ongoing ventilatory effort [1]

Apnea-hypopnea index (# of apnea and hypopneas/h sleep) >5 and excessive daytime sleepiness [1]

Predisposing/Comorbid Conditions

ASTHMA
ATRIAL FIBRILLATION [22]
CHRONIC OBSTRUCTIVE PULMONARY DISEASE (EMPHYSEMA)
CORONARY ARTERY DISEASE
DEPRESSION
DIABETES MELLITUS
END STAGE RENAL DIS [18]
HEART FAILURE [24]
HYPERTENSION – SYSTEMIC ARTERIAL
HYPOTHYROIDISM [19]
OBESITY
POST-TRAUAMATIC STRESS DISORDER

Demography

M > F
Age <35 years: more common in African Americans

Pathophysiology

Possible mechanisms [likely multiple involved]:

Pharyngeal anatomy
Abnormal muscle tone of upper airway dilator muscles
Unstable ventilatory control
Lower lung volumes
Arousal threshold
Asynchronous activation of upper airway muscles and diaphragm

Other possible factors:

> Resting BP/HR variability
> Oxidative stress
> Insulin resistance
> Increased risk of thrombosis
> Intrathoracic press changes

Signs/Symptoms

ARTERIAL PRESSURE, VARIABILITY – DECR [15]
BEHAVIOR – BIZARRE/CHANGED [5]
BLOOD PRESSURE, ARTERIAL – INCREASED/ ELEVATED [3] [16]
BREATHING, NOCT – GASPING
BREATHING, NOCT – PAUSES (SLEEP APNEA)
BREATHING, NOCT – SNORING [2]
COGNITION – DEFECT, NS [6] [7]
FACE, JAW – DISPLACED, POST (RETROGNATHISM) [9]
FACE, JAW – OVERJET [8] [9]
HEART, RATE, VAR – DECR [15]
HEART, RHYTHM – IRREG [10] [16]
MENTATION – CONCENTRATION IMPAIRED [7]
MENTATION – SLEEPY (SOMNOLENCE) [7]
MOOD – DEPRESSED [7]
MOUTH, PALATE – LOW LYING
MOUTH, PHARYNX – NARROW. LAT
MOUTH, TONSILS, SIZE – INCR [9]
MOUTH, UVULA, SIZE – INCR [9]
NECK, SIZE – INCR [9]
TONGUE, SIZE – INCR (MACROGLOSSIA) [9]

Differentiation

Central Sleep Apnea
Hypothyroidism [19]

Major depression [7]
Other causes of Systemic Arterial Hypertension
Other causes of excessive daytime sleepiness [21]

Complications

AMI [1] [11]
AF [1] [23]
Cor Pulmonale
Growth Impairment
Nocturnal Angina
Nocturnal arrhythmias [10]
Pulmonary Arterial Hypertension [14]
Stroke [1]
Sudden Death [17]

Laboratory

BLOOD, ART, PCO2 – INCR (HYPERCAPNIA) [19]

ECG

AV COND – 2ND DEGREE BLOCK, MOBITZ I
    (WENCKEBACH)
DYSRHYTHMIAS – ATRIAL (PACS/OTHERS)
DYSRHYTHMIAS – VENTRICULAR (PVCS/
    OTHERS)
FIBRILLATION WAVES, ATRIAL

Imaging

NS/VAR WITH COMORBID [ESP HTN]

Other Tests

Polysomnography

Treatment: Nonpharmacologic

Continuous positive pressure [22]
Oral appliances
Sleep posture: lateral
Weight loss

Treatment: Pharmacologic

Antihypertensives

Treatment: Surgical/Invasive

Adenotonsillectomy [13]
Uvulopalatopharyngoplasty

Prevention

Maintain normal body weight

Course

Variable depending on comorbidities

Notes

[1] OSA: independent risk factor for Ischemic Stroke for patients with AF; appears to be under-diagnosed

[2] Almost all patients with OSA

[3] Occurs in >50 % of patients with OSA

[4] Occurs in estimated 30 % of patients with Systemic Arterial Hypertension (often undiagnosed in this population)

[5] Especially children

[6] May be lifelong; learning disabilities in children

[7] Mental changes of major depression and OSA overlap

[8] Maxilla extrudes forward in relation to mandible

[9] 1 or more findings of oropharyngeal narrowing, especially tongue and lateral pharyngeal enlargement; occur in most patients with OSA

[10] Most common:

> NSVT
> 2nd degree AV block
> PVCS
> Sinus arrest
>
> Bradyarrhythmias most common and often occur during sleep with apneic episodes
> Significant number of patients with AF have OSA

[11] Especially nocturnal AMI

[12] Numerous congenital maxillofacial, soft tissue, neuromuscular, and inflammatory conditions associated with OSA

[13] Mainstay of treatment in children

[14] Usually mild and may be associated with other pulmonary disorders (eg, COPD); causal effect uncertain

[15] Daytime at rest; associated with poorer outcomes, greater likelihood of Systemic Arterial Hypertension

[16] Often resistant to antihypertensive medications

[17] Most common during sleep

[18] OSA may occur as often as 40–60 % in patients with end-stage renal disease

[19] OSA and Hypothyroidism have similar clinical features and may be causally linked

[20] Transient during apneic episodes; persistent elevation suggests associated COPD

[21] Periodic limb movements of sleep, rotating shift work, narcolepsy, respiratory disease, severe GERD

[22] From ACCF/AHA 2013 Guidelines for Management of Heart Failure (Sec 7.3.1.4. Treatment of Sleep Disorders):

> "The primary treatment for obstructive sleep apnea is nocturnal continuous positive airway pressure. In a major trial, continuous positive airway pressure for obstructive sleep apnea was effective in decreasing the apnea–hypopnea index, improving nocturnal oxygenation, increasing LVEF, lowering norepinephrine levels, and increasing the distance walked in 6 min; these benefits were sustained for up to 2 years. Smaller studies suggest that continuous positive airway pressure can improve cardiac function, sympathetic activity, and HRQOL in patients with HF and obstructive sleep apnea."

[23] OSA predisposition to AF multifactorial, including:

Atrial Stretch
Autonomic imbalance
Inflammation
Oxidative stress

[24] From ACCF/AHA 2013 Guidelines for Management of Heart Failure:

> "Sec 7.3.1.4. Treatment of Sleep Disorders Sleep disorders are common in patients with HF. A study of adults with chronic HF treated with evidence-based therapies found that 61 % had either central or obstructive sleep apnea. Despite having less sleep time and sleep efficiency compared with those without HF, patients with HF, including those with documented sleep disorders, rarely report excessive daytime sleepiness. Thus, a high degree of suspicion for sleep disorders should be maintained for these patients. The decision to refer a patient to a sleep study should be based on clinical judgment."

Guidelines

Diagnosis of Obstructive Sleep Apnea in Adults: A Clinical Practice Guideline From the American College of Physicians
Ann Intern Med. 2014;161:210–20. http://annals.org/article.aspx?articleid=1892620.

2013 ESH/ESC Guidelines for the management of arterial hypertension
Eur Heart J. 34;2199. http://eurheartj.oxfordjournals.org/content/34/28/2159.full.pdf.

Position paper on the management of patients with obstructive sleep apnea and hypertension: Joint recommendations by the European Society of Hypertension, by the European Respiratory Society and by the members of European COST
J Hypertension. 2012;30:633–46. http://journals.lww.com/jhypertension/Abstract/2012/04000/Position-paper-on-the-management-of-patients-with.1.aspx.

Patient Information

AHA

http://circ.ahajournals.org/content/132/6/e114.full.

ASSA

http://www.sleepapnea.org/learn/sleep-apnea/obstructive-sleep-apnea.html.

Boston Childrens: OSA in Children

http://www.childrenshospital.org/conditions-and-treatments/conditions/obstructive-sleep-apnea-osa.

Images

http://www.nlm.nih.gov/medlineplus/ency/imagepages/9701.htm.

Mayo Clinic

http://www.mayoclinic.org/diseases-conditions/obstructive-sleep-apnea/basics/definition/con-20027941.

Medlineplus

ENGLISH

http://www.nlm.nih.gov/medlineplus/ency/article/000811.htm.

ESPANOL

http://www.nlm.nih.gov/medlineplus/spanish/ency/article/000811.htm.

Merck

http://www.merckmanuals.com/home/lung-and-airway-disorders/sleep-apnea/sleep-apnea.

National Sleep Foundation

https://sleepfoundation.org/sleep-disorders-problems/sleep-apnea.

University of Maryland

http://umm.edu/health/medical/reports/articles/obstructive-sleep-apnea.

Professional Information

AHA Scientific Statement

http://circ.ahajournals.org/content/118/10/1080.full.pdf+html.

Review

Eur Heart J. 2013;34:809–15. http://eurheartj.oxfordjournals.org/content/34/11/809.

Acute Myocardial Infarction

Chest. 2009;135:1488–95. http://journal.publications.chestnet.org/article.aspx?articleid=1089845.

Acute Myocardial Infarction: Nocturnal AMI

J Am Coll Cardiol. 2008;52:343–6. http://content.onlinejacc.org/article.aspx?articleid=1139082&resultClick=3.

Atrial Fibrillation/Obesity

J Am Coll Cardiol. 2007;49:565–71. http://content.onlinejacc.org/article.aspx?articleid=1188673&resultClick=3.

Atrial Fibrillation/Stroke

Am J Cardiol. 2015;115:461–5. http://www.sciencedirect.com/science/article/pii/S0002914914021687.

Asthma

JAMA. 2015;313:156–64. http://jama.jamanetwork.com/article.aspx?articleid=2089354.

Children

Anesthesia Cl. 2014;32:237–61. http://www.sciencedirect.com/science/article/pii/S1932227513000827.

CPAP

Sleep Med Clin. 2010;5:383–92. http://www.sciencedirect.com/science/article/pii/S1556407X10000585.

CPAP: HTN/CAD: Long-Term Effects

Am J Hypertens. 2015;28:300–6. http://ajh.oxfordjournals.org/content/28/3/300.full?etoc.

CPAP: Prevention of a FIB Recurrence

JACCCEP. 2015;1:41–51. http://electrophysiology.onlinejacc.org/article.aspx?articleID=2277227.

CPAP: Atrial Fibrillation Recurrence Post-ablation

Heart Rhythm. 2013;10:331–7. http://www.ncbi.nlm.nih.gov/pubmed/23178687.

CPAP: Atrial Fibrillation Recurrence Post-ablation

J Am Coll Cardiol. 2013;62:300–5. http://content.onlinejacc.org/article.aspx?articleID=1685125.

Depression

Sleep Med Rev. 2009;13:437–44. http://www.sciencedirect.com/science/article/pii/S1087079209000392.

Endothelial Dysfunction

Heart. 2013;99:30–4. http://heart.bmj.com/content/99/1/30.abstract.

Heart Failure

J Am Coll Cardiol. 2011;57:119–27. http://www.acc.org/latest-in-cardiology/journal-scans/2011/01/03/15/21/obstructive-sleep-apnea-in-heart-failure?w-nav=S.

Oropharynx Abnormalities

Am J Resp Crit Care Med. 2000;162:740–8. http://www.atsjournals.org/doi/full/10.1164/ajrccm.162.2.9908123#.VMauGWfwuwV.

Post-traumatic Stress Disorder

Chest. 2016;149:483–90. http://journal.publications.chestnet.org/article.aspx?articleID=2430456.

Pulmonary Arterial Hypertension

Am J Cardiol. 2009;104:1300–6. http://www.sciencedirect.com/science/article/pii/S0002914909012806#.

Sudden Cardiac Death

J Am Coll Cardiol. 2013;62:610–6. http://content.onlinejacc.org/article.aspx?articleid=1699335&resultClick=3.

Systemic Arterial Hypertension

Curr Hypertens Rep. 2007;9:529–34. http://www.ncbi.nlm.nih.gov/pubmed/18367017.

Underdiagnosis

Heart. 2015;101:1288–92. http://heart.bmj.com/content/101/16/1288? etoc.

Updates and More

https://clinicalguidecvd.com/osa

Chapter 72
Orthostatic Hypotension

ICD-10 Code

I95.1

Alternate Names/Abbreviation

BRADBURY-EGGLESTON SYNDROME
NEUROGENIC HYPOTENSION
POSTURAL HYPOTENSION
PRIMARY AUTONOMIC INSUFFICIENCY

Description/Etiology

Defined by American Autonomic Society and American
  Academy of Neurology as a reduction in systolic BP of
  ≥20 mmHg or diastolic BP of ≥10 mmHg within 3 min
  of undergoing orthostatic stress.
Can cause transient cerebral hypoperfusion after posture
  change, with symptoms such as dizziness, weakness,
  blurred vision, or syncope.
Common condition with prevalence of up to 30 % in older
  home-dwelling persons
Possible risk factor for CVD [17]

V.E. Friedewald, *Clinical Guide to Cardiovascular Disease*,   963
DOI 10.1007/978-1-4471-7293-2_72,
© Springer-Verlag London 2016

Causes (see PREDISPOSING/COMORBID
CONDITIONS):

Neurogenic [1]
Non-neurogenic [1]

Predisposing/Comorbid Conditions

ACUTE MYOCARDIAL INFARCTION
ADRENAL INSUFFICIENCY
ALCOHOL USE/EXCESS [10]
AMYLOIDOSIS
ANEMIA
AORTIC STENOSIS [9]
ATRIAL FIBRILLATION
ATRIOVENTRICULAR HEART BLOCK [9]
AUTOIMMUNE/CONNECTIVE TISSUE DISEASE [2]
B12 DEFICIENCY [10]
BLOOD LOSS [7]
BOTULISM
CARCINOID SYNDROME/TUMOR
CARDIOMYOPATHY – RESTRICTIVE [9]
CEREBROVASCULAR DISEASE
CONSTRICTIVE PERICARDITIS [9]
CORONARY ARTERY DISEASE
DEHYDRATION [7]
DIABETES INSIPIDUS
DIABETES MELLITUS [2]
DIARRHEA [7]
DIURETICS [7]
DOPAMINE BETA-HYDROLASE DEFICIENCY
DRUGS [8]
FAMILIAL DYSAUTONOMIA [2]
FRAILTY
GUILLAIN BARRE SYNDROME [5]
HEART FAILURE
HIV [10]
HYPERGLYCEMIA – ACUTE

HYPERTENSION – SYSTEMIC ARTERIAL
HYPOALDOSTERONISM
HYPOKALEMIA
HYPOTHYROIDISM
LEWY BODY DEMENTIA
LUMBAR SYMPATHECTOMY
MULTIPLE MYELOMA
MULTIPLE SCLEROSIS
MULTIPLE SYSTEM ATROPHY (MSA) [19]
NEUROTOXINS [10]
OLIVOPONTOCEREBELLAR ATROPHY
PARANEOPLASTIC SYNDROME [3]
PARKINSON DISEASE [2]
PHEOCHROMOCYTOMA
PHYSICAL DECONDITIONING
PORPHYRIA CUTANEA TARDA [10]
PREGNANCY
PROLONGED BED REST
PULMONARY HYPERTENSION
PURE AUTONOMIC FAILURE
RENAL FAILURE (UREMIA)
SHY-DRAGER SYNDROME
SINUS NODE DYSFUNCTION
SPINAL CORD DIS/TRANSECTION [10]
STROKE
SUBACUTE COMBINED SCLEROSIS [10]
SYMPATHECTOMY
SYRINGOMYELIA [10]
SYSTEMIC MASTOCYTOSIS
TACHYARRHYTHMIAS
TOXIC   AUTONOMIC   NEUROPATHY   [HEAVY
    METALS, DRUGS]
VALVULAR HEART DISEASE
VENOUS INSUFFICIENCY
VOMITING [7]
WERNICKE KORSAKOFF SYNDROME

Demography

Increased prevalence in:

Advanced age
Males
Persons in institutions

Pathophysiology

When body assumes upright posture, gravity causes downward displacement of 500–1000 mL of blood to lower limbs and abdomen, resulting in decreased venous return to heart and about 20 % decrease in cardiac output. Medulla control centers act to compensate for BP drop by increasing sympathetic and reducing parasympathetic nervous system output, causing reflex tachycardia and increased total peripheral resistance. In heathy persons, orthostatic stabilization is achieved within 1 min of standing

Orthostatic hypotension is due to failure of any of the normal compensatory systems for maintaining upright BP.

Signs/Symptoms [20]

ARTERIAL PRESSURE – HIGHLY VARIABLE
ARTERIAL PRESSURE, POSTPRANDIAL – DECR (POSTPRANDIAL HYPOTENSION) [21]
ARTERIAL PRESSURE, PRONE – INCR [6]
ARTERIAL PRESSURE, UPRIGHT – DECR (ORTHOSTATIC HYPOTENSION) [1]
BOWEL MOVEMENTS – CONSTIPATION [MAY BE SEVERE]
CONSCIOUSNESS – LOSS, SUDDEN (SYNCOPE)
DIZZY/LIGHTHEADED/PRESYNCOPE
EYES, VISION – BLURRED
EYES, VISION, UPRIGHT – ALTERED, NS

FATIGUE
GENITALS, PENIS, ERECTION – DECR (ERECTILE
  DYSF)
HEART, RATE, RESPONSE – DECR
  (CHRONOTROPIC INCOMPETENCE)
NAUSEA
SWEATING – DECR (ANHIDROSIS)
SWEATING, FACE – INCR [4]
URINATION – NOCTURNAL (NOCTURIA) [22]
URINATION – RETENTION

Differentiation

Other causes of presyncope/syncope

Complications

DVT – Lower Extremity
Trauma secondary to fall

Laboratory

ASSESS FOR COMORBIDS, EG,
PHEOCHROMOCYTOMA, DIABETES

ECG

N/NS ABN
NS/VAR PER COMORBIDITY(S)

Imaging

NS/VAR WITH COMORBID

Other Tests

Autonomic function tests [6]
Supine/standing plasma norepinephrine
Thermoregulatory sweat test
24-h urinary sodium

Treatment: Nonpharmacologic [16]

Do:

Change positions slowly/carefully
Dorsiflex feet several times before standing
Eat small/frequent meals
Elevate head of bed 5–20°/6-9 in.
Increase salt/fluid intake (unless contraindicated, eg, HF)
Maintain hydration
Perform activities in afternoons, especially regular exercise, such as:

Bicycling
Rowing
Swimming

Wear abdominal binder/compression waist-high stockings

Avoid:

Alcohol
Coughing spells
Dehydration
Hot baths/environment
Hyperventilation
Large meals
Rapid ascent to high altitude
Standing:

Motionless
Rapidly
With legs crossed

Straining with urination or defecation
Working with arms above shoulders

Treatment: Pharmacologic [11] [16]

DC causative/contributory agents when possible (eg, apha-
  blockers, diuretics)
Adrenergic agonists prn [13]
Droxidopa [18]
Fludrocortisone (to increase intravascular volume) [12]
Splanchnic vasoconstrictor [14]
Treatment combinations [15]

Treatment: Surgical/Invasive

NA

Prevention

See above NONPHARMACOLOGICAL TREATMENT

Course

Usually benign but may be risk factor for CVD [17]
Frequently transient in adolescents

Notes

[1] Neurogenic causes include:

AIDS
Alcoholic polyneuropathy
Guillain-Barré syndrome
Multiple Sclerosis

Multiple system atrophy
Pure autonomic failure
Tabes Dorsalis

Non-neurogenic causes include:

Adrenal insufficiency,
AMI
Diabetes Insipidus
Dysrhythmias
HF
Intravascular volume depletion
Myocarditis
Pericarditis
Postprandial
Prolonged sitting/standing (venous pooling)
Sepsis/other acute infectious process
Venous obstruction

[2] Autonomic Neuropathy, also termed Neurogenic Orthostatic Hypotension
[3] Small Cell Lung Carcinoma, Monoclonal Gammopathies, Light Chain Disease, Amyloidosis
[4] May be compensatory for general anhidrosis
[5] Especially post-infection, eg Influenza, Zika virus
[6] Refer patients to specialized autonomic dysfunction center
[7] Due to volume loss
[8] Including:

Alpha-blockers
Antianginal agents
Antiarrhythmics
Anticholinergics
Antihyperensives
Diuretics
Dopamine agonists
Narcotics
Neuroleptics
Sedatives

Tricyclic antidepressants
Vasodilators
Venodilators

[9] Due to decreased cardiac output
[10] Peripheral neuropathy
[11] Derived from Table 1, ASH position statement (GUIDELINES)
[12] Fludrocortisone 0.1-0.3 mg/D
[13] Midodrine 2.5-10 mg; pyridostigmine 60 mg; pseudo-ephedrine 30 mg; atomoxetine 18 mg
[14] Octreotide 12.5-25 mg (subcutaneous)
[15] Fludrocortisone 0.1-0.3 mg each AM and midodrine 5–10 mg; midodrine 5–10 mg or pseudoephedrine 30 mg with 16 oz water bolus
[16] Treatment should be undertaken only after search for underlying cause and its correction (eg, hypovolemia, anemia)
[17] Including CAD, Stroke, HF, all-cause death
[18] Droxydopa specific indications include orthostatic symptoms due to:

Dopamine beta-hydroxylase deficiency
Multiple System Atrophy
Non-diabetic Autonomic Neuropathy
Parkinson Disease
Pure Autonomic Failure

[19] Progressive neurodegenerative disease manifest by clinical features related to autonomic nervous system and movement
[20] Many patients are asymptomatic; when symptoms occur, more likely to be in AM after arising and exacerbated (in part due to venous pooling) by:

Alcohol ingestion
Dehydration
Heat
Immobilization
Post-exercise
Urination

[21] Especially with large meals/carbohydrate-rich food, caused by:

Gastric distention
Release of vasodicvlatory peptides
Splanchnic blood pooling

[22] Due to peripheral blood redistribution to central areas during recumbency/forced natriuresis with concomitant supine hypertension; this nocturnal intravascular volume loss further contributes to AM hypotension

Guidelines

ASH Position Paper
J Clin Hypertension. 2013;15:147–53. http://onlinelibrary.wiley.com/doi/10.1111/jch.12062/abstract.
EFNS guidelines on the diagnosis and management of orthostatic hypotension
Eur J Neurol. 2006;13:930–6. http://onlinelibrary.wiley.com/doi/10.1111/j.1468-1331.2006.01512.x/full.

Patient Information

Medlineplus

http://www.nlm.nih.gov/medlineplus/ency/article/007278.htm.

Genetics Home Reference: Familial Dysautonomia

http://ghr.nlm.nih.gov/condition/familial-dysautonomia.

Mayo Clinic

http://www.mayoclinic.org/diseases-conditions/orthostatic-hypotension/basics/definition/con-20031255.

Espanol

http://www.nlm.nih.gov/medlineplus/spanish/ency/article/007278.
htm.

Professional Information

Review

J Am Coll Cardiol. 2015;66:848–60. http://content.onlinejacc.org/
article.aspx?articleID=2423750.

Review

J Clin Neurol. 2015;11:220–6. http://thejcn.com/DOIx.php?id=
10.3988/jcn.2015.11.3.220#B9.

Review

N Engl J Med. 2008;358:615–24. http://www.nejm.org/doi/
full/10.1056/NEJMcp074189.

Review

Am Fam Physician. 2011;84:527–36. http://www.aafp.org/
afp/2011/0901/p527.html#afp20110901p527-b10.

Review

Clin Auton Res. 2008;18(Suppl 1):8–13. http://www.ncbi.nlm.nih.gov/
pubmed/18368301.

Age-Related Changes

Circulation. 2014;130:1780–9. http://circ.ahajournals.org/content/130/20/1780.full.

Deep Vein Thrombosis

Am J Hypertens. 2016;29:634–40. http://ajh.oxfordjournals.org/content/29/5/634.abstract?etoc.

Droxidopa: Parkinsons

Neurology. 2014;83:328–35. http://www.neurology.org/content/83/4/328.long.

Heart Failure Risk Factor

J Gerontol A Biol Sci Med Sci. 2014;69:223–30. http://www.ncbi.nlm.nih.gov/pubmed/23846416.

Mortality Risk

Heart. 2014;100:406–13. http://heart.bmj.com/content/100/5/406.abstract.

Neurogenic Orthostatic Hypotension

N Engl J Med. 2008;358:615–24. http://www.nejm.org/doi/full/10.1056/NEJMcp074189.

Parkinson Disease

Vasc Health Risk Manag. 2014;10:169–76. http://www.ncbi.nlm.nih.
gov/pubmed/24729712.

Prognosis in Older Adults

Arch Intern Med. 1999;159:273–80. http://www.ncbi.nlm.nih.gov/
pubmed/9989539.

Treatment: Neurogenic Orthostatic Hypotension

Lancet Neurol. 2008;7:451–8. http://www.sciencedirect.com/science/
article/pii/S1474442208700887.

Updates and More

https://clinicalguidecvd.com/orthohyp

Chapter 73
Papillary Fibroelastoma

Management Keys

Papillary adenomas should be surgically resected when possible as they are associated with increased risk of stroke and mortality

Surgical excision has high likelihood of valve preservation and low recurrence rate when performed at a high-volume tertiary care center

Surgical excision associated with high frequency of valve preservation when performed in high-volume centers

Aggressive surgical approach requires significant experience/expertise

Anticoagulant/antiplatelet therapy should be considered in patients not undergoing surgical resection

ICD-10 Code

D15.1

Alternate Names/Abbreviation

PFE
PAPILLOMA
PAPILLARY FIBROMA

V.E. Friedewald, *Clinical Guide to Cardiovascular Disease*, 977
DOI 10.1007/978-1-4471-7293-2_73,
© Springer-Verlag London 2016

Description/Etiology

Pedunculated, avascular tumor

Most common benign cardiac neoplasm of adulthood

>90 % arising from cardiac valves (AV > MV > TV > PV) or cardiac wall (LV most often) [7]

Clinical manifestations depend on location; often detected only at autopsy or incidentally during echo, cardiac catheterization, cardiac surgery

Etiology unknown but some cases appear related to prior cardiac surgery or radiation

Predisposing/Comorbid Conditions

ATRIAL FIBRILLATION
CARDIAC SURGERY
RADIATION

Demography

All ages, increasing with age and most often >50 yrs

Pathophysiology

Avascular tumor with fibroelastic tissue surrounded by endocardium

Non-embolic physiologic effects, if any, vary according to location, usually due to MV or AV flow obstruction

Signs/Symptoms [1]

BREATHING – DIFF (DYSPNEA)
CHEST – PAIN, EFFORT (ANGINA PECTORIS)
CONSCIOUSNESS – LOSS, SUDDEN (SYNCOPE)
FEVER [2]
HEART – MURMUR, NS

HEART, LSB, MID – MURMUR, SYS [4]
HEART, LV, APEX – MURMUR, DIAS [5]

Differentiation

Antiphospholipd antibodies
AS
CAD
Infective Endocarditis
MV Stenosis
Systemic Lupus Erythematosus
Other causes of acute CNS ischemia
Other types of cardiac tumors

Complications

Acute Pulmonary Embolism
AMI
Heart block
SCD
Systemic embolus:

Ischemic Stroke [3]
Mesenteric ischemia/infarction
Renal infarction
Retinal artery [3]
TIA [3]

Laboratory

NS

ECG

AV COND – 3RD DEGREE BLOCK
DYSRHYTHMIAS – ATRIAL (PACS/OTHERS) [6]

Imaging [9] [10] [11]

AV – MASS
LA, INTRACAVITY – MASS
LV, INTRACAVITY – MASS
MV – MASS
PV – MASS
TV – MASS

Other Tests

Cardiac catheterization

Treatment: Nonpharmacologic

NS

Treatment: Pharmacologic

Antiplatelet agents

Treatment: Surgical/Invasive

Surgical resection [8]

Management of smaller, nonmobile masses not well
defined

Course

Post-surgical recurrence: 1.6 % for echo-detected recurrence by up to 6 years post-resection

Notes

[1] Often asymptomatic or only with features due to complications, especially TIA/stroke as initial manifestation
[2] Rare
[3] Cerebral embolus; >50 % initially present with acute neurological features
[4] AV location
[5] MV location
[6] Especially AF
[7] Tumor resembles Sea Anemone
[8] Highly effective in large tertiary centers with valve preservation and low recurrence rate
[9] Seen on echo; 90 % on AV or MV; valve dysfunction rare; appears as round/oval/irregular well-demarcated mass
[10] Sonographer familiarity with echo features of Papillary Fibroadenoma very important
[11] As many as 25 % of lesions can be detected by TEE but less often with TTE

Guidelines

NS

Professional Information

Acute Myocardial Infarction: Case Report

Eur Heart J. 2014;35:1970. http://eurheartj.oxfordjournals.org/content/35/29/1970.

Angina Pectoris: Case Report

Circulation. 2014;129:1714. http://circ.ahajournals.org/content/129/16/1714.full.

Angina Pectoris/Syncope in Teen: Case Report

Circulation. 2014;130:520–2. http://circ.ahajournals.org/content/130/6/520.full.

Aortic Valve

Circulation. 2007;115:e3–e6. http://circ.ahajournals.org/content/115/1/e3.full?sid=4463ee99-fe80-48ad-9369-7e0bdae36047.

Clinical and Echo Features

Circulation. 2001;103:2687–93. http://circ.ahajournals.org/content/103/22/2687.full?sid=4463ee99-fe80-48ad-9369-7e0bdae36047.

Images: Ventricular Papilary Fibroelastoma

J Am Coll Cardiol. 2014;63:2170. http://content.onlinejacc.org/article.aspx?articleID=1859525.

Imaging (Case Report)

Am J Med. 2013;126:964–5. http://www.sciencedirect.com/science/article/pii/S0002934313006220.

Left Atrial Free Wall

Circulation. 2001;104:e87–e88. http://circ.ahajournals.org/content/104/17/e87.full?sid=4463ee99-fe80-48ad-9369-7e0bdae36047.

Left Ventricle

Tex Heart Inst J. 2006;33:63–5. http://www.ncbi.nlm.nih.gov/pmc/articles/PMC1413617/.

Mitral Valve

Circulation. 1998;98:1251–2. http://circ.ahajournals.org/content/98/12/1251.full?sid=4463ee99-fe80-48ad-9369-7e0bdae36047.

Multiple Sites

Circulation. 2012;126:242–3. http://circ.ahajournals.org/content/126/2/242.full?sid=49f03f95-f2a4-4e6b-a2d8-03bd1a2c74b9.

Prognosis/Bioepidemiology

J Am Coll Cardiol. 2015;65:2420–9. http://content.onlinejacc.org/article.aspx?articleID=2300733.

Surgical Resection

Tex Heart Inst J. 2016;43:148–51. http://thij.org/doi/full/10.14503/THIJ-14-4889.

Tricuspid Valve

Circulation. 2008;117:e190–e191. http://circ.ahajournals.org/content/117/11/e190.full?sid=4463ee99-fe80-48ad-9369-7e0bdae36047.

Updates and More

https://clinicalguidecvd.com/pfe

Chapter 74
Patent Ductus Arteriosus (PDA)

Management Keys (Adults)

Routine follow-up recommended for patients with small PDA without evidence of left-sided heart volume overload; recommended every 3–5 years for patients with small PDA without evidence of left heart volume overload

Consultation with adult congenital heart disease interventional cardiologists recommended before surgical closure selected as method of repair for patients with calcified PDA

Surgical repair by a surgeon experienced in CHD surgery is recommended when:

PDA is too large for device closure
Distorted ductal anatomy precludes device closure

ICD-10 Code

Q25.0

Alternate Names/Abbreviation

PDA

V.E. Friedewald, *Clinical Guide to Cardiovascular Disease*,
DOI 10.1007/978-1-4471-7293-2_74,
© Springer-Verlag London 2016

Description/Etiology

Persistent congenital communication between aorta and PA occurring alone or associated with other congenital lesions, most often ASDs and VSDs

PDA associated with several genetic syndromes, including:

Chromosomal aberrations [12]
Single-gene mutations such as Holt-Oram syndrome
X-linked mutations

Small PDAs: usually asymptomatic and detected in adults during evaluation of heart murmur found during routine cardiac examination or by echo, CT, or chest MRI for unrelated condition

Moderate PDAs: tolerated well in childhood and patients often remain completely asymptomatic in early adulthood but usually develop exercise intolerance/symptoms of LV failure beginning in third decade

No single gene defect specific for PDA identified

Predisposing/Comorbid Conditions

ANEURYSMS-OSTEOARTHRITIS SYNDROME
ANOMALOUS CORONARY ARTERY
ATRIAL SEPTAL DEFECT - SECUNDUM
BICUSPID AORTIC VALVE
CANTU SYNDROME
CHAR SYNDROME [11]
MATERNAL RUBELLA [6]
MATERNAL VALPROIC ACID EXPOSURE [18]
NOONAN SYNDROME
OTHER FORMS OF CONGENITAL HEART DISEASE
TREACHER COLLINS SYNDROME [19]
VENTRICULAR SEPTAL DEFECT

Demography

Females 2–3:1
High altitude persistence: 6x incidence than at sea level [20]
Family history

Pathophysiology

Ductus arteriosus: vascular channel connecting junction of
main/left PA with descending aorta immediately distal
to left subclavian artery origin during fetal life; normal
anatomical closure occurs within 2–3 weeks after birth

Failure of duct closure termed Persistent Ductus Arteriosus
after 3 months in term infants and by 1 year in premature infants

L-R shunt varies in magnitude according to size of ductus,
PVR, LV function

R-L shunt occurs with onset of PAH

Signs/Symptoms [21]

ARTERIAL PULSE - DOUBLE (BISFERIENS)
ARTERIAL PULSE PRESSURE – INCR [15]
ARTERIAL PULSE, FALL – RAPID
ARTERIAL PULSE, RISE – RAPID
BREATHING – DIFF (DYSPNEA)
CHEST – PAIN
CHEST, ANT, L – BULGE
EXTREM, LOWER, DIGITS – CLUBBING
EXTREM, LOWER, DIGITS, COLOR – BLUE
  (CYANOSIS)
EXTREM, UPPER, L, DIGITS – CLUBBING
EXTREM, UPPER, L, DIGITS, COLOR – BLUE
  (CYANOSIS) FATIGUE
HEART, LSB, UPPER – MURMUR, CONT [1]
HEART, LSB, UPPER – THRILL, CONT [13]

HEART, LV, APEX – MURMUR, DIAS [14]
HEART, LV, APEX, IMP – FORCEFUL/SUSTAINED [15]
HEART, LV, APEX, IMP – TRIPLE
HEART, P2, INTENSITY – INCR
HEART, S2, SPLIT – REVERSED (PARADOXICAL)
HEART, S3 LV [14]
STERNUM, CURV – ANT (PECTUS CARINATUM)

Differentiation

Aortopulmonary collateral
Coronary Arteriovenous Fistula
Other causes of PAH
Other causes of wide pulse pressure [2]
Ruptured sinus of Valsalva
VSD with AR

Complications

Ductus aneurysm [9]
Ductus rupture
HF
Infective endarteritis/endocarditis
PAH
Pulmonary artery aneurysm
Recurrent pulmonary infections

Laboratory

NS

ECG [3] [7]

DYSRHYTHMIAS – ATRIAL (PACS/OTHERS)
AV COND – 1ST DEGREE BLOCK

P WAVE – FLAT
P WAVE – TALL/PEAKED [4]
P WAVE, DUR – INCR
QRS – BVH PATTERN
QRS – LVH PATTERN
QRS – RVH PATTERN [4]

Imaging [7] [10]

CARDIOMEGALY [17]
DUCTUS ARTERIOSUS – CALCIUM [5]
LA, CHAMBER, SIZE – INCR [16]
LV, CHAMBER, SIZE – INCR [16]
PA, MAIN, SIZE – INCR
PA, PRESS – INCR
PUL, VASCULARITY – INCR [17]

Genomics

NS

Other Tests

Cardiac catheterization [22]

Treatment: Nonpharmacologic

NS

Treatment: Pharmacologic

COX inhibitors (newborns) [23]

Ibuprofen
Indomethacin

Treatment: Surgical/Invasive

Percutaneous closure [8]
Surgical closure [8]

Prevention

Prematernal Rubella immunization

Course

Varies with magnitude of shunt, intervention, comorbidities, presence of PH

Notes

[1] Left infraclavicular area; peak intensity around S2; radiates to LSB/left interscapular area; if PAH present, murmur may be systolic only; murmur may be absent in Eisenmenger because of minimal shunting
[2] Eg, Hyperthyroidism, AR
[3] May be normal; LVH/LA enlargement indicate moderate or large PDA; RVH/RA enlargement indicate advanced stage of Pulmonary Hypertension
[4] In presence of PAH
[5] Calcification associated with increased risk of rupture during surgical repair
[6] Also cataracts, deafness, mental retardation, low birth weight, failure to thrive
[7] May be normal with small shunts
[8] Adult intervention for PDA: ACC/AHA 2008 Guidelines for Adults With CHD (J Am Coll Cardiol 2008;52:e185)

"Surgical closure of PDA in the adult may pose some problems due to the friability and/or calcification of the ductus, atherosclerosis, and aneurysm formation, as well as the presence of other unrelated comorbid conditions, such as coronary atherosclerosis or renal disease, that may adversely affect the perioperative risk. Adults with PDA are better suited for percutaneous closure with either the occlusion device or coils because of its high success and few complications. If the PDA is associated with other conditions that require surgical correction, the ductus may be closed during the same operation, although percutaneous closure of the PDA before other cardiac surgery may decrease the risk of cardiopulmonary bypass."

[9] Usually L-R shunt
[10] Also visualize ductus by echo, which is diagnostic
[11] Char Syndrome: autosomal disorder comprising:

> PDA
> Facial Dysmorphism
> Hand anomalies

[12] Esp Trisomy 21
[13] Thrill indicates moderate/large shunt
[14] Diastolic rumbling murmur/S3 due to increased LA-LV blood flow consistent with moderate/large shunt
[15] Indicates moderate/large shunt
[16] LA/LV dilatation (LA:aorta ratio >1.3) on echo indicates moderate/large shunt
[17] CXR heart size/pulmonary vascularity may be normal with small shunt; if shunt volume is moderate to large, CXR shows increased pulmonary vascular markings with prominent ascending aorta and cardiomegaly with prominent LA and LV; peripheral pruning of vascular markings with large PA shadow and right PA indicates severe PH; calcified ductus may appear in some older adults, especially in lateral CXR view

[18] Fetal Valproate Syndrome:

> Valproic acid: anticonvulsant drug
> Rare congenital disorder due to fetal exposure to valproic acid (Dalpro, Depakene, Depakote, Depakote sprinkle, Divalproex, Epival, Myproic acid) during first 3 months of pregnancy
> Clinical features include, in addition to rare occurrences of PDA:
>
> > Spina bifida
> > Distinctive facial features
> > Musculoskeletal abnormalities

[19] Treacher Collins Syndrome:

> Caused by mutations in TCOF1, POLR1C, POLR1D
> Associated with multiple defects, including (in addition to rare PDA):
>
> > Cleft palate
> > Hearing loss/ear deformities
> > Ocular/visual abnormalities
> > Normal mental development

[20] Due to exposure to low pO_2

[21] Clinical manifestations primarily determined by volume of extra blood recirculating in PA, capillaries, pulmonary veins, LA, LV, ascending aorta, and defect duration

[22] Cardiac catheterization for diagnosis not indicated for uncomplicated PDA with adequate noninvasive imaging; in adults with PDA cardiac catheterization is performed at time of planned percutaneous closure in patients meeting criteria after initial evaluation by TTE

[23] Cox inhibitor treatment for PDA closure:

> Newborns: IV indomethacin and IV ibuprofen lysine are equally effective in closure of PDA, with closure rates of 75–93 %; IV ibuprofen lysine may be associated with decreased incidence of adverse events, especially renal toxicity; IV ibuprofen lysine may have less significant impact on cerebral blood flow and mesenteric blood flow

Adults: adult ductal tissue has no response to COX inhibitors like indomethacin; thus, primary modes of PDA closure for PDA in adults are percutaneous and surgical

Guidelines

ACC/AHA 2008 guidelines for the management of adults with congenital heart disease
J Am Coll Cardiol. 2008;52:e143–263. http://content.onlinejacc.org/article.aspx?articleid=1188032#tab1
ESC guidelines for the management of grown-up congenital heart disease (new version 2010)
Eur Heart J. 2010;31:2915–57. http://www.escardio.org/guidelines-surveys/esc-guidelines/Pages/grown-up-congenital-heart-disease.aspx.

Patient Information

Images

https://www.nlm.nih.gov/medlineplus/ency/imagepages/1056.htm.
https://www.nlm.nih.gov/medlineplus/ency/presentations/100012-1.htm.

Medlineplus

ENGLISH

http://www.nlm.nih.gov/medlineplus/ency/article/001560.htm.

ESPANOL

https://www.nlm.nih.gov/medlineplus/spanish/ency/article/001560.htm.

Cleveland Clinic

http://my.clevelandclinic.org/heart/disorders/patent-ductus-arteriousis-adults.aspx.

Genetics Home Reference

http://ghr.nlm.nih.gov/search?query=patent+ductus+arteriosus

Mayo Clinic

http://www.mayoclinic.org/diseases-conditions/patent-ductus-arteriosus/basics/definition/con-20028530.

Texas Heart Institute

http://www.texasheart.org/HIC/Topics/Cond/pda.cfm.

Professional Information

Early Descriptions

Seminars in Perinatology. 2012;36:89–91. http://www.sciencedirect.com/science/article/pii/S0146000511001637.

Review

Circulation. 2006;114:1873–82. http://circ.ahajournals.org/content/114/17/1873.long.

Review

Cardiology Clinics. 2013;31:417–30. http://www.sciencedirect.com/science/article/pii/S0733865113000349

Review

Seminars in Perinatology. 2012;36:146–53. http://www.sciencedirect.
com/science/article/pii/S0146000511001716.

Review: Ligation in Premature Infants

Journal of Surgical Research. 2014;190:613–22. http://www.sciencedi-
rect.com/science/article/pii/S0022480414001164..

Review: Transcatheter Closure

Archives of Cardiovascular Diseases. 2014;107:122–32. http://www.
sciencedirect.com/science/article/pii/S1875213614000242.

Anomalous Coronary Artery

Res Cardiovasc Med. 2013;2:190–92. http://www.ncbi.nlm.nih.gov/
pubmed/25478523.

Char Syndrome

Circulation.   1999;99:3036–42.   http://circ.ahajournals.org/content/
99/23/3036.full?sid=ab458ca5-62bd-4ff1-be87-5392c85b4fe5.

Eisenmenger (Case Report)

Heart, Lung and Circulation. 2013;22:968–69. http://www.sciencedi-
rect.com/science/article/pii/S1443950613001716.

Indomethacin

J Cardiovasc Thorac Res. 2014;6:257–59. http://www.ncbi.nlm.nih.
gov/pubmed/25610559.

Infective Endarteritis

Am J Cardiol. 2004;93:513–15. http://www.sciencedirect.com/science/article/pii/S0002914903016217

Post-ligation Coronary Perfusion/LV Function

J Thor Cardiovasc Surg. 2012;143:1271–78. http://www.sciencedirect.com/science/article/pii/S0022522311011548.

Pulmonary Artery Aneurysm

Curr Cardiol Rev. 2015;11:163–66. http://www.ncbi.nlm.nih.gov/pubmed/25545802.

Transcatheter Occlusion: Followup

Circulation. 1991;84:2313–17. http://circ.ahajournals.org/content/84/6/2313.abstract?sid=ce18dc36-05ee-442a-b607-2428b8c7a019.

Transcatheter Occlusion: Preterm Infants

JACC: Cardiovascular Interventions. 2010;3:550–55. http://www.sciencedirect.com/science/article/pii/S1936879810001743.

Transcatheter Occlusion with Reversible PAH

Heart. 2007;93:514–18. http://heart.bmj.com/content/93/4/514.abstract.

Treacher Collins Syndrome

Int J Pediatr Otorhinolaryngol. 2014; 78:893–98. http://www.ncbi.nlm.nih.gov/pubmed/24690222.

Updates and More

https://clinicalguidecvd.com/pda

Chapter 75
Pericarditis: Acute

Management Keys [26]

Treat with aspirin or NSAIDs as first-line therapy, with gastro-protection

Treat with colchicine as first-line therapy as adjunct to aspirin/NSAID therapy

Use serum CRP as guide to treatment length and for assessing response to therapy

Corticosteroids are not recommended as first-line therapy for acute pericarditis

Consider treatment with low-dose corticosteroids:

   Contraindication/failure of aspirin/NSAIDs and colchicine

   When infectious cause has been excluded

   When there is a specific indication such as autoimmune disease

Consider exercise restriction for non-athletes until resolution of symptoms and normalization of CRP, ECG, echocardiogram

For athletes, duration of exercise restriction should be considered until resolution of symptoms and normalization of CRP, ECG and echocardiogram for at least 3 months

V.E. Friedewald, *Clinical Guide to Cardiovascular Disease*, 999
DOI 10.1007/978-1-4471-7293-2_75,
© Springer-Verlag London 2016

ICD-10 Code

I30.9

Description/Etiology

Inflammatory pericardial syndrome with or without pericardial effusion

Causes:

Idiopathic [1]
Adjacent structure dis
Cancer

Metastatic [16]
Primary cardiac

Connective tissue disease/vasculitis
Drugs
Infection
Metabolic disease
Post-injury syndrome (especially AMI)
Radiation
Trauma [21]

Non-penetrating
Penetrating

Predisposing/Comorbid Conditions

ANOREXIA NERVOSA
INFLAMMATORY BOWEL DISEASE
ACUTE MYOCARDIAL INFARCTION
ACUTE PANCREATITIS
ACUTE PULMONARY EMBOLISM
AMYLOIDOSIS
ANKYLOSING SPONDYLITIS
AORTIC DISSECTION

BEHCET SYNDROME
CANCER [16]
CARDIAC CONTUSION
CHURG-STRAUSS SYNDROME
DERMATOMYOSITIS
DRUGS [4]
EMPYEMA
FAMILIAL MEDITERRANEAN FEVER
GIANT CELL ARTERITIS
GOUT
HORTON DISEASE
HYPEREOSINOPHILIC SYNDROME
HYPOTHYROIDISM
INFECTION [2] [3]
LEUCOCYTOCLASTIC VASCULITIS
LOEFFLER SYNDROME
PNEUMONIA – COMMUNITY-ACQUIRED
POLYARTERITIS
POLYMYOSITIS
POST-MYOCARDIAL INFARCTION SYNDROME
POST-THORACOTOMY/PERICARDIOTOMY
    SYNDROME [17]
RADIATION [18]
REITER SYNDROME
RENAL DIALYSIS
RENAL FAILURE (UREMIA)
RHEUMATIC FEVER
RHEUMATOID ARTHRITIS
SARCOIDOSIS
SCLERODERMA
SCURVY
SJOGREN SYNDROME
STEVENS-JOHNSON SYNDROME
SYSTEMIC INFLAMMATORY DISEASE
SYSTEMIC LUPUS ERYTHEMATOSUS
TAKAYUSU DISEASE
TEMPORAL ARTERITIS

THROMBOHEMOLYTIC THROMBOCYTOPENIC
  PURPURA
TRAUMA
TUMOR   NECROSIS   FACTOR   RECEPTOR-
  ASSOCATED PERIODOC SYNDROME
WEGENER GRANULOMATOSIS
WHIPPLE DISEASE

Demography

More common in males and adults

Pathophysiology

Acute inflammatory changes of pericardium, often extend-
ing into superficial myocardium and pleura

Signs/Symptoms

ABDOMEN – PAIN
BREATHING – DIFF (DYSPNEA)
CHEST – PAIN [5]
CHEST, POST – PAIN, PLEURITIC
CONSCIOUSNESS – LOSS, SUDDEN (SYNCOPE)
COUGH
FATIGUE
FEVER [20]
HEART, LSB, LOWER – FRICTION RUB [7]
HEART, LSB, MID – FRICTION RUB [7]
HICCUPS
MENTATION – WEAKNESS (MALAISE) [20]
MUSCLES – PAIN (MYALGIA) [20]
SWALLOWING – DIFFICULT (DYSPHAGIA)

Differentiation

Acute Pulmonary Embolism
AMI
Aortic Dissection
Costochondritis
Gastroesophageal Reflux Disease
Pneumonia

Complications

Cardiac Tamponade [24]
Dysrhythmias (especially AF)
Pericarditis – Constrictive
Recurrent pericarditis

Laboratory

BLOOD, CKMB – INCR
BLOOD, CRP – INCR
BLOOD, ESR – INCR
BLOOD, TROPONIN – INCR
BLOOD, WBC – INCR (LEUKOCYTOSIS)

ECG

DYSRHYTHMIAS – ATRIAL (PACS/OTHERS) [10]
PR SEGMENT – DEPRESSED [9]
ST SEGMENT – ELEV [11]
T WAVE – INVER, ABN [12]
VOLTAGE, GEN – DECR [8]

Imaging

CARDIOMEGALY [LARGE EFFUSION]
PERICARD – FLUID
PLEURA – FLUID

Other Tests

Pericardiocentesis [14]
Pericardial biopsy

Treatment: Nonpharmacologic

Activity restrictions [27]

Treatment: Pharmacologic

Antibiotics: suspected/proven bacterial etiology
Colchicine [25]
NSAIDS
Corticosteroids [28]:

Severe cases without adequate response to colchicine/
NSAIDS
Tuberculosis-related etiology

Treatment: Surgical/Invasive

Pericardiocentesis [14]

Prevention

NS

Course

Usual resolution in 2–6 weeks [15]
Indicators of poor prognosis:

Fever (>38° C)
Large effusion/tamponade
Pneumonia
NSAID/ASA/colchicine failure (1 week)
Sepsis
Subacute course
Trauma

Notes

[1] Majority of cases
[2] Including:

Bacterial
Fungal
Leptospiral
Mycoplasma
Parasitic
Rickettsial
Tuberculosis
Viral, especially:

Adenovirus
Cytomegalovirus
Enterovirus
Herpes simplex
HIV
Influenza

[3] In immunocompromised patients: Herpes complex and
Cytomegalovirus are especially important
[4] Including:

Diphenylhydantoin

     Doxorubicin
     Hydralazine
     Isoniazid
     Penicillin
     Procainamide

[5] May radiate to left or right shoulder, arms, elbows, trapezius area (due to common phrenic nerve innervation), jaw, throat, ear, occipital area, interscapular area

[6] Exacerbated by reclining position/relieved by leaning forward

[7] Often absent; presence/character may vary between exams; best heard at end-expiration/patient leaning forward; monophasic/biphasic/triphasic

[8] When pericardial effusion present

[9] Best seen in ECG leads II, AVR, AVF, V4-6

[10] <10 %: AF/A Flutter most common

[11] Most characteristic ECG feature; due to subepicardial inflammation; diffuse; saddle-shaped/concave upward

[12] After ST segments return to baseline

[13] About 25 %; usually on left

[14] Primarily for drainage or when underlying pathology suspected, eg, cancer/infection

[15] For idiopathic/viral cause

[16] Usually secondary, via local invasion/lymphatic/hematogenous spread; >60 % of cardiac metastases involve pericardium

[17] Reported in up to 20 % of patients post-CABG; mean 4 weeks

[18] Especially breast cancer, mediastinal tumors (eg, Hodgkins)

[19] Differentiate from AMI by:

     Absence of Q wave/R wave loss in pericarditis
     QRS prolongation/QT shortening in leads with ST elevation in AMI but not pericarditis

[20] Prodromal of fever, myalgia, malaise often precedes onset

[21] Prior cardiac surgery most common

[22] Lung adenocarcinoma most common

[23] Criteria for diagnosis of Acute Pericarditis (from 2015 ESC Guidelines)

1. Chest pain (85–90 % of cases) – typically sharp and pleuritic, improved by sitting up and leaning forward
2. Pericardial friction rub (≤33 % of cases) superficial scratchy or squeaking sound best heard with diaphragm of stethoscope over LSB
3. ECG changes (up to 60 % of cases) – new widespread ST elevation or PR depression in acute phase
4. Pericardial effusion (up to 60 % of cases, generally mild)

Additional signs and symptoms may be present according to underlying etiology or systemic disease (i.e., signs and symptoms of systemic infection such as fever and leucocytosis, or systemic inflammatory disease or cancer)

[24] Acute tamponade rare in acute idiopathic pericarditis; more common with specific underlying causes such as cancer, tuberculosis, purulent pericarditis

[25] Colchicine: 15–30 % of patients not treated with colchicine develop recurrent or incessant disease, while colchicine decreases recurrence rate by 50 %

[26] Derived from 2015 ESC Guidelines

[27] Activity restrictions:

Consider exercise restriction for non-athletes until resolution of symptoms and normalization of CRP, ECG, echocardiogram

For athletes, duration of exercise restriction should be considered until resolution of symptoms and normalization of CRP, ECG and echocardiogram for at least 3 months

[28] Use corticosteroids in HIV pts as may increase risk of malignancy

Guidelines

2015 ESC guidelines for the diagnosis and management of pericardial diseases

Eur Heart J. 2015;36:2921–64. http://eurheartj.oxfordjournals.org/content/36/42/2921.

American Society of Echocardiography clinical recommendations for multimodality cardiovascular imaging of patients with pericardial disease: endorsed by the Society for Cardiovascular Magnetic Resonance and Society of Cardiovascular Computed Tomography

J Am Soc Echocardiogr. 2013;26:965–1012. http://www.sciencedirect.com/science/article/pii/S0894731713005336.

Patient Information

Images

http://www.nlm.nih.gov/medlineplus/ency/imagepages/18081.htm.
http://www.nlm.nih.gov/medlineplus/ency/imagepages/18151.htm.

Medlineplus

ENGLISH

http://www.nlm.nih.gov/medlineplus/ency/article/001103.htm.

ESPANOL

http://www.nlm.nih.gov/medlineplus/spanish/ency/article/001103.htm.

Mayo Clinic

http://www.mayoclinic.org/diseases-conditions/pericarditis/basics/definition/con-20035562.

Cleveland Clinic

http://my.clevelandclinic.org/services/heart/disorders/pericarditis.

MERCK

http://www.merckmanuals.com/home/heart-and-blood-vessel-disorders/pericardial-disease/acute-pericarditis.

http://www.merckmanuals.com/home/heart-and-blood-vessel-disorders/pericardial-disease/chronic-pericarditis.

AHA

http://www.heart.org/HEARTORG/Conditions/More/Symptoms-and-Diagnosis-of-Pericarditis-UCM-444932-Article.jsp.

Texas Heart Institute

http://www.texasheart.org/HIC/Topics/Cond/pericard.cfm.

Cardiosmart

https://www.cardiosmart.org/Heart-Conditions/Pericarditis

Professional Information

Review

N Engl J Med. 2014;371:2410–16. http://www.nejm.org/doi/full/10.1056/NEJMcp1404070?query=cardiology.

Review

J Nurse Pract. 2015;11:146–48. http://www.sciencedirect.com/science/article/pii/S1555415514007508

Review

Am Fam Physician. 2014;89:553–60. http://www.aafp.org/afp/2014/0401/p553.html.

Review

Lancet. 2004;363:717–27. http://www.sciencedirect.com/science/article/pii/S0140673604156481.

Review: Treatment

Circulation.   2013;127:1723–26.   http://circ.ahajournals.org/content/127/16/1723.full.

Atrial Flutter/Fibrillation

Heart. 2015;101:1463–67. http://heart.bmj.com/content/101/18/1463?etoc

Clinical Profiles/Outcomes Hospitalized Patients

Circulation.   2014;130:1601–06.   http://circ.ahajournals.org/content/130/18/1601.full?sid=94c2fb71-9fbe-443d-8f15-79263d7ce758.

Colchicine

N Engl J Med. 2013;369:1522–28. http://www.nejm.org/doi/full/10.1056/NEJMoa1208536.

Colchicine: Prevention of Post-Pericardiotomy Syndrome

Eur Heart J. 2010;31:2749–54. http://eurheartj.oxfordjournals.org/content/31/22/2749.

Colchicine: Prevention of Post-Pericardiotomy Syndrome

JAMA. 2014;312:1016–23. http://jama.jamanetwork.com/article.
aspx?articleid=1900482.

Corticosteroids

Circulation. 2008;118:667–71. http://circ.ahajournals.org/content/
118/6/667.full.

Cystic Tuberculous Pericarditis (Case Report)

J Am Coll Cardiol. 2013;62:1393–93. http://content.onlinejacc.org/
article.aspx?articleID=1729179.

ECG (New Criteria): Acute Pericarditis Vs AMI

Am J Med. 2014;27:233–39. http://www.sciencedirect.com/science/
article/pii/S0002934313009753.

Etiology

Am J Med. 2015;128:784.e1–784.e8. http://www.sciencedirect.com/
science/article/pii/S0002934315001771.

Hydatid Cyst Rupture (Case Report)

Circulation. 2013;128:2073–4. http://circ.ahajournals.org/content/128/
18/2073.full.

Metastatic Cancer

Circulation. 2013;128:1790–4. http://circ.ahajournals.org/content/128/16/1790.full

Prognosis

Circulation. 2013;128:42–9. http://circ.ahajournals.org/content/128/1/42.full.

Prognosis: Indicators

Circulation. 2007;115:2739–44. http://circ.ahajournals.org/content/115/21/2739.full.

Triage/Management

Int J Cardiol. 2007;118:286–94. http://www.sciencedirect.com/science/article/pii/S0167527306008862.

Tuberculosis

Heart. 2014;100:135–9. http://heart.bmj.com/content/100/2/135abstract

Updates and More

http://www.cormt.com/acperi
https://clinicalguidecvd.com/aaa

Chapter 76
Pericarditis: Constrictive

Management Keys

Differentiate from Restrictive Cardiomyopathy
Perform pericardiectomy when not responding to medical
therapy

ICD-10 Code

I31.1

Description/Etiology

Thick, adherent, fibrotic pericardium causing decreased
pericardial compliance and limited diastolic filling
Occurs after many diverse pericardial disease processes

Most common reported causes in developed countries:

Viral and idiopathic: 42–49 %
Post-cardiac surgery: 11–37 %
Post-radiation: 9–31 % [13]
Connective tissue/inflammatory disorder (3–7 %) [8]
Post-infectious (TB or purulent pericarditis): (3–6 %) [15]
Miscellaneous causes: 10 % [14]

V.E. Friedewald, *Clinical Guide to Cardiovascular Disease*,   1013
DOI 10.1007/978-1-4471-7293-2_76,
© Springer-Verlag London 2016

Risk of progression:

> Viral and idiopathic pericarditis: <1 %
> Immune-mediated pericarditis and neoplastic pericardial diseases: 2–5 %
> Bacterial pericarditis (especially purulent pericarditis): 20–30 %

Rarely follows recurrent pericarditis
Clinical features due to volume overload and decreased cardiac output

Predisposing/Comorbid Conditions

> ACUTE PERICARDITIS [ESP INF]
> AUTOIMMUNE/CONNECTIVE TISSUE DISEASE [8]
> BLUNT CHEST TRAUMA
> CANCER
> CARCINOID HEART DISEASE
> CARDIAC SURGERY
> CHRONIC RENAL FAILURE
> HEART TRANSPLANT
> INFECTIVE   ENDOCARDITIS   [ESP   WITH INCOMPLETE DRAINAGE]
> LUNG TRANSPLANT
> RADIATION

Demography

Variable according to etiology

Pathophysiology

Anatomical: prominent pericardial thickening and calcifications; however, constriction may be present with normal pericardial thickness in up to 20 % of cases

Physiological:

> Restrictive filling and intracardiac-intrathoracic pressure dissociation
>
> Decreased venous filling of RV and ventricular interdependence lead to right heart volume overload and decreased LVSV [10]

Signs/Symptoms

ABDOMEN–DISTENSION
ABDOMEN–FLATULENCE
ABDOMEN–FLUID (ASCITES)
ABDOMEN–FULLNESS [ESP POSTPRANDIAL]
ABDOMEN–PAIN
APPETITE–DECR (ANOREXIA)
ARTERIAL PULSE–PARADOXICAL
   (PARADOXICAL PULSE)
ARTERIAL PULSE PRESSURE–DECR
BREATHING–DIFF (DYSPNEA)
BREATHING–DIFF, RECLINING FLAT
   (ORTHOPNEA)
BREATHING–RAPID (TACHYPNEA)
EXTREM, HANDS, PALMS, COLOR–RED (PALMAR
   ERYTHEMA)
EXTREM, LOWER, BILAT–EDEMA
EYES/SKIN–YELLOW (JAUNDICE)
FATIGUE
GENITALS, SCROTUM–SWOLLEN (EDEMA)
HEART–PERICARD KNOCK
HEART, LV, APEX, IMP–DECR/ABSENT
HEART, LV, APEX, IMP–RETRACTION, SYS
HEART, RATE–RAPID (TACHYCARDIA)
HEART, S2, SPLIT–WIDE
HEART, SOUNDS, INTENSITY–DECR
HYPOTENSION (BLOOD PRESSURE–
   DECREASED/LOW)
LIVER–ENLARGED (HEPATOMEGALY)

LIVER–PULSATION, PRESYS
LIVER–PULSATION, SYS
MUSCLES–ATROPHY
NECK, JVP–ELEV
NECK, JVP–INSP RISE (KUSSMAUL SIGN)
NECK, JVP, Y DESCENT–RAPID
SKIN–SPIDER ANGIOMAS
SKIN, COLOR, EFFORT–BLUE (CYANOSIS)
SPLEEN, SIZE–INCR (SPLENOMEGALY)
WEIGHT–LOSS

Differentiation

Cardiac Tamponade
Hypertrophic Cardiomyopathy
Hepatic disease
Intraabdominal malignancy
Nephrotic Syndrome
Other causes of HF
Other causes of systemic venous congestion
RA Myxoma
Restrictive Cardiomyopathy
SVC obstruction
TV regurgitation
TV stenosis

Complications

AF [1]
Cardiac Tamponade
Circulatory collapse
Effusive Constrictive Pericarditis
Heart block
HF
Hepatic dysfunction
Protein-losing Enteropathy

Laboratory

BLOOD, NT-PROBNP–INCR

ECG [6]

AV COND–1ST DEGREE BLOCK
AV COND–3RD DEGREE BLOCK
DYSRHYTHMIAS–ATRIAL (PACS/OTHERS)
P WAVE, DUR–INCR [2]
Q WAVE–ABN [3]
QRS–LONG, NS
QRS–RVH PATTERN
QRS–SLURRED
QRS, AMP–DECR
QRS, AXIS–R
RATE–INCREASED (SINUS TACHYCARDIA)
ST-T WAVE–ABN, NS
T WAVE–INVER, ABN
VOLTAGE, GEN–DECR

Imaging [5]

ABDOM–FLUID (ASCITES)
IVS, MOTION, DIAS–ABN [4]
LA, CHAMBER, SIZE–INCR
LIVER, SIZE–INCR (HEPATOMEGALY)
LV, FILLING–DECR/RESTRICTED
PERICARD–CALCIUM
PERICARD–FLUID
PERICARD–THICK
PLEURA–FLUID
RA, CHAMBER, SIZE–INCR
RV, FILLING–RESTRICTED

SPLEEN, SIZE–INCR (SPLENOMEGALY)
VEINS, HEPATIC, SIZE–INCR [WITH RESTRICTED RESP FLUCTUATIONS]
VENA CAVA, INF, SIZE–INCR [WITH RESTRICTED RESP FLUCTUATIONS]

Other Tests

Tests to rule out non-idiopathic causes
Cardiac catheterization [11]

Treatment: Nonpharmacologic

NS

Treatment: Pharmacologic

Treatment of congestion/supportive [9]
Treatment of inflammation [7]
Treatment of specific etiologies [16]

Treatment: Surgical/Invasive

Pericardiectomy [12]

Prevention

Treatment of underlying causes before progression to Constrictive Pericarditis [16]

Course

Variable per underlying etiology

Worse prognosis in patients with mixed disease (ie, underlying restrictive Cardiomyopathy, liver disease, prior radiation)

Notes

[1] 1/3 of patients

[2] Also may be notched, resembling P mitrale

[3] "Pseudoinfarction" pattern

[4] Termed septal bounce: "dip-plateau" phenomenon: abnormal early outward/inward IVS diastolic motion; also occurs in Cardiac Tamponade

[5] Transthoracic echocardiography recommended in all patients with suspected Constrictive Pericarditis; CXR (frontal/lateral views) recommended in all patients with suspected Constrictive Pericarditis; CT/CMR indicated as second-level imaging techniques to assess calcifications, pericardial thickness, degree/extension of pericardial involvement

[6] Can be normal

[7] May reverse transient constriction (occurs in 10–20 % of cases) within a few months, as a temporary measure during resolution of pericarditis; elevated CRP and imaging evidence of pericardial inflammation by contrast enhancement on CT/CMR may help identify patients with potentially reversible forms of constriction for whom empiric anti-inflammatory therapy should be considered, preventing need for pericardiectomy

[8] Including:

Amyloidosis
Behcet Disease
Familial Mediterranean Fever
Inflammatory Bowel Disease

> Rheumatoid Arthritis
> Sarcoidosis
> Sjogren Syndrome
> Systemic Lupus Erythematosus
> Temporal Arteritis
> Whipple Disease

[9] Especially diuretics, aimed at controlling symptoms of congestion in advanced cases and when surgery is high risk/contraindicated; medical therapy should never delay surgery

[10] Both ventricles cannot expand/fill at same time due to noncompliant pericardium; expansion of RV causes LV compression

[11] Cardiac catheterization indicated when non-invasive diagnostic methods do not provide a definite diagnosis; used to evaluate for ventricular interdependence, equalization of ventricular end-diastolic pressure, dissociation of intrathoracic/intracardiac pressures

[12] Nontrivial morbidity/mortality, but may be only definitive treatment in subset of patients

[13] Most cases due to Hodgkin's disease or breast cancer

[14] Includes malignancy, trauma, drug-induced, Asbestosis, Sarcoidosis, uremia

[15] Tuberculosis as a cause, however, may be increasing among immigrants from underdeveloped nations and in patients with HIV

[16] Especially tuberculosis, to prevent progression to constriction; antituberculous antibiotics may decrease risk of constriction from >80 % to <10 %

Guidelines

2015 ESC guidelines for the diagnosis and management of pericardial diseases
Eur Heart J. 2015;36:2921–64. http://eurheartj.oxfordjournals.org/content/36/42/2921.
American Society of Echocardiography Clinical Recommendations for multimodality cardiovascular imaging of patients with pericardial disease: endorsed by the Society for Cardiovascular

Magnetic Resonance and Society of Cardiovascular Computed Tomography

J Am Soc Echocardiogr. 2013;26:965–1012. http://www.sciencedirect.com/science/article/pii/S0894731713005336.

Patient Information

Images

http://www.nlm.nih.gov/medlineplus/ency/imagepages/18081.htm.
http://www.nlm.nih.gov/medlineplus/ency/imagepages/18151.htm.

Medlineplus

ENGLISH

http://www.nlm.nih.gov/medlineplus/ency/article/001103.htm.

ESPANOL0

http://www.nlm.nih.gov/medlineplus/spanish/ency/article/001103.htm.

Mayo Clinic

http://www.mayoclinic.org/diseases-conditions/pericarditis/basics/definition/con-20035562.

Cleveland Clinic

http://my.clevelandclinic.org/services/heart/disorders/pericarditis.

MERCK

http://www.merckmanuals.com/home/heart-and-blood-vessel-disorders/pericardial-disease/acute-pericarditis.
http://www.merckmanuals.com/home/heart-and-blood-vessel-disorders/pericardial-disease/chronic-pericarditis.

AHA

http://www.heart.org/HEARTORG/Conditions/More/Symptoms-and-Diagnosis-of-Pericarditis-UCM-444932-Article.jsp.

Texas Heart Institute

http://www.texasheart.org/HIC/Topics/Cond/pericard.cfm.

Cardiosmart

https://www.cardiosmart.org/Heart-Conditions/Pericarditis.

Professional Information

Review

Lancet. 2004;363:717–27. http://www.thelancet.com/journals/lancet/article/PIIS0140-6736(04)15648-1/abstract.

Antiinflammatory Therapy

Circulation.   2011;124:1830–7.   http://circ.ahajournals.org/content/124/17/1830.full?sid=3316db6d-3b55-4bc2-bc34-148c5f4022e1.

Imaging: Fungal Effusive Constrictive Pericarditis (Case Report)

Am J Med. 2013;126:25–6. http://www.sciencedirect.com/science/article/pii/S0002934312008017.

Pericardiectomy

Ann Thorac Surg. 2013;96:571–6. http://www.sciencedirect.com/science/article/pii/S0003497513008746.

Septal Bounce

Heart. 2013;99:1376. http://heart.bmj.com/content/99/18/1376.extract.

Syncope (Case Report)

Eur Heart J. 2013;34:1817. http://eurheartj.oxfordjournals.org/content/34/24/1817.

Thoracic Radiation

J Am Coll Cardiol. 2013;61:2319–28. http://content.onlinejacc.org/article.aspx?articleID=1679522.

Updates and More

https://clinicalguidecvd.com/conperi

Chapter 77
Peripheral Extremity Arteriovenous Fistula

ICD-10 Code

I77.0 ACQUIRED

Alternate Names/Abbreviation

A-V MALFORMATION
ARTERIOVENOUS MALFORMATION [2]

Description/Etiology

Abnormal vascular connection between peripheral artery
and peripheral vein
Acquired and congenital forms

Predisposing/Comorbid Conditions

ANEURYSM
DEEP VEIN THROMBOSIS
HEMODIALYSIS SHUNT
HEREDITARY TELANGIECTASIA [CONGEN
FORM]

V.E. Friedewald, *Clinical Guide to Cardiovascular Disease*, 1025
DOI 10.1007/978-1-4471-7293-2_77,
© Springer-Verlag London 2016

PERIPHERAL ARTERY DISEASE
SURGERY
TRAUMA [1]

Demography

All populations, with variances according to etiology

Pathophysiology

Local effects due to blood shunting from high press artery (s) to low pressure vein (s) with resulting distal ischemia and impingement on adjacent tissue (bone, nerve, skin)

Signs/Symptoms [3]

ARTERIAL PULSE PRESSURE – INCR
BLOOD PRESSURE, ARTERIAL – INCREASED/ ELEVATED [SYS]
BRANHAM SIGN – POS [4]
BREATHING – DIFF (DYSPNEA)
EXTREM, LOCAL – BRUIT
EXTREM, LOCAL – MASS, PULSATILE
EXTREM, LOCAL – THRILL
EXTREM, UNILAT – DEFORMED [6]
EXTREM, UNILAT – EDEMA
EXTREM, UNILAT – ISCHEMIA, DISTAL
EXTREM, UNILAT – PAIN
EXTREM, UNILAT – PARESTHESIA
EXTREM, UNILAT, COLOR – BLUE (CYANOSIS)
FATIGUE
HEART, LV, APEX – MURMUR, SYS [5]

HEART, RATE – RAPID (TACHYCARDIA)
HEART, S3 LV
HEART, S4 LV
SKIN, COLOR – RED (ERYTHEMA)
SKIN, COLOR, LOCAL – HYPERPIGMENTATION
SKIN, LOCAL – ULCER
SKIN, TEMP, LOCAL – INCR
VEINS, SUPERFICIAL – DIL

Differentiation

Arterial aneurysm
Atherosclerotic occlusive disease
DVT

Complications

Bacterial endarteritis
Bone destruction
Cellulitis
HF (high output)
Hemorrhage
Infection/gangrene
Limb deformity
Pulmonary embolism

Laboratory

NS

ECG

QRS – LVH PATTERN

Imaging

CARDIOMEGALY [7]
DUPLEX ULTRASOUND FOR DX
LV, CHAMBER, SIZE – INCR
LV, WALL MOTION – INCR/HYPERDYNAMIC [8]

Other Tests

Angiography

Treatment: Nonpharmacologic

NS

Treatment: Pharmacologic

NS

Treatment: Surgical/Invasive

Embolization
Surgical resection

Course

Variable according to site/size of fistula

Notes

[1] Penetrating injuries, eg, gunshot; most often to thigh
[2] Angiographic classification of A-V malformations

Group 1: predominantly arterial or arteriovenous
Group 2: predominantly capillaries and small vessels
Group 3: predominantly venous

[3] Highly variable according to fistula duration, location
[4] Temporary occlusion of proximal artery causes transient reflex slowing of HR
[5] Due to increased cardiac output
[6] Congenital; limb may be elongated
[7] More often present with involvement of liver and lungs
[8] Severe shunts

Guidelines

NS

Patient Information

Medlineplus

ENGLISH

http://www.nlm.nih.gov/medlineplus/arteriovenousmalformations. html.

ESPANOL

http://www.nlm.nih.gov/medlineplus/spanish/arteriovenousmalfor- mations.html.

Mayo Clinic

http://www.mayoclinic.org/diseases-conditions/arteriovenous- fistula/basics/definition/con-20034876.

AANS

http://www.aans.org/Patient%20Information/Conditions%20
and%20Treatments/Arteriovenous%20Malformations.aspx.

ASA

http://www.strokeassociation.org/STROKEORG/AboutStroke/
TypesofStroke/HemorrhagicBleeds/What-Is-an-Arteriovenous-
Malformation-AVM-UCM-310099-Article.jsp.

Johns Hopkins

http://www.hopkinsmedicine.org/neurology-neurosurgery/centers-
clinics/cerebrovascular/conditions/arteriovenous-malformations-
avm.html.

Stanford

https://stanfordhealthcare.org/medical-conditions/brain-and-nerves/
arteriovenous-malformation.html.

NORD

https://rarediseases.org/rare-diseases/arteriovenous-malformation/.

UCSF

http://www.ucsfhealth.org/conditions/arteriovenous-malformation/.

Professional Information

Anterior Tibial Artery (Case Report)

J Vasc Surg. 2007;45:1076–9. http://www.sciencedirect.com/science/article/pii/S0741521406022634.

Imaging

Am J Roentgen. 2009;193:1425–33. http://www.ajronline.org/doi/abs/10.2214/AJR.09.2631.

Mechanisms of High Output HF

Am J Kidney Dis. 2004;43:e17–22. http://www.sciencedirect.com/science/article/pii/S0272638604001519.

Trauma Series

Surgery. 1975;78:817–28. http://www.surgjournal.com/article/0039-6060(75)90209-3/abstract.

Updates and More

https://clinicalguidecvd.com/peavf

Chapter 78
Pheochromocytoma (Chromaffin Tumor/ Paraganglioma)

Management Keys

Suspect in patients with paroxysmal hypertension, tachycardia, diaphoresis, panic attacks

Avoid beta-blockade prior to alpha-blockade; may exacerbate alpha effect of catecholamine surge

Treat acute episodes with alpha-blocker and volume expansion, followed by beta-blocker/related agents after adequate alpha-blockade

Avoid any form of sympathetic stimulation [7]

Involve endocrinologist or hypertension expert in management decisions for patients with suspected pheo

ICD-10 Code

C74.10

V.E. Friedewald, *Clinical Guide to Cardiovascular Disease*,
DOI 10.1007/978-1-4471-7293-2_78,
© Springer-Verlag London 2016

Alternate Names/Abbreviation

Pheo
PCC
PPGL (Pheochromocytoma And Paraganglioma)
Chromaffin Paraganglioma
Chromaffin Tumor
Chromaffinoma
Medullary Paraganglioma

Description/Etiology

Catecholamine secreting tumor that may cause life-threatening hypertension episodes/cardiac arrhythmias
Pheochromocytoma: tumor arising from adrenomedullary chromaffin cells that:

Commonly produces one or more catecholamines: epinephrine, norepinephrine, and dopamine
Are rarely biochemically silent

Paraganglioma: tumor derived from extra-adrenal chromaffin cells of thoracic/abdominal/pelvic sympathetic paravertebral ganglia; also arise from parasympathetic ganglia located along glossopharyngeal and vagal nerves in neck and at base of skull, but these do not produce catecholamines
Occur in both sporadic (75 %) and hereditary forms (25 %)

Predisposing/Comorbid Conditions

CARDIOMYOPATHY–DILATED
CARDIOMYOPATHY–HYPERTROPHIC
CARDIOMYOPATHY–TAKOTSUBO
MULTIPLE ENDOCRINE NEOPLASIA TYPE 2 [5]
NEUROFIBROMATOSIS [5]
VON HIPPEL-LINDAU DISEASE [5]
WERMER SYNDROME [9]

Demography

All ages affected, with first manifestations, usually:

Hereditary form: childhood/young adult
Sporadic form: 40–50 years

Pathophysiology

85–90 % located in adrenal medulla; 98 % intraabdominal; less often in sympathetic ganglia (paraganglioma); rarely intracardiac

10 % malignant

Clinical manifestations caused by secretion of excess catecholamines and enhanced sympathetic activity and resultant effects (HTN, tachycardia)

Increased sensitivity to normal sympathetic activity; any sympathetic stimulation to patient with pheo can cause hypertension crisis [7]

Signs/Symptoms

ABDOMEN–PAIN
ARTERIAL PRESSURE–HIGHLY VARIABLE [22]
ARTERIAL PRESSURE, UPRIGHT–DECR (ORTHOSTATIC HYPOTENSION)
BLOOD PRESSURE, ARTERIAL–INCREASED/ELEVATED [1]
BOWEL MOVEMENTS–CONSTIPATION [15]
CHEST–PAIN
CHEST–PALPITATIONS [2]
EXTREM, HANDS–TREMOR
EYES, RETINA–RETINOPATHY, HTN
EYES, VISION–BLURRED
FEVER [16]
FLANK–PAIN

HEADACHE [2]
HEART, RATE–RAPID (TACHYCARDIA) [3]
HYPOTENSION   (BLOOD   PRESSURE–
   DECREASED/LOW) [11]
MENTATION–FEELING OF DOOM
MOOD–ANXIOUS
MUSCLES–WEAK
NAUSEA
SKIN, COLOR–PALE (PALLOR) [23]
SLEEP–DISTURBED (INSOMNIA)
SWEATING–INCR (DIAPHORESIS/
   HYPERHIDROSIS) [2] [4]
VOMITING (EMESIS)
WEIGHT–LOSS [6]

Differentiation

Acute Intermittent Porphyria
Anxiety disorders
Alcohol withdrawal
Autonomic seizure disorder
Carcinoid
Chemical abuse [8]
Cluster headaches
CAD
Hyperthyroidism
Illicit drug use (ie, cocaine)
Mastocytosis
Menopausal Syndrome
Migraine
MVP
Panic attacks
Paroxysmal tachyarrhythmias
Poems Syndrome
Polypharmacy
Other causes of Orthostatic Hypotension

Complications [12]

Acute abdomen [10]
Acute Pulmonary Edema
AMI
DCM
Dysrhythmias – Supraventricular
Dysrhytmias – Ventricular
Encephalopathy
HCM
HF
Hypercalcemia
Ischemic Colitis
Lactic Acidosis
Postop Hypotension [21]
Postop Hypoglycemia [21]
Renal Failure
Shock
Stroke
Tumor rupture

Laboratory

BLOOD, ARTERIAL PH–DECREASED (ACIDOSIS)
BLOOD, CALCIUM–INCR [14]
BLOOD, GLUCOSE–INCR (HYPERGLYCEMIA) [13]
BLOOD, HGB/HCT–INCR [24]
BLOOD, LACTATE–INCR
BLOOD, WBC–INCR (LEUKOCYTOSIS) [24]

ECG [17]

DYSRHYTHMIAS–ATRIAL (PACS/OTHERS)
DYSRHYTHMIAS–VENTRICULAR (PVCS/OTHERS)
P WAVE, DUR–INCR
PR INTERVAL–SHORT

QRS–LVH PATTERN
QRS, AXIS–L
QT/QTC INTERVAL–LONG
RATE–INCREASED (SINUS TACHYCARDIA) [3]
ST-T WAVE–ABN, NS [17]

Imaging

IVS, MOTION–PARADOX [18]
LV,   MYOCARD,   WALL   THICKNESS–INCR
  (HYPERTROPHY)
MV, LEAFLETS, MOTION, SYS–ANT [18]

Genomics

FP/TMEM127
RET (Multiple Endocrine Neoplasia type IIa OMIM 171400)
SDHB
SDHC
SDHA (Paragangliomas 5 OMIM 614165)
SDHAF2 (Paragangliomas 2 OMIM 601650)
SDHD (Paragangliomas 1 OMIM 168000)

Other Tests

Urine (24 h)

   Norepinephrine
   Epinephrine
   Normetanephrine
   Metanephrine [19]
   VMA

Blood

   Noradrenaline
   Adrenaline
   Normetanephrine
   Metanephrine [19]

Treatment: Nonpharmacologic

Avoid sympathetic stimulation [8]

Treatment: Pharmacologic [20]

Alpha - blockers
Beta-blockers
CCBs
Methyl paratyrosine

Treatment: Surgical/Invasive

Tumor excision [21]

Notes

[1] May be constantly (50 %) or part-time (95 %) elevated
[2] Triad of headache, palpitations, diaphoresis on background of hypertension is highly suggestive of pheo; may be precipitated by ingestion of tyramine-containing foods
[3] May be inappropriately increased for level of BP
[4] May be profound
[5] Hereditary forms
[6] Despite normal appetite
[7] Eg, pain, emotional upset, intubation, anesthesia, abdominal trauma
[8] Eg, cocaine, amphetamines, alcohol, MAO inhibitors
[9] Hyperparathyroidism, pituitary adenoma, pancreatic islet cell tumors
[10] Due to numerous causes, eg, tumor necrosis, bowel infarction/obstruction, cholecystitis
[11] Patients may present with hypotension rather than hypertension

[12] This is a partial list as pheos cause many diverse adverse effects on many organ systems

[13] Usually mild and occurs during acute hypertensive state

[14] Uncommon

[15] Due to catecholamine-induced intestinal hypomobility

[16] Due to hypercatabolic state; patients may present with fever of unknown origin

[17] Acute myocardial ischemic changes may also occur during hypertensive crisis

[18] During hypertensive crisis

[19] Metanephrines recommended for screening with >95 % sensitivity

[20] Significantly reduce perioperative mortality

[21] Preoperative and postoperative precautions, eg, pre-op alpha-blockers and post-op monitoring for hypotension and hypoglycemia; example: 2-week course of phenoxybenzamine or doxazosin with progressive dosage escalation until patient is orthostatic; CCBs also effective

[22] Variability is an added independent risk for CV morbidity and mortality

[23] Especially face/upper torso

[24] Due to hemoconcentration

Guidelines

Pheochromocytoma and paraganglioma: an endocrine society clinical practice guideline

J Clin Endocrinol Metab. 2014;99:1915–42. http://press.endocrine.org/doi/10.1210/jc.2014-1498?url_ver=Z39.88-2003&rfr_id=ori%3Arid%3Acrossref.org&rfr_dat=cr_pub%3Dpubmed&.

Patient Information

Mayo

http://www.mayoclinic.org/diseases-conditions/pheochromocytoma/basics/definition/con-20030435.

Medlineplus

https://www.nlm.nih.gov/medlineplus/ency/article/000340.htm.

MERCK

https://www.merckmanuals.com/home/hormonal-and-metabolic-disorders/adrenal-gland-disorders/pheochromocytoma.

UCSF

https://www.ucsfhealth.org/conditions/pheochromocytoma/?gclid=CjwKEAjwyPW5BRCC3JaM7qfW_FwSJACM3jz9WBX_04Tioz1S7CPeAqvm-W8E9UqeWKfdSkYBfKe E6xoC3aHw_wcB.

Professional Information

Review/Update

Circulation. 2014; 130: 1295–8. https://circ.ahajournals.org/content/130/15/1295.full.pdf+html.

Review

Lancet. 2005;366:665–75. http://www.thelancet.com/journals/lancet/article/PIIS0140-6736(05)67139-5/abstract.

Catecholamine Metabolism

Pharmacol Rev. 2004;56:331–49. http://pharmrev.aspetjournals.org/content/56/3/331.

Cardiovascular Manifestations

J Hypertens. 2011;29:2049–60. http://journals.lww.com/jhyperten-sion/pages/articleviewer.aspx?year=2011&issue=11000&article=00001&type=abstract.

Clinical Experience

Ann Surg. 1999;229:755–64. http://journals.lww.com/annalsofsur-gery/pages/articleviewer.aspx?year=1999&issue=06000&article=00001&type=abstract.

Genetics

Horm Metab Res. 2012;44:328–33. https://www.thieme-connect.de/DOI/DOI?10.1055/s-0031-1301302.

Metanephrines

J Clin Endocrinol Metab. 1998;83:2175–85. http://press.endocrine.org/doi/10.1210/jcem.83.6.4870.

Metastatic

Horm Metab Res. 2012;44:390–9. https://www.thieme-connect.de/DOI/DOI?10.1055/s-0031-1299707.

MRI

Eur Radiol. 2008;18:2885–92. http://link.springer.com/article/10.1007%2Fs00330-008-1073-z.

Overlooked Diagnosis

Am J Surg. 2000;179:212–5. http://www.americanjournalofsurgery.com/article/S0002-9610(00)00296-8/abstract.

Perioperative Morbidity/Mortality Factors

J Clin Endocrinol Metab. 2001;86:1480–6. http://press.endocrine.org/doi/abs/10.1210/jcem.86.4.7392.
Preoperative Apha Blockade In Normotensive Patients
J Hypertens. 2011;29:2429–32. http://journals.lww.com/jhypertension/pages/articleviewer.aspx?year=2011&issue=12000&article=00020&type=abstract.

Updates and More

https://clinicalguidecvd.com/pheo

Chapter 79
Primary Aldosteronism (Conn Syndrome)

ICD-10 Code

E26.09

Alternate Names/Abbreviation

CONN SYNDROME

Description/Etiology

Constellation of physiological abnormalities due to increased autonomous secretion of aldosterone, most often clinically manifest by Systemic Arterial Hypertension and its effects

Causes:

Adrenal Hyperplasia

Unilateral
Bilateral

Adrenal Carcinoma [2]
Adrenocortical Adenoma (Aldosteronoma) [1]
Ectopic tumors
Familial/hereditary [3]

V.E. Friedewald, *Clinical Guide to Cardiovascular Disease*, 1045
DOI 10.1007/978-1-4471-7293-2_79,
© Springer-Verlag London 2016

Predisposing/Comorbid Conditions

HYPERTENSION – SYSTEMIC ARTERIAL
HYPOKALEMIA [SYMPTOMATIC]

Demography

Rare in children
Usual initial presentation age 30–50 years

Pathophysiology

Increased levels of serum aldosterone with:

Decreased renin
Increased BP
Increased sodium resorption/K excretion

Direct effects on CV system beyond hypertension-related
pathology [12]

Signs/Symptoms

BLOOD PRESSURE, ARTERIAL – INCREASED/
ELEVATED [7]
EXTREM – PAIN, SHOOTING (PARESTHESIAS) [5]
MUSCLES – CRAMPS [4]
MUSCLES – SPASM (TETANY) [5]
MUSCLES – WEAK [5]
URINATION – INCR (POLYURIA) [4]
URINATION – NIGHTTIME (NOCTURIA) [4]

Differentiation

Other causes of increased BP, especially (idiopathic)
Systemic Arterial Hypertension
Other causes of Hypokalemia

Complications [6]

AF
AMI
LVH
STROKE
SCD

Laboratory

BLOOD, ALDOSTERONE: RENIN RATIO – INCR [13]
BLOOD, GLUCOSE – INCR (HYPERGLYCEMIA) [8]
BLOOD, POTASSIUM (K) – DECR (HYPOKALEMIA)
   [16]
BLOOD, RENIN – DECR
URINE, POTASSIUM – INCR

ECG [11]

AV COND – 1ST DEGREE BLOCK
AV COND – 2ND DEGREE BLOCK, MOBITZ I
   (WENCKEBACH)
AV CONDUCTION – AV DISSOCIATION, COMPLETE
DYSRHYTHMIAS – ATRIAL (PACS/OTHERS)
DYSRHYTHMIAS – VENTRICULAR (PVCS/
   OTHERS) [9]
QRS – LONG, NS
QRS – LVH PATTERN
ST SEGMENT – DEPR
T WAVE, AMP – DECR/FLAT
U WAVE – PROMINENT

Imaging

DEFINE RENAL ANATOMY
EXCLUDE ADRENAL CARCINOMA
LOCALIZE ADRENAL VEINS FOR SAMPLING

Genomics

ATP1A1 [SPORADIC FORM OF ADENOMA]
ATP2B3 [SPORADIC FORM OF ADENOMA]
CACNA1D [SPORADIC FORM OF ADENOMA]
CYP11B1 [FAMILIAL TYPE 1]
CYP11B2 [FAMILIAL TYPE 1]
KCNJ5 [FAMILIAL TYPE 111 OMNI 613677]

Other Tests

Adrenal vein sampling [14]
Confirmatory testing [15]

Captopril challenge
Fludrocortisone suppression
Oral sodium loading
Saline infusion

Treatment: Nonpharmacologic

NS

Treatment: Pharmacologic

Aldosterone antagonists
Eplerenone
Spironolactone

Treatment: Surgical/Invasive

Adrenalectomy

Notes

[1] Small, benign
[2] Rare; often secrete other adrenal hormones; locally invasive/metastatic
[3] Types:

> FH 1:   Glucocorticoid-Remedial Aldosteronism (autosomal dominant)
> FH 2:   Non-glucocorticoid   Remediable Aldosteronism (5x more common than FH 1)
> FH 3:   Paradox worsening of HTN with Dexamethasone

[4] Due to hypokalemia
[5] Severe hypokalemia
[6] All significantly more frequent than in patients with essential hypertension
[7] Usually moderate-severe increase; occasionally normal
[8] With glucose load
[9] PVCS, VT
[10] AF, PAT with block
[11] Changes mainly due to hypokalemia/LVH
[12] Fibrosis, inflammation, remodeling, LVH
[13] Preferred screening test for Primary Aldosteronism; positive test: >20 ng/dl per ng/m/h with aldosterone >10 mg/dl
[14] Differentiates between unilateral disease and bilateral disease before adrenalectomy as CT alone may be inadequate
[15] After adrenal vein sampling
[16] May be normal in absence of diet high in sodium or when not taking diuretics
[17] 1/3 of patients with this disease achieve normal BP after adrenalectomy; factors associated with normal BP post-surgery include negative family history of hypertension, <3 antihypertensive agents

Guidelines

Case detection, diagnosis, and treatment of patients with primary aldosteronism: an endocrine society clinical practice guideline
J Clin Endocrinol Metab. 2008;93:9. http://press.endocrine.org/doi/full/10.1210/jc.2008-0104.

2013 ESH/ESC guidelines for the management of arterial hypertension
Eur Heart J. 2014;34:2159–219. http://www.escardio.org/guidelines-surveys/esc-guidelines/Pages/arterial-hypertension.aspx.

The 2012 Canadian Hypertension Education Program recommendations for the management of hypertension: blood pressure measurement, diagnosis, assessment of risk, and therapy
Can J Cardiol. 2012;28:277. http://www.sciencedirect.com/science/article/pii/S0828282X12001365#.

NICE: hypertension in adults: diagnosis and management (2011)
http://www.nice.org.uk/guidance/cg127/chapter/1-recommendations#choosing-antihypertensive-drug-treatment-2.

JNC 7: seventh report of the Joint National Committee on prevention, detection, evaluation, and treatment of high blood pressure
Hypertension. 2003;42:1206–12. http://hyper.ahajournals.org/content/42/6/1206.long.

Patient Information

Images

http://www.nlm.nih.gov/medlineplus/ency/imagepages/1093.htm.
http://www.nlm.nih.gov/medlineplus/ency/imagepages/8719.htm.

Medlineplus

ENGLISH

http://www.nlm.nih.gov/medlineplus/ency/article/000330.htm.

ESPANOL
http://www.nlm.nih.gov/medlineplus/spanish/ency/article/000330.htm.

Mayo Clinic

http://www.mayoclinic.org/diseases-conditions/primary-aldosteronism/basics/definition/con-20030194.

Professional Information

Review

Postgrad Med J. 2001;77:639–44. http://pmj.bmj.com/content/77/912/639.full.

Review

N Engl J Med. 2007;356:601–10. http://www.nejm.org/doi/full/10.1056/NEJMcp065470.

Review

Trends in Endocrinology & Metabolism. 2013;24:421–30. http://www.sciencedirect.com/science/article/pii/S1043276013000829.

Review: Genetic/Autoimmune Triggers

Hypertension. 2015;66:248–53. http://hyper.ahajournals.org/content/66/2/248.full.

Adrenal Hypertension

Arch Intern Med. 1974;133:1001–6. http://archinte.jamanetwork.com/article.aspx?articleid=583081.

Adrenalectomy

Am J Hypertens. 2015;28:312–8. http://ajh.oxfordjournals.org/content/28/3/312.abstract.

Adrenalectomy

J Am Coll Surg. 2011;213:106–12. http://www.sciencedirect.com/science/article/pii/S1072751511001876.

Adrenocortical Function Assessment

N Engl J Med. 1971;285:735–9. http://www.nejm.org/doi/full/10.1056/NEJM197109232851306.

Aldosterone-Renin Ratio

JAMA.   2014;312:184–5.   http://jama.jamanetwork.com/article.aspx?articleid=1886170.

Atrial Fibrillation

Eur Heart J. 2011;33:2098–108. http://eurheartj.oxfordjournals.org/content/33/16/2098.

Complications

J Am Coll Cardiol. 2005;45:1243–8. http://content.onlinejacc.org/article.aspx?articleid=1136490.

Cardioavascular Outcomes Post-treatment

Arch Intern Med. 2008;168:80–5. http://archinte.jamanetwork.com/article.aspx?articleid=413688.

Differentiation of Unilateral from Bilateral Adrenal Disease

Ann Intern Med. 2009;151:329–37. http://annals.org/article.aspx?arti cleid=744703&resultClick=24.

Familial

Endocrinol Metab Clin North Am. 2011;40:343–68. http://www.sci encedirect.com/science/article/pii/S0889852911000089.

Medical Threapy

J Hypertension. 2001;19:353–61. http://www.ncbi.nlm.nih.gov/pubme d/?term=11288803%5Buid%5D.

Post-Surgery BP

Ann Intern Med. 2001;135:258–61. http://annals.org/article.aspx?arti cleid=714690&resultClick=24.

Updates and More

https://clinicalguidecvd.com/aldo

Chapter 80
Pulmonary Arteriovenous Fistula

ICD-10 Code

Q25.72 CONGENITAL
I28.0 ACQUIRED

Alternate Names/Abbreviation

Pulmonary AV Fistula
Pulmonary Arteriovenous Malformations (PAVMs)

Description/Etiology

Abnormal direct high flow, low-resistance fistulous connection between pulmonary artery and vein
Usually congenital with autosomal dominance, most often
Hereditary Hemorrhagic Telangiectasia, but may be
acquired [1]
R-L shunt can cause dyspnea but most patients are
asymptomatic
Paradoxical emboli can cause stroke and brain abscess and
acute events in other organs

V.E. Friedewald, *Clinical Guide to Cardiovascular Disease*, 1055
DOI 10.1007/978-1-4471-7293-2_80,
© Springer-Verlag London 2016

PAVMs in hepatopulmonary syndrome: due to failure of hepatic clearance of vasoactive substances (eg, prostaglandins); may be mechanism of PAVM development in children following shunt procedures for congenital cardiac anomalies

Predisposing/Comorbid Conditions

HEPATIC CIRRHOSIS
HEREDITARY HEMORRHAGIC TELANGIECTASIA
[CONGEN FORM] [1]
HISTORY: CHEST SURGERY
INFECTION [4]
PENETRATING CHEST TRAUMA
PULMONARY AMYLOIDOSIS
PULMONARY METASTASIS

Demography

F > M [2]
All ages [3]

Pathophysiology

Anatomic types:

Simple: single segmental artery feeding malformation; feeding segmental artery may have multiple subsegmental branches feeding malformation
Complex: multiple segmental feeding arteries

Lesions: >50 % lower lobes and right middle lobe; 70 % unilateral; may be multiple
Depending on shunt size, cardiac/circulatory hemodynamics may be normal (most cases); large shunts may cause significant arterial O_2 desaturation

Signs/Symptoms [1] [5] [9]

BOWEL MOVEMENTS, STOOL–BLOOD (HEMATOCHEZIA) OR BLACK (MELENA) [1]

BREATHING–DIFF (DYSPNEA)

BREATHING–DIFF, UPRIGHT (PLATYPNEA)

CHEST–PAIN

CHEST, LOCAL–MURMUR, SYS [6] [14]

CHEST, LOCAL–THRILL [6] [14]

CHEST. LOCAL–MURMUR, CONT [6] [14]

CONSCIOUSNESS–LOSS, SUDDEN (SYNCOPE) [1] [9]

COUGH

DIZZY/SPINNING (TRUE VERTIGO) [1] [9]

EXTREM, DIGITS–CLUBBED

EXTREM, DIGITS, NAILS–TELANGIECTASIA [1] [12]

EYES, RETINA–TELANGIECTASIA [1] [12]

HEADACHE [1]

HEART, P2, INTENSITY–INCR

LIPS–BLEEDING [1]

LIPS–TELANGIECTASIA [1] [12]

MENTATION–CONFUSION [1] [9]

MOUTH, MUCOUS MEMBRANES–TELANGIECTASIA [1] [12]

NOSE–BLOOD (EPISTAXIS) [1]

NOSE, MUCOSA–TELANGIECTASIA [1] [12]

SKIN–TELANGIECTASES [1] [10] [12]

SKIN, COLOR–BLUE (CYANOSIS)

SPUTUM–BLOOD (HEMOPTYSIS) [7]

SWALLOWING–DIFFICULT (DYSPHAGIA) [1] [9]

TONGUE–TELANGIECTASIA [1] [12]

URINE–BLOOD (HEMATURIA) [1]

VOMITING–BLOOD (HEMATEMESIS) [1]

Differentiation

Atelectasis
CNS Disease
Coagulation disorders
Lung benign and malignant masses
Primary Polycythemia Vera
Pulmonary embolism
Pulmonary Hypertension
Pulmonary infarction

Complications

Cerebral abscess [8] [9]
Hemothorax
Massive hemoptysis [7]
Meningitis [8] [9]
PAH [8]
Seizures [8] [9]
Stroke [8] [9]

Laboratory

BLOOD, ART, PO2–DECR/WORSENS IN UPRIGHT
    POSITION (ORTHODEOXIA)
BLOOD, ARTERIAL PCO2–DECREASED [11]
BLOOD, ARTERIAL PO2–DECREASED (HYPOXIA)
    [11] [15]
BLOOD, HGB/HCT–INCR [11]
BLOOD, RBC COUNT–INCR [11]
BLOOD, RETICULOCYTE COUNT–INCR [11]

ECG

N/NS ABN

Imaging

CARDIOMEGALY   [LARGE   FISTULAE;
OTHERWISE N SIZE]
CONTRAST ECHO/CT
LUNG DENSITY(S) [CHEST X-RAY] [13]

Other Tests

Pulmonary arteriography

Treatment: Nonpharmacologic

NS

Treatment: Pharmacologic

NS

Treatment: Surgical/Invasive

Embolization [16]
Surgical resection [16]

Course

Highly variable due to associated malformations

Notes

[1] Hereditary Hemorrhagic Telangiectasia (Rendu-Osler-Weber syndrome); >80 % of cases; many clinical features due to CNS involvement, which may be caused by A-V fistulae in brain, paradoxical embolism, or severe polycythemia; other organs (kidneys, GI tract) may also be involved with A-V fistulae causing the listed signs and symptoms

[2] Ratio varies among reports, from about 1:1 up to 2:1 female predominance

[3] Defect present at birth expands with age and usually clinically first manifest age 20–40 years

[4] Including Schistosomiasis, Actinomycosis

[5] Includes features of Hereditary Hemorrhagic Telangiectasia

[6] Over A-V malformation sites, which are usually peripheral in lower lobes and right middle lobe; louder during systole and with deep inspiration

[7] Usually due to fistula rupture; rarely due to endobronchial telangiectasia

[8] May be more common in acquired form

[9] CNS signs and symptoms are presenting manifestations in many patients

[10] Skin lesions are fragile and bleed easily, especially with sunlight exposure

[11] Blood indices correct after definitive treatment of pulmonary fistulae

[12] Small clusters of ruby red lesions

[13] Oval, round, homogeneous lesions; single or multiple; unilateral or bilateral; most often lower lobes and right middle lobe; usually peripheral

[14] May disappear during pregnancy due to diaphragm elevation

[15] Does not correct with pure O_2 inhalation

[16] Historically treated with surgical resection but endovascular embolization now treatment standard, using coils and detachable occlusion balloons; >95 % success rate with embolization but recanalization can occur

Guidelines

NS

Patient Information

Medlineplus

ENGLISH

http://www.nlm.nih.gov/medlineplus/ency/article/001090.htm.

ESPANOL

http://www.nlm.nih.gov/medlineplus/spanish/ency/article/001090.htm.

Mayo Clinic

http://www.mayoclinic.org/diseases-conditions/arteriovenous-fistula/basics/symptoms/con-20034876.

Professional Information

First Description: Churton

Br Med J. 1897;1:1223.

Review

Semin Intervent Radiol. 2011;28:24–31. http://www.ncbi.nlm.nih.gov/pmc/articles/PMC3140246/.

Review

Postgrad Med J. 2002;78:191–97. http://pmj.bmj.com/content/78/918/191.

Review

Am J Resp Crit Care Med. 1998;158:643–61. http://www.atsjournals. org/doi/full/10.1164/ajrccm.158.2.9711041#.Vzs_HvMUV1s.

Review: Hereditary Hemorrhagic Telangiectasia

N Engl J Med. 1995;333:918–24. http://www.nejm.org/doi/ full/10.1056/NEJM199510053331407.

Case Report: Hereditary Complex Av Fistula

BMJ Case Reports. 2014. doi:10.1136/bcr-2014-205939. http://caser-eports.bmj.com/content/2014/bcr-2014-205939.abstract.

Case Series

Chest. 1963;43:449–55. http://journal.publications.chestnet.org/arti-cle.aspx?articleid=1055734.

Cavo-Pulmonary Shunt (Children)

Circulation. 1995;92:309–14. http://circ.ahajournals.org/con-tent/92/9/309.full?sid=28b1b275-ef73-45d4-b159-76c7c813e4a8.

Images

N Engl J Med. 2009;360:1769. http://www.nejm.org/doi/full/10.1056/ NEJMicm0803889.

Neurological Manifestations

Circulation. 1970;41:123–28. http://circ.ahajournals.org/content/41/1/123. abstract?sid=6831653d-5534-4f24-bd0b-bf8bb3b92815.

Pulmonary Amyloidosis

Am J Respir Crit Care Med. 2014;190:e14–5. http://www.ncbi.nlm. nih.gov/pubmed/25127313.

Pulmonary Amyloidosis

Chest. 1989;96:1435–6. http://journal.publications.chestnet.org/article.aspx?articleid=1062488&resultClick=3.

Surgery: Children

J Pediatr Surg. 2008;43:1365–367. http://www.ncbi.nlm.nih.gov/pubmed/18639698.

Transcatheter Coil Closure

J Interv Cardiol. 2004;17:23–6. http://onlinelibrary.wiley.com/doi/10.1111/j.1540-8183.2004.00287.x/abstract;jsessionid=A0FD3 515BFFD722686A689300670D2BF.f01t03.

Transcatheter Occlusion

Heart. 2011;97:A1550. doi:10.1136/heartjnl-2011-300867.451. http://heart.bmj.com/content/97/Suppl_3/A155.1.abstract?sid=12 a8325b-4b29-430a-8c29-266d7ac8aa45.

Updates and More

https://clinicalguidecvd.com/pavf

Chapter 81
Pulmonary Hypertension

ICD-10 Code

I27.0

Alternate Names/Abbreviation

CTPH (CHRONIC THROMBOEMBOLIC PULMONARY HYPERTENSION)
PH (PULMONARY HYPERTENSION)
PAH (PULMONARY ARTERIAL HYPERTENSION)

Description/Etiology

- Pulmonary Hypertension: pulmonary arterial pressure ≥ 25 mmHg (mean) at rest measured by right heart catheterization [31]
- Pulmonary Arterial Hypertension: PH characterized hemodynamically by presence of pre-capillary PH, defined by a pulmonary artery wedge pressure ≤15 mmHg and PVR >3 Wood units (WU) in absence of other causes of pre-capillary PH such as PH due to lung diseases, CTEPH, or other rare diseases

V.E. Friedewald, *Clinical Guide to Cardiovascular Disease*,
DOI 10.1007/978-1-4471-7293-2_81,
© Springer-Verlag London 2016

Symptoms: non-specific and mainly related to progressive RV dysfunction

2013 Updated Classification [31]

Group 1: Pulmonary Arterial Hypertension

1.1 Idiopathic PAH
1.2 Hereditable PAH

1.2.1 BMPR2
1.2.2 Alk-1, Eng, Smad9, Cav1, Kcnk3
1.2.3 Unknown

1.3 Drug and toxin induced [32]
1.4 Associated with:

1.4.1 Connective tissue disease
1.4.2 HIV infection
1.4.3 Portal Hypertension
1.4.4 Congenital heart disease
1.4.5 Schistosomiasis

1' Pulmonary Veno-Occlusive Disease and/or Pulmonary Capillary Hemangiomatosis
1' Persistent Pulmonary Hypertension of the Newborn (PPHN)

Group 2: Pulmonary Hypertension due to left heart disease

2.1 Left ventricular systolic dysfunction
2.2 Left ventricular diastolic dysfunction
2.3 Valvular disease
2.4 Congenital/acquired left heart inflow/outflow tract obstruction and congenital cardiomyopathies

Group 3: Pulmonary Hypertension due to lung disease and/or hypoxia

3.1 Chronic Obstructive Pulmonary Disease

3.2 Interstitial Lung Disease

3.3 Other pulmonary diseases with mixed restrictive and obstructive pattern

3.4 Sleep-disordered breathing

3.5 Alveolar hypoventilation disorders

3.6 Chronic exposure to high altitude

3.7 Developmental lung disease

Group 4: Chronic Thromboembolic Pulmonary Hypertension (CTEPH)

Group 5: Pulmonary Hypertension with unclear multifactorial mechanisms [29]

5.1 Hematologic disorders:

Chronic hemolytic anemia
Myeloproliferative disorders
Splenectomy

5.2 Systemic disorders:

Sarcoidosis
Pulmonary Histiocytosis
Lymphangiomyomatosis

5.3 Metabolic disorders:

Glycogen Storage Disease
Gaucher Disease
Thyroid Disorders (including Hyperthyroidism, Graves Disease)

5.4 Others:

Tumoral obstruction
Fibrosing Mediastinitis
Chronic renal failure
Segmental PH

Predisposing/Comorbid Conditions

[SEE DISEASES LISTED IN 2013 UPDATED CLASSIFICATION]

Demography

Highly variable according to etiology

Pathophysiology

PH: abnormal cell signaling pathways within alveolar-pulmonary arteriole-right ventricular axis causes increased PVR, which leads to RV dysfunction

PAH: among the many etiologies and varying complex pathogeneses, common mechanisms that trigger abnormal vascular remodeling include:

Aberrant vascular wall cell proliferation
Bone morphogenetic protein receptor type 2 gene mutations
Endothelial dysfunction
Inflammation

Signs/Symptoms [4]

ABDOMEN – DISTENSION [15]
ABDOMEN – FLUID (ASCITES) [15]
APPETITE, SATIETY – EARLY [15]
ARTERIAL PULSE PRESSURE – DECR
ARTERIAL PULSE, AMP – DECR/ABS
BREATHING – DIFF (DYSPNEA)
BREATHING – DIFF, NOCTURNAL (DYSPNEA, NOCT)
BREATHING – DIFF, RECLINING FLAT (ORTHOPNEA)
CHEST – PAIN

CHEST – PAIN, EFFORT (ANGINA PECTORIS) [16]
CONSCIOUSNESS – LOSS, SUDDEN (SYNCOPE)
EXTREM, LOWER, BILAT – EDEMA
FATIGUE
HEART, LSB, LOWER – IMP, SYS
HEART, LSB, LOWER – MURMUR, SYS [6]
HEART, LSB, UPPER – CLICK, SYS
HEART, LSB, UPPER – MURMUR, DIAS [7]
HEART, P2 – PALPABLE
HEART, P2, INTENSITY – INCR
HEART, RATE – RAPID (TACHYCARDIA)
HEART, RSB, LOWER – HEAVE
HEART, S2, SPLIT – FIXED [3]
HEART, S2, SPLIT – REVERSED (PARADOXICAL) [3]
HEART, S2, SPLIT – WIDE
HEART, S3 RV [UNCOMMON]
HEART, S4 RV
HYPOTENSION (BLOOD PRESSURE – DECREASED/
   LOW)
LIVER – ENLARGED (HEPATOMEGALY)
LIVER – PULSATION, PRESYS
MENTATION – WEAKNESS (MALAISE)
NECK, JVP, A WAVE – INCR/LARGE (CANNON
   WAVE)
NECK, JVP, C WAVE – INCR/LARGE
NECK, JVP, V WAVE – INCR/LARGE
NECK, SENSATION – PULSATIONS
SKIN, COLOR – BLUE (CYANOSIS)
SKIN, COLOR, EFFORT – BLUE (CYANOSIS)
SKIN, TEMP, HANDS/FEET – DECR
SPUTUM – BLOOD (HEMOPTYSIS) [17]
SWALLOWING – DIFFICULT (DYSPHAGIA)
VOICE – HOARSE [33]

Differentiation

Chronic Obstructive Pulmonary Disease
Myxoma – Right Ventricle
Other causes of right heart failure

Other causes of cyanosis

Complications [4]

Pneumonia
Pulmonary artery dissection/rupture with Cardiac Tamponade
RV failure
Sudden Death

Laboratory [4] [37]

BLOOD, NT-PROBNP – INCR [18]
BLOOD, PLATELETS – DECR (THROMBO CYTOPENIA) [21]
BLOOD, PLATELETS – INCR (THROMBOCYTOSIS) [21]
BLOOD, ST2 – INCR [PAH]
BLOOD, TROPONIN – INCR [SEVERE]
BLOOD, URIC ACID – INCR [20]

ECG [4] [34] [37]

P WAVE – TALL/PEAKED
QRS – RVH PATTERN [26]
QRS, AXIS – R
T WAVE – INVER, ABN [25]

Imaging [4] [8] [35] [37]

LA, CHAMBER, SIZE – INCR [27]
RA, CHAMBER, SIZE – INCR
PA, BRANCHES, SIZE – DECR
PA, MAIN, PRESS – INCR [12]

PA, MAIN, SIZE – INCR
PERICARD – FLUID [13]
PV, FLOW – REGURG
RV, CHAMBER, SIZE – INCR

Genomics [37]

ALK-1
CAV1
EF2AK4
ENDOGIN
KCNK3
SMAD9
BMPR2 [>80 % OF FAMILIAL CASES of PAH]

Other Tests [8] [37]

Pulse oximetry [19]
Ventilation/perfusion scan for detecting chronic thrombo-
    embolic PH
Right heart catheterization/pulmonary angiography: con-
    firm diagnosis; assess hemodynamic severity and vaso-
    reactivity of pulmonary circulation [28]
Coronary angiography: assess for comorbid CAD
6 min walk test [36]

Treatment: Nonpharmacologic [4] [37]

Avoid pregnancy
Exercise rehabilitation
Low sodium diet for volume overload with RV failure
O_2
Smoking cessation

Treatment: Pharmacologic [4] [37]

Antiarrhythmics [10]
Anticoagulants
CCBs
Diuretics
Pulmonary artery vasodilators

Treatment: Surgical/Invasive [4] [37]

Atrial septostomy [11]
Lung transplant
Pulmonary artery denervation (investigational for PAH)

Prevention

Tobacco avoidance/cessation
Vaccination:

Pneumococcal
Viral

Course

Variable according to category

Notes

[1] Initial symptoms (mainly dyspnea with effort) usually do
not appear until disease is advanced
[2] Higher incidence in males reported in Japan
[3] With severe RV dysfunction
[4] Not including specific manifestations/treatment for associated conditions (eg, Sarcoidosis, Heart Failure, Thyroid

disease, Pulmonary Thromboembolic disease), which must be individualized

[5] Occur mainly in advanced cases

[6] Pansystolic; due to TR

[7] Pulmonary regurgitation; due to dilated main PA, usually due to long-standing increased PA press

[8] Normal CXR does not rule out PH; may assist in differential diagnosis of PH by showing features of lung or left heart disease; may help distinguish between arterial PH (increased artery-vein ratio) and venous PH (decreased artery-vein ratio)

[9] Autoimmune thyroid disease common in group 5

[10] Maintenance of sinus rhythm if possible

[11] Palliative/bridging

[12] Doppler echo estimate of PA systolic pressure correlates well with direct measure

[13] Presence of pericardial fluid correlates with poorer survival

[14] Heart Failure: most common cause of PH; occurs in >80 % of HF patients

[15] Due to abdominal venous congestion

[16] Believed due to decreased right coronary flow to hypertrophied RV causing myocardial ischemia

[17] Hemoptysis uncommon; presence should prompt search for other causes, such as Pulmonary Embolism, Mitral Stenosis

[18] May be sign of impending/overt RV failure, suggesting need for more aggressive treatment

[19] In PAH: normal/low; marked desaturation with exercise suggests possible cardiac shunt

[20] Clubbing uncommon except in Eisenmenger and hypoxic lung disease

[21] Increased platelets: risk factor for PH

[22] Decreased platelets: suggests possible autoimmune disease, hypersplenism, cirrhosis

[23] Increased BNP common in PH: degree correlates with RVH severity/poorer outcomes

[24] Mechanism of increased uric acid uncertain

[25] Anterior leads, may extend to inferior leads

[26] Insensitive but highly specific for RVH secondary to PH

[27] LA dilatation suggests pulmonary venous hypertension rather than PAH

[28] Agents for testing pulmonary vasoreactivity include:

Adenosine
Epoprostenol
Iloprost
Nitric oxide

[29] Also: Hereditary Hemorrhagic Telangiectasia

[30] In PAH and experimental PH, KCNK3 expression/activity strongly reduced in pulmonary artery smooth muscle cells and endothelial cells

[31] Normal mean PA resting pressure: 14 ± 3 mmHg with upper limit of normal about 20 mmHg; clinical significance of PA resting pressure of 21–24 mmHg uncertain but patients with pressures in this range should be followed closely

[31] Clinical classification of Pulmonary Hypertension derived from J Am Coll Cardiol 2004;43 (Suppl 1): S5–S12

[32] Drug/toxin causes of PAH:

Definite

Aminorex
Fenfluramine
Dexfenfluramine
Toxic rapeseed oil
Benfluorex
Selective serotonin reuptake inhibitors

Likely

Amphetamines
Dasatinib
L-tryptophan
Methamphetamines

Possible

    Cocaine
    Phenylpropanolamine
    St John's Wort
    Amphetamine-like drugs
    Interferon α and β
    Some chemotherapeutic agents such as alkylating agents

       Mytomycine C
       Cyclophosphamide

[33] Due to PA dilatation compressing left recurrent laryngeal nerve

[34] Normal ECG does not rule out PH

[35] ESC/ERS Guideline: Echocardiography should always be performed when PH is suspected and may be used to infer a diagnosis of PH in patients in whom multiple different echocardiographic measurements are consistent with this diagnosis

[36] ESC/ERS Guideline: 6 min walk test is most widely used exercise test in PH centers; test is easy to perform, inexpensive and familiar to patients and centers; as with all PH assessments, test results must always be interpreted in clinical context; distance is influenced by several factors, including sex, age, height, weight, comorbidities, need for O_2, learning curve, motivation

[37] Listed diagnostics and treatments are generic; management of patients with PH/PAH should be conducted by experts in these conditions whenever possible, with careful attention/adherence to most current guidelines

Guidelines

2015 ESC/ERS guidelines for the diagnosis and treatment of pulmonary hypertension

Eur Heart J. 2016;37:67–119. http://eurheartj.oxfordjournals.org/content/37/1/67.

Pharmacologic therapy for pulmonary arterial hypertension in adults: CHEST guideline and expert panel report
Chest 2014;146:449–75. http://journal.publications.chestnet.org/article.aspx?articleid=1881654.

Executive summary: expert consensus statement on the diagnosis and treatment of paediatric pulmonary hypertension. The European Paediatric Pulmonary Vascular Disease Network, endorsed by ISHLT and DGPK
Heart. 2016;102:ii86–100. doi:10.1136/heartjnl-2015-309132. http://heart.bmj.com/content/102/Suppl-2/ii86?etoc.

Patient Information

Genetics Home Reference

http://ghr.nlm.nih.gov/condition/pulmonary-arterial-hypertension.

Medlineplus

ENGLISH
http://www.nlm.nih.gov/medlineplus/pulmonaryhypertension.html

ESPANOL
http://www.nlm.nih.gov/medlineplus/spanish/pulmonaryhypertension.html.

Cleveland Clinic

http://my.clevelandclinic.org/lungs-breathing-allergy/departments-centers/pulmonary-hypertension.aspx.

Mayo Clinic

http://www.mayoclinic.org/diseases-conditions/pulmonary-hypertension/basics/definition/con-20030959.

NHLBI

http://www.nhlbi.nih.gov/health/health-topics/topics/pah.

AHA

http://www.heart.org/HEARTORG/Conditions/HighBloodPressure/
AboutHighBloodPressure/What-is-Pulmonary-Hypertension-
UCM-301792-Article.jsp.

ALA

http://www.lung.org/lung-disease/primary-pulmonary-hypertension
/?referrer=https://www.google.com/"style='text-decoration
:none;"target="_blank">https://www.google.com/"style="text-
decoration:none;"target="_blank">http://www.lung.org/lung-
disease/primary-pulmonary-hypertension/?referrer=https://
www.google.com/.

MERCK

http://www.merckmanuals.com/home/lung-and-airway-disorders/
pulmonary-hypertension/pulmonary-hypertension.

CDC-Fact Sheet

http://www.cdc.gov/dhdsp/data-statistics/fact-sheets/fs-pulmonary-
hypertension.htm.

Professional Information

Review: Chronic Thromboembolic Pulmonary Hyertension

J Am Coll Cardiol. 2013;62(25-S):doi:10.1016/j.jacc.2013.10.024.
http://content.onlinejacc.org/article.aspx?articleID=1790594.

Review: Clinical Syndrome

Circulation Res. 2014;115:115–30. http://circres.ahajournals.org/content/115/1/115.full?sid=e47ded1f-302b-4d47-bab4-9476a19b6193.

Review: Current Management

Circulation Res. 2014;115:131–47. http://circres.ahajournals.org/content/115/1/131.full?sid=e47ded1f-302b-4d47-bab4-9476a19b6193.

Review: Genetics

Circulation Res. 2014;115:189–202. http://circres.ahajournals.org/content/115/1/189.full?sid=e47ded1f-302b-4d47-bab4-9476a19b6193.

Review: Metabolic Theory

Circulation Res. 2014;115:148–64. http://circres.ahajournals.org/content/115/1/148.full?sid=e47ded1f-302b-4d47-bab4-9476a19b6193.

Review: Molecular Basis of PAH

Circulation. 2015;131:1691–702. http://circ.ahajournals.org/content/131/19/1691.full.

Review: Pathogenesis: Inflammation/Immunity

Circulation Res. 2014;115:165–75. http://circres.ahajournals.org/content/115/1/165.full?sid=e47ded1f-302b-4d47-bab4-9476a19b6193.

Review: Pathophysiology

Handb Exp Pharmacol. 2013;218:231. http://www.ncbi.nlm.nih.gov/pubmed/24092335.

Review: Pediatric Pulmonary Hypertension

J Am Coll Cardiol. 2013;62(25-S):doi:10.1016/j.jacc.2013.10.028. http://content.onlinejacc.org/article.aspx?articleID=1790598.

Review: Thromboembolic PAH

Circulation.   2014;130:508–18.   http://circ.ahajournals.org/content/130/6/508.full.

Updated Classification

J Am Coll Cardiol. 2013;62:D34–41. http://content.onlinejacc.org/article.aspx?articleid=1790599&resultClick=3.

Beta-Thalassemia: Prevalence/Risk Factors

Circulation.   2014;129:338–45.   http://circ.ahajournals.org/content/129/3/338.full.

Chest Pain

Am J Med. 2014;127:605–07. http://www.sciencedirect.com/science/article/pii/S0002934314002782.

Chronic Thromboembolic Pulmonary Hypertension: Long-Term Outcomes

Circulation.   2016;133:859–71.   http://circ.ahajournals.org/content/133/9/859.full.

Clinical Diagnosis

Circulation. 2014;130:1820–30. http://circ.ahajournals.org/content/130/20/1820.full.

Congenital Heart Disease

Eur Heart J. 2014;35:691–700. http://eurheartj.oxfordjournals.org/content/35/11/691.

Congenital Heart Disease

Circulation. 2015;131:200–10. http://circ.ahajournals.org/content/131/2/200.extract?etoc.

CCR5: Treatment Target

Circulation. 2014;130:880–91. http://circ.ahajournals.org/content/130/11/880.full

Fibrosing Mediastinitis

Medicine. 2015;94:e1800. http://journals.lww.com/md-journal/Fulltext/2015/11030/Pulmonary-Hypertension-Complicating-Fibrosing.18.aspx.

Genomics: BMPR2

Circulation: Cardiovascular Genetics. 2012;5:511–18. http://circgenetics.ahajournals.org/content/5/5/511.abstract?sid=7011c5d8-884a-4297-afa7-b94138d6b7b6.

Genomics: KCNK3

Circulation. 2016;133:1371–85. http://circ.ahajournals.org/content/133/14/1371.abstract.

Heart Failure

Eur Heart J. 2016;37:942–54. http://eurheartj.oxfordjournals.org/content/37/12/942.full?etoc.

Hereditary Hemorrhagic Telangeictasia

Chest. 2016;149:362–71. http://journal.publications.chestnet.org/article.aspx?articleID=2411213.

High Altitude Pulmonary Vascular Disease

Circulation. 2015;131:582–90. http://circ.ahajournals.org/content/131/6/582.extract?etoc.

Imaging: Noninvasive

Circulation. 2015;131:899–913. http://circ.ahajournals.org/content/131/10/899.extract?etoc.

NT-PROBNP

Eur Respir J. 2005;25:509–13. http://erj.ersjournals.com/content/25/3/509.full.

Pathophysiology: Parenchymal Lung Disease

Am J Med. 2016;129;366–71. http://www.sciencedirect.com/science/article/pii/S0002934315300255.

Pulmonary Arterial HTN: HIV

Circulation. 2015;131:1361–70. http://circ.ahajournals.org/content/s131/15/1361.extract?etoc.

Pulmonary Arterial HTN: LV Cardiomyocyte Contractile Dysfunction

J Am Coll Cardiol. 2014;64:28–37. http://content.onlinejacc.org/article.aspx?articleID=1886831.

Pulmonary Arterial HTN: RV Diastolic Impairment

Circulation. 2013;128:2016–25. http://circ.ahajournals.org/content/128/18/2016.full.

Pulmonary Arterial HTN: ST2

Int J Cardiol. 2013;168:1545–7. http://www.sciencedirect.com/science/article/pii/S0167527312016609.

Pulmonary Arterial HTN: Survival in Children

J Am Coll Cardiol. 2014;63:2159–69. http://content.onlinejacc.org/article.aspx?articleID=1851431.

Predicting Survival

Circulation. 2010;122:164–72. http://circ.ahajournals.org/content/122/2/164.full.

Right Coronary Blood Flow Decrease

Eur Heart J. 2008;29:120–27. http://eurheartj.oxfordjournals.org/content/29/1/120.full.

Pulmonary Artery Denervation

J Am Coll Cardiol. 2013;62:1092–100. http://content.onlinejacc.org/article.aspx?articleID=1710960.

Right Ventricle

Circulation Research. 2014;115:176–88. http://circres.ahajournals.org/content/115/1/176.full?sid=e47ded1f-302b-4d47-bab4-9476a19b6193.

Scleroderma

Circulation.   2013;127:141–42.   http://circ.ahajournals.org/content/127/1/141.full.

Uric Acid

Chest. 2000;117:19–24. http://journal.publications.chestnet.org/article.aspx?articleID=1078557.

Updates and More

https://clinicalguidecvd.com/ph

Chapter 82
Pulmonary Stenosis: Supravalvular

ICD-10 Code

Q25.6

Alternate Names/Abbreviation

PULMONARY ARTERY STENOSIS

Description/Etiology

Narrowing (single/combination) of:

Main pulmonary trunk
Pulmonary artery bifurcation
Primary/intrapulmonary artery branches

Variant: hourglass pattern, similar to SupraAS; technically a form of valvular PS as it is due to stenosis at valve commissural ridge

All forms can cause RVOT obstruction and subsequent RV dysfunction/RHF

V.E. Friedewald, *Clinical Guide to Cardiovascular Disease*,
DOI 10.1007/978-1-4471-7293-2_82,
© Springer-Verlag London 2016

Lesions:

> Range from single focal to diffuse hypoplastic to overt occlusion
> May be secondary to previous pulmonary artery band placement
> Arteries distal to patent stenotic lesions often dilated (poststenotic dilation)

Membranous forms of obstruction both above/below pulmonary valve may occur

Comorbid Conditions

AORTIC STENOSIS – SUPRAVALVULAR
ALAGILLE SYNDROME [10]
BEHCET DISEASE
CONGENITAL RUBELLA
EHLERS-DANLOS SYNDROME
KEUTEL SYNDROME [11]
SCARRING AT SITE OF PREVIOUS PA BAND OR AORTICOPULMONARY SHUNT
SILVER SYNDROME [12]
SYSTEMIC VASCULITIS
TAKAYASU ARTERITIS
WILLIAMS SYNDROME

Demography

GENDER EQUAL

Pathophysiology

Lesions: fibrous intimal proliferation with varying degrees of medial hyperplasia and elastic fibers loss
Hemodynamics: hypertension in proximal PA with secondary pulmonary regurgitation leading to:

RV pressure/volume overload
RV dilatation
TR
RV dysfunction/RH failure

Progresses to loss of distal lung parenchyma by adulthood

Peripheral PA stenoses often occur in multiple PA tertiary branches and are progressive

Signs/Symptoms

BREATHING – DIFF (DYSPNEA)
CHEST – PAIN [3]
CHEST, LAT – BRUIT [4]
CHEST, LAT – MURMUR, CONT [4]
CHEST, POST – BRUIT [4]
CHEST, POST – MURMUR, CONT [4]
HEART, RSB, UPPER – MURMUR, DIAS [7]
HEART, S4 RV
NECK, JVP, A WAVE – INCR/LARGE (CANNON WAVE)
NECK, VENOUS PULSE – AWARE [5]
SKIN, COLOR – BLUE (CYANOSIS) [6]
SPUTUM – BLOOD (HEMOPTYSIS) [1]

Differentiation

Myxoma – Right Ventricle
Pulmonary Hypertension [8]
Pulmonary Stenosis – Valvular

Complications

Infective Endocarditis [2]
HF
RV infarction

Laboratory

NS

ECG

QRS – RVH PATTERN
QRS, AXIS – R

Imaging

[MRI/CT SUPERIOR TO ECHO IN IDENTIFYING LESIONS]
PA, MAIN, SIZE – INCR [POSTSTENOTIC DILATATION]
PV, FLOW – REGURG
RV, PRESS, SYS – INCR
RV, WALL THICKNESS – INCR

Genomics

BSCL2
ELASTIN
JAG1
MGP

Other Tests

Cardiac catheterization with contrast angiography: definitive for lesions and severity of PAH [8].

Treatment: Nonpharmacologic

NS

Treatment: Pharmacologic

NS

Treatment: Surgical/Invasive [13]

Balloon angioplasty
Stenting
Surgical patch enlargement
Lung transplant [9]

Notes

[1] Due to rupture of thin-walled aneurysm in areas of post-stenotic dilatation

[2] At sites of jet lesions distal to obstruction

[3] Uncommon; may be due to RV myocardial ischemia or PA thrombosis

[4] Increases with inspiration

[5] Correlates with cannon A waves

[6] Increased RA pressure with R-L interatrial shunt

[7] Pulmonary regurgitation

[8] Many adult patients are referred with incorrect diagnosis of Primary Pulmonary Hypertension

[9] Severe peripheral pulmonary stenosis with large loss of lung parenchyma

[10] Dominant inherited multisystem disease involving pulmonary arteries, liver, vertebrae (butterfly), eye, facial dysmorphism

[11] Rare autosomal dominate recessive disease comprising:

Brachytelephalangism
Cartilage calcification
Characteristic physiognomy
Hearing loss
Mental retardation (mild)
Peripheral pulmonary stenosis

[12] Hereditary spastic paraplegia with progressive muscle stiffness

[13] ACC/AHA 2008 Guidelines:

"Percutaneous interventional therapy is recommended as the treatment of choice in the management of appropriate focal branch and/or peripheral pulmonary artery stenosis with greater than 50 % diameter narrowing, an elevated RV systolic pressure greater than 50 mmHg, and/or symptoms

In patients with the above indications for intervention, surgeons with training and expertise in CHD should perform operations for management of branch pulmonary artery stenosis not anatomically amenable to percutaneous interventional therapy"

Guidelines

ACC/AHA 2008 guidelines for the management of adults with congenital heart disease

J Am Coll Cardiol. 2008;52:e143–263. http://content.onlinejacc.org/article.aspx?articleid=1188032.

ESC guidelines for the management of grown-up congenital heart disease (new version 2010)

Eur Heart J. 2010;31:2915–57. http://www.escardio.org/guidelines-surveys/esc-guidelines/Pages/grown-up-congenital-heart-disease.aspx.

Patient Information

Images

http://www.nlm.nih.gov/medlineplus/ency/imagepages/9380.htm.

Medlineplus

ENGLISH

http://www.nlm.nih.gov/medlineplus/ency/imagepages/9380.htm.

ESPANOL
http://www.nlm.nih.gov/medlineplus/spanish/ency/article/001096.
   htm.

Genetics Home Reference

http://ghr.nlm.nih.gov/condition/supravalvular-aortic-stenosis.

Mayo Clinic

http://www.mayoclinic.org/diseases-conditions/pulmonary-valve-
   stenosis/basics/definition/con-20013659.

URMC

https://www.urmc.rochester.edu/encyclopedia/content.aspx?Conten
   tTypeID=90&ContentID=P01815.

Professional Information

Alagille Syndrome

Circulation. 2004;109:1354–8. http://circ.ahajournals.org/content/109/11/
   1354.full?sid=311e721c-e2ba-4de5-9604-1194f13518c9.

Auscultation (PERLOFF)

Br Heart J. 1969;31:314–21. (NO DIRECT LINK)

Balloon Angioplasty

Circulation.   2001;103:2165–70.   http://circ.ahajournals.org/con-
   tent/103/17/2165.full?sid=a88156b1-6649-498e-94d8-88b6a23f7db2.

RVOT Lesions

Circulation. 2007;115:1933–47. http://circ.ahajournals.org/content/115/14/1933.full?sid=7dc432e9-ff2f-4bfd-acb6-5225a7d615e1.

Supravalvular AS/PS

J Am Coll Cardiol. 1990;15:1625–30. http://www.ncbi.nlm.nih.gov/pubmed/2345244?dopt=Abstract.

Surgical Reconstruction

J Thorac Cardiovasc Surg. 2013;145:476–81. http://www.ncbi.nlm.nih.gov/pubmed/23228407?dopt=Abstract.

Transcatheter Therapy: Outcomes

Circulation: Cardiovasc Interv. 2013;6:460–7. http://circinterventions.ahajournals.org/content/6/4/460.full.

Williams Syndrome

Circulation. 2013;127:2125–134. http://circ.ahajournals.org/content/127/21/2125.full?sid=de7dc6e9-1e41-4b94-97e6-e55568419dca.

Updates and More

https://clinicalguidecvd.com/pssupra

Chapter 83
Pulmonary Stenosis: Valvular

Management Keys

- Balloon valvotomy recommended for asymptomatic patients with domed pulmonary valve and peak instantaneous Doppler gradient >60 mmHg or mean Doppler gradient >40 mmHg (in association with less than moderate PV regurgitation)

- Balloon valvotomy recommended for symptomatic patients with domed PV and peak instantaneous Doppler gradient >50 mmHg or mean Doppler gradient >30 mmHg (in association with less than moderate pulmonic regurgitation)

- Surgical therapy recommended for patients with severe PS and associated hypoplastic pulmonary annulus, severe pulmonary regurgitation, subvalvular PS, or supravalvular PS; surgery also preferred for most dysplastic pulmonary valves and when there is associated severe TR or need for surgical Maze procedure

- Surgeons with training and expertise in congenital heart disease should perform operations for RVOT and pulmonary valve

V.E. Friedewald, *Clinical Guide to Cardiovascular Disease*, 1093
DOI 10.1007/978-1-4471-7293-2_83,
© Springer-Verlag London 2016

ICD-10 Code

Q22.1

Alternate Names/Abbreviation

PS

Description/Etiology

Usually isolated lesion, occurring in approximately 7–12 % of all cases of congenital heart disease

80–90 % of all lesions that cause RVOT obstruction

Inheritance rate low (1.7–3.6 %)

Approximately 20 % have a dysplastic valve

If part of Noonan syndrome, patients have autosomal dominant trait with variable penetrance that has been mapped to chromosome 12

Congenital (usual)

Most common:

Isolated
Tetralogy Of Fallot [4]

Others:

Complete Atrioventricular Septal Defect
Double-Outlet RV
Univentricular Atrioventricular Connection

Acquired

Carcinoid
Rheumatic Fever (rare)

Usually presents with asymptomatic systolic murmur; sometimes with exercise intolerance

Rarely progressive when initial gradient is mild, but moderate PS can progress due to progressive valve stenosis or reactive infundibular hypertrophy

Mild forms well-tolerated

Predisposing/Comorbid Conditions

ARTERIOHEPATIC DYSPLASIA
CARCINOID SYNDROME/TUMOR
CONGENITAL RUBELLA
NOONAN SYNDROME
TETRALOGY OF FALLOT
WILLIAMS SYNDROME

Demography

Gender equal
Familial uncommon/rare

Pathophysiology

Morphologic types:

1. Typical dome-shaped:

   Narrow central opening with preserved, mobile valve mechanism

   Three rudimentary raphes are usually present without clear-cut commissures

   Pulmonary trunk dilated, mostly due to inherent medial abnormality

   Jet from stenotic valve tends to favor flow to left PA branch

   Calcification of valve sometimes occurs in older adults

2. Dysplastic pulmonary valve:

   Less common
   Leaflets poorly mobile
   Marked myxomatous thickening with no commissural fusion
   Pulmonary annulus and outflow tract may be narrowed
   Frequent component of Noonan syndrome.

3. Unicuspid or bicuspid PV:

   Usually a feature of Tetralogy of Fallot
   May or may not create significant obstruction

Other morphologic/physiologic abnormalities due to associated conditions
Severity based on peak gradient across valve:

   Mild: <30 mmHg
   Moderate: 30–50 mmHg
   Severe: >50 mmHg.

RV pressure overload/wall stress progresses to RVH/RV failure in advanced stage

Signs/Symptoms [8]

ABDOMEN – FLUID (ASCITES)
ABDOMEN – FULLNESS
ABDOMEN – PULSATION, PRESYS
BREATHING – DIFF (DYSPNEA)
CHEST – PAIN, EFFORT (ANGINA PECTORIS)
CHEST – RV LIFT
CONSCIOUSNESS – LOSS, SUDDEN (SYNCOPE)
EXTREM, LOWER, BILAT – EDEMA
HEART – PULMONARY EJECTION SOUND [6]
HEART, LSB, LOWER – IMP, SYS
HEART, LSB, UPPER – MURMUR, SYS [3]
HEART, LSB, UPPER – THRILL, SYS

HEART, P2, INTENSITY – DECR/ABSENT
HEART, S2 – SINGLE [SEVERE; ONLY A2 AUDIBLE]
HEART, S2, SPLIT – WIDE
HEART, S4 RV
LIVER – ENLARGED (HEPATOMEGALY)
LIVER – PULSATION, PRESYS
NECK, JVP, A WAVE – INCR/LARGE (CANNON WAVE)
NECK, SUPRASTERNAL NOTCH – MURMUR, SYS
NECK, SUPRASTERNAL NOTCH – THRILL, SYS

Differentiation

Myxoma – Right Ventricle
Other causes of RVOT obstruction [7]

Complications

Right heart failure

Laboratory

NS

ECG [9]

P WAVE – TALL/PEAKED
QRS – RVH PATTERN
QRS, AXIS – R

Imaging [10]

CHEST X-RAY: VASC FULLNESS L>R LUNG BASE [1]

PA, MAIN, SIZE – INCR [2]
PV, PRESS – GRADIENT
PV, FLOW – REGURG
PV, LEAFLETS – THICK
PV. LEAFLETS – FUSED
PV/LEAFLETS – DOMED
RA, CHAMBER, SIZE – INCR
RV, CHAMBER, SIZE – INCR
RV, WALL THICKNESS – INCR
TV, FLOW – REGURG

Other Tests

Cardiac catheterization:

Rarely needed for diagnosis
Distinguish valvular from extravalvular stenosis

Treatment: Nonpharmacologic

NS

Treatment: Pharmacologic

NS
IE prophylaxis not indicated

Treatment: Surgical/Invasive [12]

Balloon valvotomy [5] [11]
Surgical valvotomy
Valve replacement

Prevention

NA

Course

Variable according to severity/associated defects

Notes

[1] Chen Sign, due to preferential flow to left lung in PS
[2] Dome-type PS
[3] Crescendo/decrescendo occurring later in systole with increased severity; may obscure A2
[4] When associated with Tetralogy of Fallot, most often bicuspid with variable degrees of annular hypoplasia
[5] Except patients with dysplastic valves (Noonan Syndrome)/Subvalvular Stenosis, who should receive surgical valvotomy
[6] Decreased intensity with inspiration; only right heart sound to do so
[7] Non-valvular causes of RVOT obstruction:

Muscular Infundibular Stenosis, associated with

Hypertrophic Cardiomyopathy
Pulmonic Valve Stenosis
Tetralogy of Fallot (usual)

Non-Muscular Infundibular Stenosis

Fibrous Tags
Coronary Sinus
Inferior Vena Cava

Membranous Septum Aneurysm
Sinus of Valsalva Aneurysm
Tricuspid Valve Tissue
Postoperative

Conduit Stenosis
Peripheral stenosis after prior arterial shunt to pulmonary arteries
Valvular

Native Valve Restenosis
Prosthetic Valve Stenosis

Subinfundibular Obstruction

Double-Chamber RV

Supravalvular Stenosis
Associations – syndromes:

Alagille
Pulmonary Artery Stenosis
Keutel
Rubella
Williams

Hourglass deformity at valve
Peripheral Pulmonary Artery Stenosis
Pulmonary Artery Membrane
Pulmonary Artery Stenosis

[8] Cardiac examination findings depend on stenosis severity, valve pathology, associated cardiac lesions

[9] ECG usually normal when RV systolic pressure <60 mmHg

[10] Cardiac size on CXR is normal unless there is associated cardiac lesion

[11] Balloon valvotomy:

Usually completely eliminates gradient with RVH regression

Mild pulmonary regurgitation post-procedure common/clinically insignificant

Comparable results to surgical valvotomy

[12] 2008 ACC/AHA Guideline recommendations:

- Balloon valvotomy is recommended for asymptomatic patients with a domed pulmonary valve and a peak instantaneous Doppler gradient greater than 60 mmHg or a mean Doppler gradient greater than 40 mmHg (in association with less than moderate pulmonic valve regurgitation). *(Level of Evidence: B)*
- Balloon valvotomy is recommended for symptomatic patients with a domed pulmonary valve and a peak

instantaneous Doppler gradient greater than 50 mmHg or a mean Doppler gradient greater than 30 mmHg (in association with less than moderate pulmonic regurgitation). *(Level of Evidence: C)*

- Surgical therapy is recommended for patients with severe PS and an associated hypoplastic pulmonary annulus, severe pulmonary regurgitation, subvalvular PS, or supravalvular PS. Surgery is also preferred for most dysplastic pulmonary valves and when there is associated severe TR or the need for a surgical Maze procedure. *(Level of Evidence: C)*
- Surgeons with training and expertise in CHD should perform operations for the RVOT and pulmonary valve. *(Level of Evidence: B)*

Class IIb

- Balloon valvotomy may be reasonable in asymptomatic patients with a dysplastic pulmonary valve and a peak instantaneous gradient by Doppler greater than 60 mmHg or a mean Doppler gradient greater than 40 mmHg. *(Level of Evidence: C)*
- Balloon valvotomy may be reasonable in selected symptomatic patients with a dysplastic pulmonary valve and peak instantaneous gradient by Doppler greater than 50 mmHg or a mean Doppler gradient greater than 30 mmHg. *(Level of Evidence: C)*

Class III

- Balloon valvotomy is not recommended for asymptomatic patients with a peak instantaneous gradient by Doppler less than 50 mmHg in the presence of normal cardiac output. *(Level of Evidence: C)*
- Balloon valvotomy is not recommended for symptomatic patients with PS and severe pulmonary regurgitation. *(Level of Evidence: C)*
- Balloon valvotomy is not recommended for symptomatic patients with a peak instantaneous gradient by Doppler less than 30 mmHg. *(Level of Evidence: C)*

Guidelines

ACC/AHA 2008 guidelines for the management of adults with congenital heart disease
J Am Coll Cardiol. 2008;52:e143–263. http://content.onlinejacc.org/article.aspx?articleid=1188032.

ESC guidelines for the management of grown-up congenital heart disease (new version 2010)
Eur Heart J. 2010;31:2915–57. http://www.escardio.org/guidelines-surveys/esc-guidelines/Pages/grown-up-congenital-heart-disease.aspx.

Patient Information

Images

http://www.nlm.nih.gov/medlineplus/ency/imagepages/9380.htm.

Medlineplus

ENGLISH
http://www.nlm.nih.gov/medlineplus/ency/imagepages/9380.htm.

ESPANOL
http://www.nlm.nih.gov/medlineplus/spanish/ency/article/001096.htm.

Mayo Clinic

http://www.mayoclinic.org/diseases-conditions/pulmonary-valve-stenosis/basics/definition/con-20013659.

AHA

http://www.heart.org/HEARTORG/Conditions/CongenitalHeartDefects/AboutCongenitalHeartDefects/Pulmonary-Valve-Stenosis-UCM-307034-Article.jsp.

Cincinnati Childrens

http://www.cincinnatichildrens.org/health/p/pvs/.

Stanford Childrens

http://www.stanfordchildrens.org/en/topic/default?id=pulmonary-stenosis-90-P01815.

Boston Childrens: Pulmonary Valve Stenosis in Children

http://www.childrenshospital.org/conditions-and-treatments/conditions/pulmonary-valve-stenosis.

MERK

http://www.merckmanuals.com/home/SearchResults?query=Pulmonic+Stenosis&icd9=424.3.

Professional Information

Review

Heart. 2013;99:339–47. http://heart.bmj.com/content/99/5/339.

Review

Cardiol Clin. 2011;29:223–7. http://www.sciencedirect.com/science/article/pii/S0733865111000130.

Review

Am J Med. 1949;6:24–40. http://www.sciencedirect.com/science/article/pii/0002934349900042#.

Balloon Valvuloplasty: Effectiveness in Adults

Am J Cardiol. 1991;68:1111–13. http://www.sciencedirect.com/science/article/pii/000291499190510R.

Balloon Valvuloplasty

N Engl J Med. 1996;335:21–5. http://www.nejm.org/doi/full/10.1056/NEJM199607043350104.

Long-Term Outcome After Repair

Int J Cardiol. 2012;156:11–5. http://www.sciencedirect.com/science/article/pii/S0167527310008867.

Long-Term Outcome After Repair

Circulation. 1988;78:1150–6. http://circ.ahajournals.org/content/78/5/|1150.full.pdf+html?sid=12160f6c-b471-4e49-be15-b1a85b63ddfd.

Regression of Infundibular Hypertrophy After Valvuloplasty

Am J Cardiol. 1988;62:977–9. http://www.sciencedirect.com/science/article/pii/0002914988909083.

Updates and More

https://clinicalguidecvd.com/psvalv

Chapter 84
Renal Artery Stenosis

ICD-10 Code

I70.1 Atherosclerotic
Q27.1 Congenital

Alternate Names/Abbreviation

RAS

Description/Etiology

Narrowing of renal arteries caused by many conditions
(see PREDISPOSING/COMORBID CONDITIONS),
most often atherosclerosis (90 % of cases)

May be present in up to 3–6 % of normotensive individuals

>40 % bilateral

In bilateral disease, may induce acute/subacute acceleration of pre-existing essential hypertension including
flash pulmonary edema

Renal Artery Stenosis should be suspected in a variety of
clinical situations, including:

- Hypertension onset before age 30 years and after 55
  years

V.E. Friedewald, *Clinical Guide to Cardiovascular Disease*, 1105
DOI 10.1007/978-1-4471-7293-2_84,
© Springer-Verlag London 2016

- Hypertension with hypokalemia, especially when receiving thiazide diuretics
- Hypertension and abdominal bruit
- Accelerated hypertension (sudden/persistent worsening of previously controlled hypertension)
- Resistant hypertension (failure of blood-pressure control despite full doses of an appropriate three-drug regimen including a diuretic)
- Malignant hypertension (hypertension with coexistent end-organ damage, i.e., acute renal failure, flash pulmonary edema, hypertensive LV failure, Aortic Dissection, new visual or neurological disturbance, advanced retinopathy)
- New azotemia or worsening renal function after administration of an ACEI or ARB
- Unexplained hypotrophic kidney
- Unexplained renal failure [17]

Predisposing/Comorbid Conditions

ABDOMINAL AORTIC ANEURYSM
ATHEROSCLEROSIS IN OTHER CV AREAS
CAROTID ARTERY STENOSIS
CONGENITAL BANDS
CORONARY ARTERY DISEASE
DIABETES MELLITUS
FIBROMUSCULAR DYSPLASIA [5]
HYPERCOAGULATION STATES
NEUROFIBROMATOSIS
PERIPHERAL ARTERY DISEASE
RADIATION
RENAL ARTERY COMPRESSION
RENAL/AORTIC ANEURYSM
RENAL/AORTIC DISSECTION
TAKAYASU ARTERITIS
THROMBOEMBOLISM
TRAUMA
WILLIAMS SYNDROME [1]

Demography

Follows traditional atherosclerotic CV risk factors
Advanced age
Females more common

Pathophysiology

Varies by etiology but all forms have common natural history of progressive loss of renal mass and function and secondary accelerated, resistant, or malignant hypertension if stenosis not treated
Atherosclerotic form (90% of cases) involves ostium/proximal 1/3 of renal artery
Hypertension primarily due to activation of RAAS in hypo-perfused kidneys
LVH more common than in Essential Hypertension [18]

Signs/Symptoms

ABDOMEN – BRUIT [4]
ABDOMEN, LUQ – BRUIT [3] [4]
ABDOMEN, RUQ – BRUIT [3] [4]
BLOOD PRESSURE, ARTERIAL – INCREASED/ELEVATED [13]
FLANK – BRUIT [3] [4]

Differentiation

Other causes of abdominal bruit
Other causes of resistant/accelerated Hypertension

Complications [2]

Aortic Dissection
CAD

Flash Pulmonary Edema [14]
LVH/HF
Renal Failure [17]
Resistant/malignant Hypertension
Stroke

Laboratory

BLOOD RENIN/ANGIOTENSIN II LEVELS – INCR [6]
BLOOD, BUN – INCR [7]
BLOOD, CREATININE – INCREASED [7]
URINE, PROTEIN – INCR (PROTEINURIA) [11]

ECG

QRS – LVH PATTERN [2] [18]

Imaging

CT ANGIO: DIAGNOSTIC [9]
ECHO/DOPPLER   SCREENING,   DEGREE   OF
    STENOSIS, PHYSIOLOGIC PATTERNS [8] [19]
MR ANGIOGRAPHY: DIAGNOSTIC [9]

Other Tests

Ambulatory BP monitoring
Angiography [10]

Treatment: Nonpharmacologic

Hypertension diet
Atherosclerosis risk modification

Treatment: Pharmacologic

Antihypertensives

> ACEIs [12]
> ARBs [12]
> CCBs

Diabetes control
Statins

Treatment: Surgical/Invasive [21]

Percutaneous angioplasty [15]
Stent [16]
Surgical revascularization [20]

Prevention

Atherosclerotic risk factor modification

Course

Data on progression of atherosclerotic RAS are inconsistent
Significant disease progression to high-grade stenosis or occlusion occurs in 1.3–11.1 % of patients
Loss of function after 2 years:

> Unilateral stenosis: 3 %
> Bilateral stenosis: 18 %
> Contralateral occlusion: 55 %

Notes

[1] Includes Supravalvular AS, PA Stenosis, RAS; "elfin" facies, teeth/jaw malformations, mental retardation, hypercalcemia, joint abnormalities, small stature, hypertension, nephrocalcinosis

[2] Incidence of many complications is disproportionate to degree of hypertension, attributed to angiotensin II inflammatory/toxic effects (eg, myocardial fibrosis, arterial medial hypertrophy, plaque rupture, endothelial cell dysfunction, smooth muscle proliferation)

[3] Depending on site of stenosis

[4] High-pitched, long, may extend into part/most of diastole

[5] Second most common cause of RAS; most often in females; involves mid-distal 2/3 of renal artery and branches

[6] Only in acute stages; normalize after a few months; NS

[7] May be normal; may increase as a sign of progressive RAS

[8] First-line screening modality; peak systolic velocity 85 % sensitivity compared to about 98 % for angiography; 92 % specificity compared to about 99 % for angiography

[9] Use contrast agents with caution with decreased renal function; MRI contrast safer but not recommended when serum creatinine clearance <30 ml/min due to risk of Nephrogenic Systemic Fibrosis

[10] Use with caution due to risk of trauma, spasm, thromboembolism

[11] Advanced disease

[12] RAAS inhibitors may transiently decrease GFR; contraindicated in bilateral RAS and RAS in patients with single functioning kidney

[13] Resistant to standard hypertension treatment

[14] Flash pulmonary edema: dramatic form of acute HF; RAS, esp when bilateral, is comman cause

[15] Preferred treatment in cases of Fibromuscular Dysplasia

[16] Angioplasty with/without stenting indications:

>60 % obstruction/symptomatic RAS secondary to atherosclerosis.
Ostial atherosclerotic RAS
RAS with impaired renal function
Unexplained recurrent CHF or sudden pulmonary edema and preserved LV systolic function

[17] Renal failure may occur with severe bilateral RAS or unilateral RAS in a single functional kidney
[18] LVH prevalence in RAS is 79 %, compared to 46 % in patients with essential hypertension, with significant effect on morbidity and mortality
[19] Duplex ultrasonography: first-line screening modality for atherosclerotic RAS; can be applied serially to assess degree of stenosis and physiological patterns, such as flow velocities and vascular resistance

Increased peak systolic velocity in main renal artery associated with post-stenotic turbulence is most frequently used to determine relevant RAS, and corresponds to ≥60 % angiographic RAS with a sensitivity and specificity of 71–98 % and 62–98 %, respectively
Several duplex criteria should be used to identify significant (60 %) stenosis, including:

Imaging of intrarenal interlobar or segmental arteries, including calculation of side difference of intrarenal resistance index
Missing early systolic peak
Retarded acceleration
Increased acceleration time

[20] Surgical revascularization indications:

Patients undergoing aorta surgical repair
Patients with complex renal artery anatomy
Failed endovascular procedure

[21] 2013 ESC Guidelines on the diagnosis and treatment of peripheral artery diseases on renal revascularization:

"The decision regarding the potential revascularization strategy should be based on the patient's individual characteristics, such as life expectancy, co-morbidities, quality of blood pressure control, and renal function. Evidence supporting the benefit of aggressive diagnosis and timing of renal revascularization remains unclear. Among patients receiving medical therapy alone, there is the risk for deterioration of kidney function with worsening morbidity and mortality. Renal artery revascularization can provide immediate improvement in kidney function and blood pressure; however, as with all invasive interventions, it may result in mortality or substantial morbidity in a small percentage of patients. This is particularly the case for renovascular lesions that pose no immediate hazard or risk of progression. There is general consensus that renal revascularization should be performed in patients with anatomically and functionally significant RAS who present with particular clinical scenarios such as sudden onset or 'flash' pulmonary oedema or congestive heart failure with preserved left ventricular function and acute oligo-/anuric renal failure with kidney ischaemia."

Guidelines

ESC guidelines on the diagnosis and treatment of peripheral artery diseases. 2013 ESH/ESC guidelines for the management of arterial hypertension
Eur Heart J. 2011;32:2851–906. http://eurheartj.oxfordjournals.org/content/ehj/32/22/2851.full.pdf.

2013 ESH/ESC guidelines for the management of arterial hypertension
Eur Heart J. 2014;34:2159–219. http://www.escardio.org/guidelines-surveys/esc-guidelines/Pages/arterial-hypertension.aspx.

JNC 7: Seventh report of the Joint National Committee on prevention, detection, evaluation, and treatment of high blood pressure
Hypertension. 2003;42:1206–52. http://hyper.ahajournals.org/content/42/6/1206.long.

NICE: Hypertension in adults: diagnosis and management (2011)
http://www.nice.org.uk/guidance/cg127/chapter/1-recommendations
#choosing-antihypertensive-drug-treatment-2.

2011 ACCF/AHA focused update of the guideline for the management of patients with peripheral artery disease (updating the 2005 guideline)
Circulation.   2011;124:2020–45.   http://circ.ahajournals.org/content/124/18/2020.long.

Patient Information

Medlineplus

ENGLISH
http://www.nlm.nih.gov/medlineplus/ency/article/000204.htm.

ESPANOL
http://www.nlm.nih.gov/medlineplus/spanish/ency/article/000204.htm.

Mayo Clinic

http://www.mayoclinic.org/diseases-conditions/renal-artery-stenosis/basics/definition/con-20036702.

MERCK

http://www.merckmanuals.com/home/SearchResults?query=Renal+Artery+Stenosis+and+Occlusion&icd9=593.81%3b440.1%3b447.3.

Cleveland Clinic

http://my.clevelandclinic.org/services/heart/disorders/renal-artery-disease.

Professional Information

Review

Mayo Clin Proc. 2011;86:649–57. http://www.mayoclinicproceedings. org/article/S0025-6196(11)60070-0/abstract.

Review

N Engl J Med. 2009;361:1972–8. http://www.nejm.org/doi/ full/10.1056/NEJMcp0809200.

Diagnosis: CTA Versus Catheterization

Radiology. 2009;252:299–305. http://pubs.rsna.org/doi/abs/10.1148/ radiol.2521081362.

Diagnosis: CTA Versus MRA

Ann Intern Med. 2004;141:674–82. http://annals.org/article. aspx?articleid=717920.

Treatment: Astral Trial (Revasc Versus Medical Therapy)

N Engl J Med. 2009;361:1953–62. http://www.nejm.org/doi/ full/10.1056/NEJMoa0905368.

Treatment: Coral Trial (Medical Therapy Versus Stent + MED RX)

J Am Coll Cardiol. 2015;66:2487–94. http://content.onlinejacc.org/ article.aspx?articleID=2473755.

Treatment: Coral Trial (Medical Therapy Versus Stent + MED RX)

N Engl J Med. 2014;370:13–22. http://www.nejm.org/doi/full/10.1056/NEJMoa1310753.

Treatment: Star Trial (Medical Therapy Versus Stent + MED RX)

Ann Intern Med. 2009;150:840–8. http://annals.org/article.aspx?articleid=744542.

Updates and More

https://clinicalguidecvd.com/ras

Chapter 85
Short QT Syndrome (SQTS)

ICD-10 Code

NS

Alternate Names/Abbreviation

SQTS

Description/Etiology

Genetically-transmitted cardiac channelopathy in structurally normal hearts associated with dysrhythmias (especially AF and VF) and SCD

Specific triggers of arrhythmic events do not occur

Associated with several mutations affecting cardiac ion channel function responsible for currents that generate cardiac action potential

Classification according to genotype: [11]

SQT1: KCNH2
SQT2: KCNQ1
SQT3: KCNJ2

V.E. Friedewald, *Clinical Guide to Cardiovascular Disease*,   1117
DOI 10.1007/978-1-4471-7293-2_85,
© Springer-Verlag London 2016

SQT4: CACNA1C
SQT5: CACNB2B

Diagnosis:

Males with QTc <330 ms and females with QTc <340 ms
even when asymptomatic

Males with QTc <360 ms and females with <370 ms
should be considered for this diagnosis only when
symptomatic or have positive family history because
these values overlap with healthy population

Predisposing/Comorbid Conditions

DYSRHYTHMIAS – ATRIAL
DYSRHYTHMIAS – VENTRICULAR

Demography

Males 2:1
Mean age of first clinical manifestation about 30 years, but
occurs in all ages, from infancy to very aged

Pathophysiology

Shortening of refractory periods and increased dispersion
of repolarization predispose to arrhythmias

Signs/Symptoms [1]

CARD ARREST [2]
CHEST – PALPITATIONS [3]
CONSCIOUSNESS – LOSS, SUDDEN (SYNCOPE)

Differentiation [6]

Acidosis
Altered autonomic tone
Digitalis
Hypercalcemia
Hyperkalemia
Hyperthermia

Complications

SCD

Laboratory

NS

ECG

DYSRHYTHMIAS – ATRIAL (PACS/OTHERS) [8]
DYSRHYTHMIAS – VENTRICULAR (PVCS/OTHERS)
J POINT-T PEAK INTERVAL – SHORT [7]
PR SEGMENT – DEPRESSED
QT INTERVAL – SHORT [4]
ST SEGMENT – ELEV [5]
ST SEGMENT – SHORT/ABSENT
T WAVE – TALL/PEAKED

Imaging

NS

Genomics [11]

CACNA1C
CACNB2b
KCNH2
KCNJ2
KCNQ1

Other Tests

Ambulatory ECG [4]
Electrophysiologic testing (controversial)
Exercise test [4]

Treatment: Nonpharmacologic

NS

Treatment: Pharmacologic [12]

Quinidine [9]
Disopyramide [9]

Treatment: Surgical/Invasive [12]

ICD [10]

Prevention

Screen family members

Course

Untreated: high mortality

Notes

[1] Often asymptomatic
[2] Often first clinical manifestation
[3] AF/flutter, PVCs
[4] Both QT length and accommodation to HR must be considered:

> Persons with SQTS have constant QT values and lack adaptation to HR, with failure to prolong adequately at slower HRs and abnormal shortening during acceleration (pseudonormalization of QT interval at rapid rates)

> Serial ECGs, ambulatory ECG monitoring and TST may help prevent unrecognition of SQTS patients with increased HR at baseline and can reduce wrong diagnosis in presence of sinus bradycardia since Bazett formula overcorrects QT interval at slow HRs

[5] Brugada-like, right precordial leads
[6] Causes of short QT interval listed
[7] Degree of shortening correlates with symptoms in affected persons
[8] Both AF and atrial flutter
[9] Both quinidine and disopyramide prolong QT interval but clinical efficacy unproven
[10] ICD: mainstay treatment for SQTS in symptomatic patients; data lacking to definitely support use in asymptomatic persons, especially those with negative family history
[11] Gene mutations not identified in all cases of Short QT Syndrome

[12] HRS/EHRA/APHRS Expert Consensus Statement on the Diagnosis and Management of Patients with Inherited Primary Arrhythmia Syndromes:

"The optimal strategy for primary prevention of cardiac arrest in SQTS is not clear given the lack of independent risk factors, including syncope, for cardiac arrest. Although intuitively it might seem reasonable to suggest that patients with the shortest QTc values are at highest risk, clinical data do not support this hypothesis. However, in a combined symptomatic and asymptomatic group (QTc <360 ms) QTc was the only risk factor for arrhythmic events."

Guidelines

HRS/EHRA/APHRS expert consensus statement on the diagnosis and management of patients with inherited primary arrhythmia syndromes
Heart Rhythm. 2013;10:1932–63.

Patient Information

Genetics Home Reference

http://ghr.nlm.nih.gov/condition/short-qt-syndrome.

Sads Foundation

http://www.sads.org/What-is-SADS/Short-QT-Syndrome#.VYVRRGfJB1s.

Professional Information

Review

Circulation Arrhythmia Electrophysiol. 2010;3:401–8. http://circep.ahajournals.org/content/3/4/401.full.

Review

Ann Noninvasive Electrocardiol. 2005;10:371–7. http://www.ncbi.nlm.nih.gov/pubmed/16029390.

Review

Cardiovasc Res. 2005;67:357–66. http://cardiovascres.oxfordjournals.org/content/67/3/357.long.

Review

Acta Cardiol. 2008;63:553–5. http://www.ncbi.nlm.nih.gov/pubmed/19013996.

Review: Genetics of Sudden Cardiac Death

Circulation Research. 2015;116:1919–36. http://circres.ahajournals.org/content/116/12/1919.full.

Children: Long-Term Follow-Up

J Am Coll Cardiol. 2013;61:1183–91. http://content.onlinejacc.org/article.aspx?articleID=1567306.

Clinical/Medical Genetics

Curr Opin Cardiol. 2008;23:192–8. http://www.ncbi.nlm.nih.gov/pubmed/18382206.

Early Repolarization: Prevalence

Heart Rhythm. 2010;7:647–52. http://www.ncbi.nlm.nih.gov/pubmed/20206319?dopt=Abstract.

Echocardiography

Heart Rhythm. 2016;12:2096–105. http://www.heartrhythmjournal.com/article/S1547-5271(15)00626-8/abstract.

Mutation: KCNJ2 Gene

Proc Natl Acad Sci USA. 2013;110:4291–6. http://www.pnas.org/content/110/11/4291.full.

Mutation: SQTS6 Gene

Eur Heart J. 2011;32:1077–88. http://eurheartj.oxfordjournals.org/content/32/9/1077.

Natural History

J Am Coll Cardiol. 2014;63:1300–13. http://content.onlinejacc.org/article.aspx?articleID=1789345.

Ventricular Arrhythmias in Channelopathies: Management

Circulation Arrhythmia Electrophysiol. 2015;8:221–31. http://circep.ahajournals.org/content/8/1/221.extract?etoc.

Updates and More

https://clinicalguidecvd.com/sqts

Chapter 86
Sinus Node Dysfunction

ICD-10 Code

I49.8

Alternate Names/Abbreviation

SND
BRADYCARDIA-TACHYCARDIA SYNDROME
CHRONOTROPIC INCOMPETENCE
SICK SINUS SYNDROME
SINOATRIAL DISEASE
SINOATRIAL DYSFUNCTION

Description/Etiology

Broad array of abnormalities in sinus node and atrial impulse formation and propagation, including:

Persistent sinus bradycardia and chronotropic incompetence without identifiable causes

Paroxysmal or persistent sinus arrest with replacement by subsidiary escape rhythms in atrium, AV junction, or ventricular myocardium

V.E. Friedewald, *Clinical Guide to Cardiovascular Disease*,
DOI 10.1007/978-1-4471-7293-2_86,
© Springer-Verlag London 2016

1125

In older persons, primary form due to senescence of sinus node and atrial muscle; same degenerative process also affects specialized conduction system, although rate of progression is slow and does not dominate clinical course

Secondary forms may occur at any age due to any condition that affects sinus node cells, such as ischemia or infarction, infiltrative disease, collagen vascular disease, surgical trauma, endocrine abnormalities, autonomic insufficiency

Bradycardia-Tachycardia Syndrome: frequent association of paroxysmal AF and sinus bradycardia or sinus brady-arrhythmias, which may oscillate suddenly from one to the other

Chronotropic incompetence: inadequate HR response to physical activity

Familial forms occur

Predisposing/Comorbid Conditions

ATRIAL FIBRILLATION
ACUTE MYOCARDIAL INFARCTION [1]
AUTOIMMUNE/CONNECTIVE TISSUE DISEASE [4]
CARDIAC AMYLOIDOSIS
CARDIAC INFILTRATIVE DISORDERS [2]
CARDIAC SURGERY [7]
CARDIOMYOPATHY – NONCOMPACTION [18]
CORONARY ARTERY DISEASE
DRUGS [5]
ELECTROLYTE ABNORMALITIES [6]
HYPOTHYROIDISM
INTRACRANIAL HYPERTENSION
MUSCULOSKELETAL DISORDERS [3]
MYOCARDITIS
OBSTRUCTIVE JAUNDICE
PARASYMPATHETIC STIMULATION
PERICARDITIS – ACUTE
STABLE ISCHEMIC HEART DISEASE

Demography

Idiopathic form: advanced age
Less common in African-Americans

Pathophysiology

Abnormal sinus node and atrial impulse formation and
propagation, presumed due to senescence of sinus node
and atrial muscle

Signs/Symptoms [8]

BREATHING – DIFF (DYSPNEA)
CHEST – PAIN, EFFORT (ANGINA PECTORIS)
CHEST – PALPITATIONS
CONSCIOUSNESS – LOSS, SUDDEN (SYNCOPE) [14]
DIZZY/LIGHTHEADED/PRESYNCOPE
FATIGUE [19]
HEART, RATE – RAPID (TACHYCARDIA)
HEART, RATE – SLOW (BRADYCARDIA)
HEART,   RATE,   RESPONSE   –   DECR
   (CHRONOTROPIC INCOMPETENCE) [16]
MENTATION – CHANGES, NS
MENTATION, MEMORY – DECR (AMNESIA)
MOOD – LETHARGIC

Differentiation

Other causes of bradycardia
Other causes of syncope
Physiologic bradycardia [21]

Complications

HF
Peripheral embolism
Progressive mental deterioration
Stroke [17] [20]
Death [20]

Laboratory

NS

ECG

AV COND – 1ST DEGREE BLOCK [13]
AV COND – 2ND DEGREE BLOCK
AV COND – 3RD DEGREE BLOCK
DYSRHY – JUNCT [12]
DYSRHYTHMIAS – ATRIAL (PACS/OTHERS) [11]
DYSRHYTHMIAS – VENTRICULAR (PVCS/ OTHERS) [15]
P WAVE – ABSENT INTERMITTENT [9]
QRS – LBBB/LBBB PATTERN [13]
QRS – LONG, NS [13]
QRS – RBBB/RBBB PATTERN [13]
RATE – DECREASED (SINUS BRADYCARDIA) [10]
RATE – INCREASED (SINUS TACHYCARDIA) [10]

Imaging

NS/VAR WITH COMORBID

Genomics

HCN4 [18]
MYH6
SCN5A

Other Tests

Ambulatory ECG monitoring
EP
Exercise test

Treatment: Nonpharmacologic

NS

Treatment: Pharmacologic [22]

Variable per etiology

Treatment: Surgical/Invasive

Pacing/ablation [23] [24]

Prevention

Variable per etiology

Course

Variable per etiology

Notes

[1] Especially Inferior AMI

[2] Eg, Amyloidosis, Hemochromatosis, tumor

[3] Eg, Duchenne Muscular Dystrophy, Myotonic Dystrophy, Friedreich Ataxia

[4] Eg, SLE, Scleroderma

[5] Eg, antiarrhythmics, sympatholytic antihypertensives, beta-blockers, CCBs, cimetidine, lithium, phenytoin

[6] Especially hyperkalemia

[7] Eg, Mustard procedure, ASD repair

[8] List does not include signs/symptoms due to associated conditions; often asymptommatic

[9] Due to sinus arrest or SA block

[10] Alternating Bradycardia-Tachycardia Syndrome, occurring in >50 %

[11] Especially AF, which fails to convert to sinus rhythm with cardioversion attempt, and may be a component of Bradycardia-Tachycardia Syndrome

[12] Escape rhythm

[13] Persistent or intermittent AV Block may occur

[14] Often due to prolonged asystole following abrupt end of run of PAT

[15] Especially in AMI

[16] Failure to reach appropriate HR for level of exercise

[17] Due to cerebral embolus or reduced cardiac output during Tachycardia/Bradycadia dysrhythmia in presence of atherosclerotic CVD

[18] Isolated reports of familial form with HCN4 mutation and Noncompaction Cardiomyopathy

[19] Easy fatigability due to chronotropic incompetence

[20] Associated with CHADS2/CHA2DS2-VASc score

[21] Especially athletic heart: may have resting HRs of 40–50 BPM while awake, with sleeping HRs as slow as 30 bpm, with sinus pauses or progressive sinus slowing accompanied by AV conduction delay (PR prolongation), some-

times culminating in type I second-degree AV block; distinction depends on correlating bradycardia with symptoms of cerebral hypoperfusion

[22] Treatment generally not indicated in asymptommatic persons; drugs causing brady arrhythmias should be DCd with care when possible

[23] **ACC/AHA/HRS 2008 Guidelines for Device-Based Therapy of Cardiac Rhythm Abnormalities**

Permanent Pacing in Sinus Node Dysfunction

CLASS I

1. Permanent pacemaker implantation is indicated for SND with documented symptomatic bradycardia, including frequent sinus pauses that produce symptoms. *(Level of Evidence: C)*

2. Permanent pacemaker implantation is indicated for symptomatic chronotropic incompetence. *(Level of Evidence: C)*

3. Permanent pacemaker implantation is indicated for symptomatic sinus bradycardia that results from required drug therapy for medical conditions. *(Level of Evidence: C)*

CLASS IIa

1. Permanent pacemaker implantation is reasonable for SND with heart rate less than 40 bpm when a clear association between significant symptoms consistent with bradycardia and the actual presence of bradycardia has not been documented. *(Level of Evidence: C)*

2. Permanent pacemaker implantation is reasonable for syncope of unexplained origin when clinically significant abnormalities of sinus node function are discovered or provoked in electrophysiological studies. *(Level of Evidence: C)*

CLASS IIb

1. Permanent pacemaker implantation may be considered in minimally symptomatic patients with chronic heart rate less than 40 bpm while awake. *(Level of Evidence: C)*

CLASS III

1. Permanent pacemaker implantation is not indicated for SND in asymptomatic patients. *(Level of Evidence: C)*
2. Permanent pacemaker implantation is not indicated for SND in patients for whom the symptoms suggestive of bradycardia have been clearly documented to occur in the absence of bradycardia. *(Level of Evidence: C)*
3. Permanent pacemaker implantation is not indicated for SND with symptomatic bradycardia due to non-essential drug therapy. *(Level of Evidence: C)*

[24] **2013 ESC Guidelines on cardiac pacing and cardiac resynchronization therapy**

Patients with persistent bradycardia

1. Sinus node disease. Pacing is indicated when symptoms can clearly be attributed to bradycardia. Class I
2. Sinus node disease. Pacing may be indicated when symptoms are likely to be due to bradycardia, even if the evidence is not conclusive. Class IIb
3. Sinus node disease. Pacing is not indicated in patients with SB which is asymptomatic or due to reversible causes. Class III

Patients with intermittent (documented) bradycardia

1. Sinus node disease (including brady-tachy form). Pacing is indicated in patients affected by sinus node disease

who have the documentation of symptomatic bradycardia due to sinus arrest or sinusatrial block. Class I

2. Intermittent asystolic paroxysmal AV block (including AF with slow ventricular conduction). Pacing is indicated in patients with intermittent/paroxysmal intrinsic third- or second degree AV block. Class I

3. Reflex asystolic syncope. Pacing should be considered in patients ≥40 years with syncopes and documented symptomatic pause/s due to sinus arrest or AV block or the combination of the two. Class IIa

4. Asymptomatic pauses (sinus arrest or AV block). Pacing should be considered in patients with history of syncope and documentation of asymptomatic pauses >6 s due to sinus arrest, sinus-atrial block or AV block. Class IIa

5. Pacing is not indicated in reversible causes of bradycardia. Class III

Guidelines

ACC/AHA/HRS 2008 Guidelines for Device-Based Therapy of Cardiac Rhythm Abnormalities
Circulation. 2008;117:e356. http://circ.ahajournals.org/content/117/21/e350.full.pdf.

2013 ESC Guidelines on cardiac pacing and cardiac resynchronization therapy
Eur Heart J. 2013;34:2285. http://eurheartj.oxfordjournals.org/content/34/29/2281.full.pdf+html?sid=0742d2bc-d672-4b4f-91c9-42e549685d2d.

Patient Information

Genetics Home Reference

http://ghr.nlm.nih.gov/condition/sick-sinus-syndrome.

Medlineplus

ENGLISH
http://www.nlm.nih.gov/medlineplus/ency/article/000161.htm.

ESPANOL
http://www.nlm.nih.gov/medlineplus/spanish/ency/article/000161.
htm.

Mayo Clinic

http://www.mayoclinic.org/diseases-conditions/sick-sinus-syndrome/
basics/definition/con-20029161.

Cleveland Clinic

http://www.clevelandclinicmeded.com/medicalpubs/diseasemanage-
ment/cardiology/cardiac-arrhythmias/.

Texas Heart Institute

http://www.texasheartinstitute.org/HIC/Topics/Cond/sicksinus.cfm.

Professional Information

Review

Circulation.   2007;115:1921–32.   https://circ.ahajournals.org/con-
tent/115/14/1921.full.

Atrial Fibrillation

Europace. 2013;15:205–11. http://europace.oxfordjournals.org/con-
tent/15/2/205.full.

Atrial Remodeling

Circulation.   2004;109:1514–22.   http://circ.ahajournals.org/content/109/12/1514.full.

Autoantibodies

Heart Rhythm. 2011;8:1788–95. http://www.heartrhythmjournal.com/article/S1547-5271(11)00787-9/abstract.

CHADS2/CHA2DS2-VASc Score

Heart.   2013;99:843–8.   http://heart.bmj.com/content/99/12/843.abstract.

Congenital Sick Sinus Syndrome

J   Clin   Invest.   2003;112:1019–28.   http://www.jci.org/articles/view/18062.

Heart Failure

Circulation.   2004;110:897–903.   http://circ.ahajournals.org/content/110/8/897.full.

Incidence/Risk Factors

J Am Coll Cardiol. 2014;64:531–8. http://content.onlinejacc.org/article.aspx?articleID=1894673.

Mutations: SCN4 Familial/LV Noncompaction

J Am Coll Cardiol. 2014;64:757–67. http://content.onlinejacc.org/article.aspx?articleID=1898539.

Stroke Predictors

J Am Coll Cardiol. 2004;43:1617–22. http://content.onlinejacc.org/article.aspx?articleid=1135557&resultClick=3.

Syncope in Paced Patients

Heart. 2014;100:842–47. http://heart.bmj.com/content/100/11/842.abstract.

Updates and More

https://clinicalguidecvd.com/snd

Chapter 87
Sinus of Valsalva Aneurysm: (Windsock Aneurysm)

ICD-10 Code

Q25.4 [ruptured]

Alternate Names/Abbreviation

SVA
WINDSOCK ANEURYSM

Description/Etiology

Congenital and acquired dilatation of aortic wall between AV annulus and sinotubular ridge, usually protruding into adjacent cardiac chamber; rupture consists of fistula via this connection

Acquired forms due to aortic degenerative disease, infection, trauma [1] [2]

Predisposing/Comorbid Conditions

ABRUPT DECELERATION INJURY [16]
ANEURYSMS-OSTEOARTHRITIS SYNDROME [13]

V.E. Friedewald, *Clinical Guide to Cardiovascular Disease*,
DOI 10.1007/978-1-4471-7293-2_87,
© Springer-Verlag London 2016

AORTIC STENOSIS – SUBVALVULAR
ATHEROSCLEROSIS IN OTHER CV AREAS [14]
ATRIAL SEPTAL DEFECT – SECUNDUM [13]
BICUSPID AORTIC VALVE [13]
CARDIAC SURGERY [16]
COARCTATION OF AORTA [13]
CORONARY ARTERY ANOMALIES [13]
CYSTIC MEDIAL NECROSIS [14]
DECELERATION TRAUMA
EBSTEIN ANOMALY [13]
EHLERS-DANLOS SYNDROME [13]
INFECTIVE ENDOCARDITIS
INTENSE PHYSICAL ACTIVITY
MARFAN SYNDROME [13]
MITRAL REGURGITATION – CHRONIC [13]
PATENT DUCTUS ARTERIOSUS [13]
SYPHILIS [15]
TETRALOGY OF FALLOT [13]
TRANSPOSITION OF GREAT ARTERIES – CORRECTED [13]
TREACHER COLLINS SYNDROME
TRICUSPID REGURGITATION [13]
TUBERCULOSIS [15]
VENTRICULAR SEPTAL DEFECT [13][17]

Demography

M 4:1
More common in Asians
Initial manifestations (eg, embolism, rupture) occur at all ages [12]

Pathophysiology

AV right coronary cusp most often involved, followed by noncoronary cusp and left coronary cusp

Unruptured (expansion) effects depend on site, including:

RVOT obstruction
LVOT obstruction
Conduction abnormalities
Coronary artery obstruction
Systemic Emboli

Hemodynamic changes with rupture depend on site; most often into:

RV (60 %) (with RV volume overload)
RA (29 %)
LA (6 %)
LV (4 %)
Pericardium (1 %)

Signs/Symptoms [19] [20]

(RUPTURED AND NONRUPTURED) [3]
ABDOMEN – FLUID (ASCITES) [7]
BREATH SOUNDS – CRACKLES (RALES) [7]
BREATHING – DIFF (DYSPNEA)
CHEST – PAIN [RUPTURE]
CHEST – PAIN, EFFORT (ANGINA PECTORIS)
CHEST – PALPITATIONS
COUGH
EXTREM, LOWER, BILAT – EDEMA
FATIGUE
HEART, LSB – MURMUR, CONT [TO-AND-FRO][4] [5]
HEART, LSB – THRILL, DIAS [5]
HEART, LSB, MID – MURMUR, DIAS [8]
HEART, LSB, MID – THRILL, SYS [5]
HEART, LV, APEX – MURMUR, DIAS [8]
HEART, RATE – RAPID (TACHYCARDIA)
HEART, RSB – MURMUR, CONT [TO-AND-FRO][4][6]
HEART, RSB – THRILL, DIAS [6]

HEART, RSB, MID – THRILL, SYS [6]
HEART, RSB, UPPER – MURMUR, DIAS
LIVER – ENLARGED (HEPATOMEGALY) [7]

Differentiation

Other causes of AV regurgitation
Other causes of heart failure
Other causes of right heart volume overload
Patent Ductus Arteriosus

Complications

(INCLUDES   BOTH   UNRUPTURED   AND
   RUPTURED)
ACUTE MYOCARDIAL INFARCTION [18]
AV BLOCK
CARDIAC TAMPONADE
DYSRHYTHMIAS
HEART FAILURE
INFECTIVE ENDOCARDITIS [19]
M Y O C A R D I A L   I S C H E M I A
   [18]'ANEURYSMS-OSTEOARTHRITIS
PERIPHERAL EMBOLISM
RV OUTFLOW OBSTRUCTION
SUDDEN DEATH
TIA/STROKE

Laboratory

NS

ECG [21]

AV COND – 3RD DEGREE BLOCK [9]

DYSRHYTHMIAS – ATRIAL (PACS/OTHERS)
DYSRHYTHMIAS – VENTRICULAR (PVCS/OTHERS)
PR INTERVAL – LONG <1ST DEGREE BLOCK
QRS – LBBB/LBBB PATTERN
QRS – LVH PATTERN [10]
QRS – RBBB/RBBB PATTERN
QRS – RVH PATTERN [10]
QRS, AXIS – R
ST-T WAVE – ABN, NS

Imaging [11]

AV, FLOW – REGURG
CARDIOMEGALY
PERICARD – FLUID
SINUS OF VALSALVA, SIZE – INCR

Other Tests

Cardiac catheterization and coronary angiography

Treatment – Nonpharmacologic

NS

Treatment – Pharmacologic

HF protocol when applicable

Treatment – Surgical/Invasive [22]

Surgical repair of aneurysm

Surgical correction of associated lesions (most often VSD, ASD, abnormal AV)
Coronary revascularization
AV repair/replacement

Course

Variable according to severity and complexity
Usual survival without surgery: about 4 years

Notes

[1] Eg, Endocarditis, Tuberculosis, Syphilis
[2] Abrupt deceleration, surgery
[3] Unruptured: usually asymptomatic; clinical onset may be abrupt or gradual, beginning with aneurysmal expansion
[4] Primary clinical sign; loud, harsh, superficial; resembles PDA except located at 3–4th ICS or xiphisternum
[5] Rupture into RV – most cases
[6] Rupture into RA
[7] Due to HF, present in 50 % of ruptured SVAs
[8] Aortic regurgitation
[9] May occur due to impingement on AV conduction
[10] Often biventricular hypertrophy
[11] With adequate quality, echo usually suffices in assessment of aneurysm size, sinus of origin, point of termination; findings highly variable depending on aneurysm severity, location, and presence of HF
[12] Rupture uncommon before puberty
[13] Congenital form
[14] Degenerative form
[15] AV endocarditis is most common cause
[16] Traumatic form
[17] Reported in 12–78 % of patients; usually associated with aneurysm of right coronary sinus

[18] Due to coronary artery compression or emboli
[19] Symptoms of occult infection may be only manifestation
[20] Symptoms due to rupture may subside, then worsen
[21] ECG almost always abnormal with rupture
[22] Definite indications for surgery (in some asymptomatic patients, surgery may be delayed according to circumstances):

Coronary ostial obstruction
Infection
Malignant arrhythmias
Rupture

Guidelines

NS.

Patient Information

Medlineplus

ENGLISH
http://www.nlm.nih.gov/medlineplus/aneurysms.html.

ESPANOL
http://www.nlm.nih.gov/medlineplus/spanish/aneurysms.html.

Professional Information

Review

Am J Cardiol 2007;99:1159–64. http://www.sciencedirect.com/science/article/pii/S0002914907000549.

Review

Semin Thorac Cardiovasc Surg 2006;9:165–76. http://www.sciencedirect.com/science/article/pii/S1092912606000159.

Giant Unruptured Aneurysm: Angina Pectoris

Eur Heart J 2013;34:1608. http://eurheartj.oxfordjournals.org/content/34/21/1608.

Giant Unruptured Aneurysm: Aortic Regurgitation

Heart 2013;99:972. http://heart.bmj.com/content/99/13/972.2.extract.

Long-Term Outcome Post-surgery

Ann Thorac Surg 2002;73:1466–71. http://www.annalsthoracicsurgery.org/article/S0003-4975(02)03493-8/abstract.

Rupture: Case Report

Eur Heart J 2014;35:2123. http://eurheartj.oxfordjournals.org/content/35/31/2123.

Rupture: Percutaneous Vs Surg Closure

Am J Cardiol 2015;115:392–98. http://www.sciencedirect.com/science/article/pii/S0002914914020876.

Rupture to Pericardium

Int Cardiovasc Res J 2014;8:74–7. http://www.ncbi.nlm.nih.gov/pubmed/24936486.

RVOT/Complete Heart Block/LVOT Protrusion (Case Report)

J Am Coll Cardiol 2013;61:e169–e169. http://content.onlinejacc.org/article.aspx?articleID=1667421.

RVOT Obstruction/RHF (Case Report)

Eur Heart J 2014;35:2721. http://eurheartj.oxfordjournals.org/content/35/39/2721.

Updates and More

https://clinicalguidecvd.com/sva

Chapter 88
Spontaneous Coronary Artery Dissection

ICD-10 Code

I25.4

Alternate Names/Abbreviation

SCAD

Description/Etiology [4]

- Nontraumatic nonathersclerotic coronary artery dissection in younger persons, usually females, presenting as Acute Coronary Syndrome, VF, or SCD
- May have genetic basis in persons with family history of SCAD
- Often associated with Fibromuscular Dysplasia [2]
- Likely under-diagnosed as coronary angiographic appearance may be normal

V.E. Friedewald, *Clinical Guide to Cardiovascular Disease*,
DOI 10.1007/978-1-4471-7293-2_88,
© Springer-Verlag London 2016

Predisposing/Comorbid Conditions

EHLERS-DANLOS SYNDROME [TYPE 4]
EXTREME PHYSICAL ACTIVITY [1]
FIBROMUSCULAR DYSPLASIA [2]
MARFAN SYNDROME
PERIPARTUM
POSTPARTUM
PSEUDOXANTHOMA ELASTICUM
STRESS [INTENSE]

Demography

More common in females
Age range 30–50 years

Pathophysiology

Dissection of coronary artery intima/media, often with hematoma, luminal stenosis/occlusion

Most often involves LAD coronary artery; multiple arterial dissections occur in 20–25 %

Most common first presentation: AMI (STEMI or NSTEMI, including Unstable Angina)

Signs/Symptoms [3]

ABDOMEN – PAIN
BLOOD PRESSURE, ARTERIAL – INCREASED/ELEVATED
BOWEL MOVEMENTS – DIARRHEA
BREATHING – DIFF (DYSPNEA)
BREATHING – RAPID (TACHYPNEA)
CHEST – FRICTION RUB

CHEST – PAIN
CHEST – PALPITATIONS
COUGH
EXTREM, UPPER – PAIN
FACE, JAW – PAIN
FATIGUE
FEVER
HEART, LV, APEX – MURMUR, SYS
HEART, LV, APEX, IMP – FORCEFUL/SUSTAINED
HEART, LV, APEX, IMP – PRESYS
HEART, RATE – RAPID (TACHYCARDIA)
HEART, RATE – SLOW (BRADYCARDIA)
HEART, RHYTHM – IRREG
HEART, RSB, LOWER – MURMUR, SYS
HEART, S2, SPLIT – REVERSED (PARADOXICAL)
HEART, S3 LV
HEART, S4 LV
HEART, SOUNDS, INTENSITY – DECR
HICCUPS
HYPOTENSION   (BLOOD   PRESSURE   –
   DECREASED/LOW)
JOINT, SHOULDER – PAIN
JOINT, WRIST – PAIN
MENTATION – CONFUSION
MENTATION – FEELING OF DOOM
MENTATION – WEAKNESS (MALAISE)
MOOD – ANXIOUS
MOOD – DEPRESSED
MOOD – RESTLESS/IRRITABLE/COMBATIVE
NAUSEA
NECK, ANT – PAIN
NECK, JVP – ELEV
SKIN, COLOR – BLUE (CYANOSIS)
SKIN, COLOR – PALE (PALLOR)
SKIN, TEMP – DECR
SWEATING   –   INCR   (DIAPHORESIS/
   HYPERHIDROSIS)
THROAT – PAIN/TIGHTNESS

VOMITING (EMESIS)

Differentiation

Other causes of Acute Coronary Syndrome

Complications

SCD
VF

Laboratory [3]

BLOOD, CKMB – INCR
BLOOD, ESR – INCR
BLOOD, GLUCOSE – INCR (HYPERGLYCEMIA)
BLOOD, TROPONIN – INCR
BLOOD, WBC – INCR (LEUKOCYTOSIS)

ECG [3]

DYSRHYTHMIAS – ATRIAL (PACS/OTHERS)
DYSRHYTHMIAS – VENTRICULAR (PVCS/OTHERS)
Q WAVE – ABN
QRS, AMP – DECR
RATE – DECREASED (SINUS BRADYCARDIA)
ST SEGMENT – DEPR
ST SEGMENT – ELEV
T WAVE – INVER, ABN

Imaging

[ALSO   FINDINGS   OF   FIBROMUSCULAR
    DYSPLASIA IN AFFECTED PTS]
LV, EF – DECR

LV, WALL MOTION, SEG – DECR/AKINETIC

Other Tests

Skin biopsy
Coronary angiography: dissection of single/multiple coronary arteries [6]

Treatment: Nonpharmacologic [5]

NS

Treatment: Pharmacologic [5]

NS

Treatment: Surgical/Invasive [5]

NS

Prevention

NS

Course

Long-term follow up excellent in most patients regardless of acute intervention

Notes

[1] Mainly males
[2] Mainly females

[3] Includes features of STEMI/NSTEMI

[4] Tests for Ehlers-Danlos, Pseudoxanthoma Elasticum, Fibrillin Missense Mutation, Fibrillin-1 gene transversion may be positive in some cases

[5] Insufficient data to support any standardized approach, but conservative measures and revascularization (PCI, CABG) all described

[6] Coronary artery tortuosity:

Characteristic of SCAD

Most often seen in left circumflex artery, followed by LAD, RCA

More common in nonculprit arteries

Peripartum-related SCAD may less often have coronary tortuosity

Predictor of recurrent SCAD when severe

May serve as marker or potential mechanism for SCAD

Guidelines

NS

Patient Information

AHA

http://circ.ahajournals.org/content/131/1/e3.extract?etoc.

Mayo Clinic

ENGLISH

http://www.mayoclinic.org/diseases-conditions/spontaneous-coronary-artery-dissection/basics/definition/con-20037794.

ESPANOL

http://www.mayoclinic.org/espanol.

Cleveland Clinic

http://my.clevelandclinic.org/services/heart/disorders/spontaneous-coronary-artery-dissection.

SCAD Research.Org

http://www.scadresearch.org/about/.

Professional Information

Review

Cardiovasc Diagn Ther. 2015;5:37–48. http://www.ncbi.nlm.nih.gov/pmc/articles/PMC4329168/.

Review

Am J Med. 2014;127:1160–3. http://www.sciencedirect.com/science/article/pii/S0002934314006743.

Review

Can J Cardiol. 2013;29:1027–33. http://www.sciencedirect.com/science/article/pii/S0828282X1300007X.

Review

Int J Cardiol. 2014;175:8–20. http://www.sciencedirect.com/science/article/pii/S0167527314008602.

Review

J Cardiol. 2014;63:119–22. http://www.sciencedirect.com/science/article/pii/S0914508713002207.

Case Series

Am J Cardiol. 2011;107:1590–6. http://www.sciencedirect.com/science/article/pii/S0002914911003870#.

Case Series

Circulation. 2012;126:579–88. http://circ.ahajournals.org/content/126/5/579.full?sid=f744ad4b-92e2-4475-b305-9bcd75454b76.

Classification

Catheter Cardiovasc Interv. 2014;84:1115–22. http://www.ncbi.nlm.nih.gov/pubmed/24227590.

Coronary Tortuosity

Circ Cardiovasc Interv. 2014;7:656–62. http://circinterventions.ahajournals.org/content/7/5/656.long.

Editorial

Circulation. 2012;126:667–70. http://circ.ahajournals.org/content/126/6/667.full?sid=f744ad4b-92e2-4475-b305-9bcd75454b76.

Extracoronary Vascular Abnormalities: Fibromuscular Dysplasia

Am J Cardiol. 2015;115:1672–7. http://www.ajconline.org/article/S0002-9149(15)00966-2/abstract.

Extracoronary Vascular Abnormalities

J Am Coll Cardiol. 2014;63: doi:10.1016/S0735-1097(14)62060-X. http://content.onlinejacc.org/article.aspx?articleid=1854882&res ultClick=3.

Familial Ocurrences

JAMA Intern Med. Published online March 23, 2015. doi:10.1001/ jamainternmed.2014.8307. http://archinte.jamanetwork.com/article.aspx?articleID=2204028&utm-source=Silverchair%20 Information%20Systems&utm-medium=email&utm-campaign=ArchivesofInternalMedicine%3AOnlineFirst03%2F 23%2F2015.

Imaging

J Am Coll Cardiol. 2013;61:589–9. http://content.onlinejacc.org/article.aspx?articleID=1559948.

Imaging

J Am Coll Cardiol 2013;62:350–350. http://content.onlinejacc.org/ article.aspx?articleID=1691040.

Imaging

Circulation. 2006;113:e403–5. http://circ.ahajournals.org/content/113/10/ e403.full?sid=f4b4b144-b136-423c-8a71-45fdb 84a77b7.

Imaging

Circulation. 1999;99:721. http://circ.ahajournals.org/content/99/5/721. full?sid=f4b4b144-b136-423c-8a71-45fdb84a77b7.

Imaging: Coronary CT Angiography

Heart. 2013;99:672–3. http://heart.bmj.com/content/99/9/672.extract.

Imaging/Ultrasound: Left Main Coronary Artery

Heart.   2004;90:e39.   http://heart.bmj.com/content/90/7/e39. full?sid=0432476b-943f-4df4-a992-1f43336f8096.

Long-Term Prognosis/Management

Am J Cardiol. 2015;116:66–73. http://www.ajconline.org/article/ S0002-9149(15)01045-0/abstract.

Optical Coherence Tomography

J Am Coll Cardiol. 2012;59:1073–9. http://content.onlinejacc.org/ article.aspx?articleID=1201201.

Postpartum with Phospholipid Antibody

Heart.   2004;90:e53.   http://heart.bmj.com/content/90/9/e53. full?sid=0432476b-943f-4df4-a992-1f43336f8096.

Pregnancy

Circulation.   2014;130:1915–20.   http://circ.ahajournals.org/con-tent/130/21/1915.full.

Pregnancy Risk

J   Am   Coll   Cardiol   2014;63(12-S).   doi:10.1016/S0735-1097(14)60005-X. http://content.onlinejacc.org/article.aspx?articl eid=1855046&resultClick=3.

Pregnancy: Scad During Delivery

Circulation.   2013;127:1530–5.   http://circ.ahajournals.org/content/127/14/1530.full.

Two Vessel Dissection (Case Report)

Heart. 2013;99:970. http://heart.bmj.com/content/99/13/970.2.extract.

Updates and More

https://clinicalguidecvd.com/scad

Chapter 89
Stable Ischemic Heart Disease

Management Keys

Shared decisions with patients about diagnostic and treatment choices including informing patients about options, risks, benefits, and costs

Emergency referral for evaluation/treatment of patients with high/intermediate risk unstable angina [29][30]

Diagnose/treat comorbid causes that may contribute to angina pectoris by increasing myocardial O_2 demand or decreasing myocardial O_2 supply [31][32][33][34]

Individualized education plan for patients with SIHD to optimize care/promote wellness

Assess LV function in all patients with SIHD as part of all medical, revascularization, and device-based strategies

Perform stress test as first line of evaluation for functional capacity in patients capable of exercise and have interpretable ECG

Perform coronary angiography based on clinical history and noninvasive test results, for both risk stratification and defining coronary artery anatomy for possible revascularization; not all patients especially those in low-moderate risk category, need coronary angiography

Follow current ACCF/AHA GDMT for medical versus surgical management of symptom relief and prevention of AMI and death

V.E. Friedewald, *Clinical Guide to Cardiovascular Disease*,
DOI 10.1007/978-1-4471-7293-2_89,
© Springer-Verlag London 2016

ICD-10 Code

I20.0

Alternate Names/Abbreviation

SIHD

Description/Etiology

Stable Ischemic Heart Disease: an established pattern of angina pectoris, a history of myocardial infarction, or presence of plaque documented by imaging (coronary arteriography, IVUS, CTA)

Etiology:

Atherosclerotic CAD (vast majority)
Coronary Artery Entrapment
Calcific Pericarditis
Coronary artery aneurysm
Coronary artery spasm
Congenital anomalies:

Anomalous origin of coronary artery
Coronary A-V fistula
Coronary Ostial Stenosis/Congenital Rubella Syndrome

Coronary (acquired) abnormalities:

Aortic Dissection
Chest radiation
Collagen-Vascular disease
Coronary Embolism
Coronary Extrinsic Compression
Kawasaki Disease
Syphilis

Trauma
Vasculitis
Vasculopathy
HIV
Transplant

Hereditary Disease:

Down Syndrome
Gargoylism
Homocystinuria
Oxaluria – Primary
Progeria
Pseudoxanthoma Elasticum

Angina Pectoris: initial manifestation in >50 % of SIHD patients [24]

Unstable Angina: new onset, or increases in frequency, intensity, duration; or occurring at rest [28]

Risk factors for SIHD:

DM
Family history of premature ischemic heart disease
History of Cerebrovascular disease
History of PAD
Hypercholesterolemia/dyslipidemia
Obesity/Metabolic Syndrome
Physical inactivity
Systemic Arterial Hypertension
Tobacco use

Comorbid Conditions [31] [32] [33] [34]

AMPHETAMINES
ANEMIA
ANXIETY/ANXIETY DISORDER
AORTIC SCLEROSIS
AORTIC STENOSIS – VALVULAR
ARTERIOVENOUS FISTULAE

ARTHRITIS
ASTHMA [7]
ATRIAL FIBRILLATION
CABG
CARDIOMYOPATHY – DILATED
CARDIOMYOPATHY – HYPERTROPHIC
CATARACT
CHRONIC KIDNEY DISEASE
CHRONIC OBSTRUCTIVE PULMONARY DISEASE
  (EMPHYSEMA)
COCAINE
DIABETES MELLITUS
DYSLIPIDEMIA
DYSRHYTHMIAS – ATRIAL
DYSRHYTHMIAS – VENTRICULAR
ENDOMETRIOSIS
FAMILY HX: ACUTE MYOCARDIAL INFARCTION
  [PRIOR]
FAMILY HX: ATHEROSCLEROSIS
GOUT
HEART FAILURE
HYPERCHOLESTEROLEMIA
HYPERGAMMAGLOBULINEMIA [8]
HYPERTENSION – SYSTEMIC ARTERIAL
HYPERTHERMIA
HYPERTHYROIDISM
HYPOTHYROIDISM
HYPOXEMIA
INTERSTITIAL PULMONARY FIBROSIS [7]
LEUKEMIA [8]
MICROVASCULAR DISEASE
OBSTRUCTIVE SLEEP APNEA
PERIPHERAL ARTERY DISEASE
PHEOCHROMOCYTOMA
PNEUMONIA – COMMUNITY-ACQUIRED [7]
POLYCYTHEMIA [8]
PORCELAIN AORTA [36]

PULMONARY ARTERIAL HYPERTENSION [7]
PULMONARY EMBOLISM
SICKLE CELL DISEASE/TRAIT
THROMBOCYTOSIS [8]
TOBACCO USE

Demography

Global

More common in males >age 40 years

All ethnicities

Under age 75 years, females with CAD usually present with angina pectoris; males usually present with AMI

Females lag 10 years behind males in terms of first CAD presentation

Pre-menopausal females: low risk of serious CAD manifestations such as AMI

Decreasing mortality and morbidity from CAD since 1975 due to improved preventive measures

Pathophysiology

Myocardial ischemia occurs due to myocardial O_2 demand beyond coronary blood supply, including either or combined:

Increased myocardial O_2 demand (eg, exercise)

Insufficient blood supply (eg, CAD)

Most common cause of angina: atherosclerotic plaque obstruction of epicardial coronary arteries

Stable coronary plaques characterized by thick fibrous capsule and calcification; in angina, pathology involves progressive luminal narrowing without plaque rupture (AMI usually caused by rupture of unstable plaques and subsequent acute thrombosis)

Signs/Symptoms

ABDOMEN – PAIN [25]

BLOOD PRESSURE, ARTERIAL – INCREASED/ELEVATED

BREATH SOUNDS – CRACKLES (RALES)

BREATHING – DIFF (DYSPNEA) [25]

CHEST – PAIN [2][24][28] [EFFORT – ANGINA PECTORIS]

CHEST – PALPITATIONS [3]

CHEST, POST – PAIN, NONPLEURITIC EFFORT (ANGINA PECTORIS) [5][25]

CONSCIOUSNESS – LOSS, SUDDEN (SYNCOPE) [3]

DIZZY/LIGHTHEADED/PRESYNCOPE [3]

EARS, BILAT, EARLOBE CREASE, DIAGONAL

EXTREM, UPPER – PAIN [4][25]

EXTREM, UPPER, SHOULDER – PAIN [25]

FACE, JAW – PAIN [25][26]

HEADACHE [25][26]

HEART, LV, APEX – IMP, DIFFUSE

HEART, LV, APEX – IMP, PARADOX

HEART, LV, APEX – MURMUR, SYS

HEART, S2, SPLIT – REVERSED (PARADOXICAL)

HEART, S3 LV

HEART, S4 LV

HEART, SOUNDS, INTENSITY – DECR

NECK, LAT – PAIN [25]

TEETH – PAIN [25][26]

THROAT – PAIN/TIGHTNESS [25]

Differentiation

AMI

Angina Pectoris – Unstable

Aortic Dissection

Cardiomyopathy

Cholecystitis

Congenital coronary artery anomalies
Costochondritis
Esophageal Reflux
Esophageal Spasm
Esophagitis
Fibromuscular Dysplasia
Fibrositis
Herpes Zoster [before rash]
Intervertebral Disc Disease
Myocarditis
Other causes of abdominal pain
Other causes of chest pain
Pericarditis – Acute
Psychogenic [eg, Anxiety, Hyperventilation, Panic Disorder, Depression]
Pulmonary Hypertension
Rib fracture
Sternoclavicular arthritis
Thoracic aortic aneurysm
Valvular heart disease (especially Aortic Stenosis – Valvular)

Complications

AMI
Dysrhythmias
HF
Major bleeding events
Sudden death

Laboratory

BLOOD, C-REACTIVE PROTEIN (CRP) – INCR [12]
BLOOD, CHOLESTEROL, HDL-C – DECR
BLOOD, CHOLESTEROL, LDL (LDL-C) – INCR
BLOOD, CHOLESTEROL, TOTAL – INCR

BLOOD, NT-PROBNP – INCR [12]
BLOOD, ST2 – INCR [37]
BLOOD, TGS – INCR
BLOOD, TRIGLYCERIDES – INCR
BLOOD, TROPONIN – INCR [39]

ECG

AV COND – 1ST DEGREE BLOCK [28]
AV COND – 2ND DEGEREE BLOCK [28]
AV COND – 3RD DEGREE BLOCK [28]
DYSRHYTHMIAS – ATRIAL (PACS/OTHERS) [28][ESP A FIB]
DYSRHYTHMIAS – VENTRICULAR (PVCS/OTHERS)
Q WAVE – ABN [27][28]
QRS – LBBB/LBBB PATTERN [28]
QRS – LVH PATTERN [28]
QRS – RBBB/RBBB PATTERN [28]
QT/QTC INTERVAL – LONG
ST SEGMENT – DEPR
ST-T WAVE – ABN, NS
T WAVE – INVER, ABN
T WAVE – NORMALIZATION
T WAVE – TALL/PEAKED
U WAVE – NEG

Imaging

ART, CAROTID, IMT – INCR
ART, CORONARY – CALCIUM
ART, CORONARY – LESION, OBS [9]
AV, LEAFLETS – CALCIUM
AV, LEAFLETS – THICK
LV, DIAS – DYSF
LV, EF – DECR

LV, SYS – DYSF
LV, WALL MOTION – DECR
LV, WALL MOTION, SEG – DECR/AKINETIC
MYOCARD, PERFUSION – DECR

Other Tests

Exercise ECG test
Exercise test with echo/nuclear MPI [10]
Pharmacological stress test with CMR
Pharmacological stress test with echo/nuclear MPI [10]
Coronary CT angiography
Coronary calcium scoring
CMR angiography
Coronary angiography
Doppler/echo assessment for:

> Abnormalities of heart valves
> Abnormalities of myocardium
> Abnormalities of pericardium
> LV systolic and diastolic function

Treatment – Nonpharmacologic [1] [15]

Patient education
Self-monitoring [13]
Lifestyle modification, including:

> Diet
> Physical activity
> Stress/depression counseling
> Weight loss/control

Cardiac rehabilitation program
Tobacco cessation
Substance abuse counseling (when applicable)

Treatment – Pharmacologic [1] [15] [40]

Prevent AMI/death

Antiplatelet Agents [16]

ASA
Clopidogrel

Beta-Blockers
RAAS Blockers [17]

ACEIs
ARBs

Symptom (angina) relief

Beta-blockers
CCBs
NTG
Ranolazine [22]
Ivabradine
Nicorandil [18]
Trimetazidine [21] [22]

Influenza vaccine

Treatment – Surgical/Invasive [1] [15]

Revascularization to improve survival – left main coronary artery obstruction

CABG
PCI

Revascularization to improve survival – non-left main coronary artery obstruction

CABG
PCI

Revascularization to improve symptoms

> CABG
> PCI

Refractory angina

> Coronary sinus reduction (investigational)
> Enhanced external counterpulsation
> Spinal cord stimulation
> Transmyocardial revascularization (controversial)

Prevention

> Atherosclerosis risk factor modification
> Statins (primary prevention)
> Control of comorbidities
>
> > DM
> > Systemic Arterial Hypertension

Course

> CAD progression may occur in absence of changes in angina character/frequency [19]

Notes

[1] Drug and interventional treatment data and outcome measures are highly dynamic, and current guidelines should be consulted for specific therapies
[2] Frequency, duration not increasing
[3] Due to arrhythmia
[4] Ulnar aspect, left more common than right
[5] Interscapular area
[6] Younger ages may occur, especially with strong risk factors

[7] Via hypoxia, usually with underlying coronary atherosclerosis

[8] Via increased blood viscosity, with/without underlying coronary atherosclerosis

[9] Multislice CCTA: high degree of concordance with coronary angiography

[10] According to current ACC/AHA guidelines: recommended for patients with intermediate-high pretest probability of ischemic heart disease with uninterpretable ECG and at least moderate physical functioning or no disabling comorbidity; pharmacologic stress test for patients who cannot exercise and patients with baseline LBBB

[11] Gender and ethnicity NS for risk

[12] Correlates with prognosis, along with other biomarkers

[13] Eg, record home BP, glucose, calorie intake, exercise

[14] Moderate-high dose in absence of contraindications or proven adverse effects

[15] Does not include treatment for comorbid conditions, which should also be addressed for optimal outcomes [31–34]

[16] ASA 75–162 mg/day or clopidogrel 75 mg/day; clinical trials of prasugrel and ticagrelor in patients with stable CAD have not been conducted; due to major bleeding risk, caution when used beyond 1 year after acute coronary event

[17] Especially patients with Systemic Arterial Hypertension, DM, LVEF ≤40 %, CKD

[18] Nitrate derivative that may be added after beta-blockers and CCBS; not FDA-approved

[19] Risk assessment for disease progression:

> Socioeconomic: advancing age, low income level
>
> CV risk factors: tobacco use, Systemic Arterial Hypertension, Dyslipidemia, FH premature CAD, obesity, sedentary lifestyle
>
> Coexisting medical conditions: DM, CKD, COPD, Cancer
>
> CV comorbidities: HF, PAD, cerebrovascular disease

Psychosocial: depression, poor social support, poverty, stress

Health status: symptoms, functional capacity, QOL

[20] COURAGE Trial
[21] Anti-ischemic metabolic modulator
[22] Improves glycemic indices in pts with DM
[23] Some genetic diseases cause accelerated atherosclerosis (eg, Down Syndrome) and others may be associated with congenital coronary artery anomalies
[24] Angina pectoris: initial clinical manifestation in at least 50 % of patients with SIHD; incidence rises continuously with age in females; peaks at age 55–65 years in males, then declines; true incidence may be greater than reported; rather than pain, angina often described as squeezing, grip-like, suffocating, heaviness, tightness, pressure
[25] May occur associated with anterior chest pain or in isolation, sometimes termed "atypical angina", more common in females and persons of advanced age
[26] Headache/craniofacial angina associated with inferior wall myocardial ischemia
[27] Abnormal Q wave presence indicates prior AMI, often silent, especially in patients with DM
[28] Indicator of worse long-term outcomes and may warrant more aggressive treatment
[29] Patients with unstable angina and high risk should receive emergency evaluation and treatment; high risk features include one or more of:

Accelerating ischemic symptoms in prior 48 h
Prolonged pain (<20 min rest)
Pulmonary edema
New/worsening MR murmur
New S3 or worsening rales
Hypotension, bradycardia, tachycardia
Age >75 years
Angina at rest with transient ECG ST segment changes >0.5 mm

BBB: new/presumed new
Sustained VT
Elevated cardiac troponin or CKMB

[30] Patients with unstable angina and intermediate risk unstable angina include one or more of the following (no high risk features present):

Prior AMI, Cerebrovasc disease, PAD, CABG
Prior ASA use
Prolonged rest angina (>20 min) with high likelihood of CAD
Rest angina relieved by TNG
Nocturnal angina
New-onset/progressive class III/IV angina in prior 2 weeks without prolonged pain but intermediate/high likelihood of CAD
ECG T wave changes
ECG pathological Q waves or resting ST depression >1 mm in multiple lead groups
Slight elevation of cardiac troponin or CK-MB

[31] Noncardiac comorbid diseases that may contribute to angina pectoris by increasing myocardial O_2 demand include:

Anxiety
Arteriovenous Fistulae
Hyperthermia
Hyperthyroidism
Sympathomimetic Toxicity (eg, cocaine)
Systemic Arterial Hypertension

[32] Cardiac comorbid diseases that may contribute to angina pectoris by increasing myocardial O_2 demand include:

Aortic Stenosis
Dilated Cardiomyopathy
Hypertrophic Cardiomyopathy
Tachycardia (Supraventricular/Ventricular)

[33] Noncardiac comorbid diseases that may contribute to angina pectoris by decreasing myocardial O_2 supply include:

> Anemia
> Asthma
> Chronic Obstructive Pulmonary Disease
> Hypergammaglobulinemia
> Hyperviscosity
> Hypoxemia
> Interstitial Pulmonary Fibrosis
> Obstructive Sleep Apnea
> Pneumonia
> Polycythemia

>> Leukemia
>> Thrombocytosis

> Pulmonary Arterial Hypertension
> Sickle Cell Disease
> Sympathomimetic   toxicity   (cocaine   use,
>> Pheochromocytoma)

[34] Cardiac comorbidities that may contribute to angina pectoris by decreasing myocardial O_2 supply include:

> Aortic Stenosis
> Coronary microvascular disease
> Hypertrophic Cardiomyopathy
> Significant coronary arterial obstruction

[35] Rare but independent predictor of death
[36] Circumferential calcification of ascending aorta due to atherosclerosis; may complicate CABG
[37] Increased ST2 may be long-term predictor of mortality outcome in stable CAD
[38] GWAS studies identifying tag SNPS in loci associated with these genes indicate possible importance in patients with CAD
[39] Baseline troponin elevation associated with increased incidence in subsequent cardiac events and mortality

[40] Optimal medical therapy proven to be as efficacious as revascularization for CAD, but has low rate of utilization

Guidelines

2012 ACCF/AHA/ACP/AATS/PCNA/SCAI/STS guideline for the diagnosis and management of patients with stable ischemic heart disease

Circulation.   2012;126:3097–137.   http://circ.ahajournals.org/content/126/25/3097.full?sid=2bbd9e2d-4dac-4385-9933-804f79b92187.

2014 focused update of ACCF/AHA/ACP/AATS/PCNA/SCAI/STS guideline for the diagnosis and management of patients with stable ischemic heart disease

Circulation.   2014;130:1749–67.   http://circ.ahajournals.org/content/130/19/1749.full.

2013 ESC guidelines on the management of stable coronary artery disease

Eur Heart J 2013;34:2949–3003. http://www.escardio.org/guidelines-surveys/esc-guidelines/Pages/stable-angina-pectoris.aspx.

2013 ACC/AHA guideline on the treatment of blood cholesterol to reduce atherosclerotic cardiovascular risk in adults

J Am Coll Cardiol. 2013. pii: S0735-1097(13)06028-2. doi: 10.1016/j.jacc.2013.11.002.   http://www.sciencedirect.com/science/article/pii/S0735109713060282.

ACC/AHA 2013 guidelines on cardiovascular risk assessment

J Am Coll Cardiol 2013. pii: S0735-1097(13)06031-2. doi: 10.1016/j.jacc.2013.11.005. [Epub ahead of print]. http://www.sciencedirect.com/science/article/pii/S0735109713060312.

Patient Information

AHA: TNG/Exercise

Circulation.   2013;127:e642–5.   http://circ.ahajournals.org/content/127/22/e642.full.

Medlineplus

ENGLISH
http://www.nlm.nih.gov/medlineplus/angina.html.

ESPANOL
http://www.nlm.nih.gov/medlineplus/spanish/angina.html.

Genetics Home Reference

http://ghr.nlm.nih.gov/glossary=angina.

Cleveland Clinic

http://my.clevelandclinic.org/heart/disorders/cad/cadsymptoms.aspx.

Professional Information

AHA scientific statement: preventing and experiencing ischemic heart disease as a woman: state of the science. Circulation. 2016;133:1302–31. http://circ.ahajournals.org/content/133/13/1302.full.

AHA Scientific Statement: Genomics

Circ Cardiovasc Genet. 2015;8:216–42. http://circgenetics.ahajournals.org/content/8/1/216.

AHA/ACC/ASH Scientific Statement: Hypertension Treatment in Patients with CAD

Hypertension. 2015;65:1372–407. http://hyper.ahajournals.org/content/65/6/1372.full.

Review

N Engl J Med. 2005;352:2524–33. http://www.nejm.org/doi/full/10.1056/NEJMcp042317.

Review: Intracoronary Imaging

Eur Heart J. 2016;37:524–35. http://eurheartj.oxfordjournals.org/content/37/6/524.abstract?etoc.

Angina due to Annomalous Origin of All 3 Coronary RTS from R Coronary Cusp

Br J Cardiol. 2015;22:39. http://bjcardio.co.uk/2015/02/anomalous-coronary-artery-origin-all-three-arising-from-right-coronary-cusp-from-separate-ostia/.

Aortic Sclerosis: Effects on CABG Outcomes

Heart. 2013;99:247–52. http://heart.bmj.com/content/99/4/247.full.

ASA: Question of Necessity (Editorial)

J Am Coll Cardiol. 2014;64:1437–40. http://content.onlinejacc.org/article.aspx?articleID=1910601.

ASA: Low Dose

N Engl J Med. 2005;353:2373–83. http://www.nejm.org/doi/full/10.1056/NEJMra052717.

Beta-Blockers: Outcomes

Heart. 2014;100:1757–61. http://heart.bmj.com/content/100/22/1757.abstract.

Biomarkers and Risk

Circulation. 2012;125:233–40. http://circ.ahajournals.org/content/125/2/233.full?sid=93b795eb-05ca-494e-bb4a-a096ae2dcfa0.

Biomarkers and Risk

Eur Heart J. 2010;31:3024–31. http://eurheartj.oxfordjournals.org/content/31/24/3024.full.

Bleeding Events (Major)

J Am Coll Cardiol. 2014;64:1430–6. http://content.onlinejacc.org/article.aspx?articleID=1910598.

CABG: History/Evolution

Eur Heart J. 2013;34:2862–72. http://eurheartj.oxfordjournals.org/content/34/37/2862.

CABG: Optimizing Outcomes

Eur Heart J. 2013;34:2873–86. http://eurheartj.oxfordjournals.org/content/34/37/2873.

Calcific Pericarditis

Circulation. 2013;128:e30–1. http://circ.ahajournals.org/content/128/3/e30.full.

Cardiac Symptoms Before Death due to CAD

Heart. 2013;99:938–43. http://heart.bmj.com/content/99/13/938.abstract.

Chronic Kidney Disease

Circulation. 2016;133:518–36. http://circ.ahajournals.org/content/133/5/518.full.

Chronic Kidney Disease

Clin J Am Soc Nephrol. 2009;4:1892–900. http://cjasn.asnjournals.org/content/4/12/1892.long.

Coronary Anomaly: LAD-Circumflex (Case Report)

Circulation. 2013;127:2465–6. http://circ.ahajournals.org/content/127/24/2465.full.

Coronary Arterial External Compression: Giant PA Aneurysm (Case Report)

Circulation. 2013;127:1340–1. http://circ.ahajournals.org/content/127/12/1340.full.

Coronary Ostial Compression: Fibrosing Mediastinitis

J Am Coll Cardiol. 2013;62:163–4. http://content.onlinejacc.org/article.aspx?articleID=1681790.

Coronary Ostial Stenosis/Congenital Rubella Syndrome

Circulation.   2013;128:2542–5.   http://circ.ahajournals.org/content/128/23/2542.full.

Coronary Sinus Aneurysm (Case Report)

Eur Heart J. 2016;37:144. http://eurheartj.oxfordjournals.org/content/37/2/144.

Coronary Sinus Reduction: Refractory Angina

N Engl J Med. 2015;372:519–27. http://www.nejm.org/doi/full/10.1056/NEJMoa1402556#t=article.

CCTA in Emergency Dept

N Engl J Med. 2012; 366:1393–403. http://www.nejm.org/doi/full/10.1056/NEJMoa1201163?query=featured-home#t=article.

CCTA in Emergency Dept

J Am Coll Cardiol. 2013;61:880–92. http://content.onlinejacc.org/article.aspx?articleid=1569174.

CT Angio: Plaque Characteristics

J Am Coll Cardiol Img. 2015;8:1–10. http://imaging.onlinejacc.org/article.aspx?articleID=2089124.

Diabetes Mellitus: Accelerated Atherosclerosis

Heart.   2013;99:743–9.   http://heart.bmj.com/content/99/10/743.extract.

Diabetes Mellitus: Angina Presence/Absence and Outcomes (BARI 2D)

J Am Coll Cardiol. 2013;61:702–11. http://content.onlinejacc.org/article.aspx?articleID=1570009.

Diabetes Mellitus: Intensive Glucose Control (ADA/ACCF/AHA Scientific Statement)

Circulation.   2009;119:351–7.   http://circ.ahajournals.org/content/119/2/351.full.

Diabetes Mellitus: Ranolazine

J Am Coll Cardiol. 2013;61:2038–45. http://content.onlinejacc.org/article.aspx?articleid=1666389&resultClick=3.

Diabetes Mellitus: Revascularization

Circulation.   2013;128:1675–85.   http://circ.ahajournals.org/content/128/15/1675.full.

Diabetes Mellitus: Revascularization

Circ Cardiovasc Interv. 2015;8:e001944. http://circinterventions.aha-journals.org/content/8/4/e001944.full.

Endometriosis

CircOutcomes. 2016;115.002224 doi: 10.1161/CIRCOUT COMES.115.002224. http://circoutcomes.ahajournals.org/content/early/2016/03/29/CIRCOUTCOMES.115.002224.abstract.

Enhanced External Counterpulsation

J Am Coll Cardiol. 1999;33:1833–40. http://content.onlinejacc.org/article.aspx?articleID=1125829.

Exercise

Am J Med. 2014;127:905–11. http://www.sciencedirect.com/science/article/pii/S0002934314003933.

Exercise: Cardiac Rehabilitation

Am J Med. 2004;116:682–92. http://www.sciencedirect.com/science/article/pii/S0002934304001238.

Genetic CAD Risk Prediction

Eur Heart J. 2016;37:561–7. http://eurheartj.oxfordjournals.org/content/37/6/561.full?etoc.

Genetics

Circulation. 2013;128:1131–8. http://circ.ahajournals.org/content/128/10/1131.full.

Gout: Increased CAD Risk

Ann Rheum Dis.2015;74:642–7. http://ard.bmj.com/content/74/4/642.full.

Headache/Craniofacial Pain due to Myocard Ischemia

J Oral Facial Pain Headache. 2014;28:317–21. http://www.ncbi.nlm.nih.gov/pubmed/25347166.

HIV and Subclinical CAD

Ann Intern Med. 2014;160:458–67. http://annals.org/article.aspx?articleid=1852867.

Hypertension: Treatment (AHA Scientific Statement)

Circulation. 2007;115:2761–88. http://circ.ahajournals.org/content/115/21/2761.full.

Inflammation and Myocardial Ischemia

Br J Cardiol. 2015;22:101–4. http://bjcardio.co.uk/2015/08/inflammation-is-associated-with-myocardial-ischaemia/.

Influenza Vaccination (ACC/AHA Science Advisory)

J Am Coll Cardiol. 2006;48:1498–502. http://content.onlinejacc.org/article.aspx?articleID=1137967.

Imaging

Ann Intern Med. 2015;162:474–84. http://annals.org/article.aspx?articleid=2214175.

Intermittent Coronary Sinus Occlusion

Heart. 2013;99:548–55. http://heart.bmj.com/content/99/8/548.abstract.

Ivabradine

Heart. 2014;100:160–6. http://heart.bmj.com/content/100/2.toc.

Ivabradine

N Engl J Med. 2014;371:1091–9. http://www.nejm.org/doi/full/10.1056/NEJMoa1406430.

Medical Therapy

Br J Cardiol. 2011;18(Suppl 3):s1–12. http://bjcardio.co.uk/2011/10/the-medical-management-of-stable-angina/.

Medical Therapy: Courage Trial

N Engl J Med. 2007;356:1503–16. http://www.nejm.org/doi/full/10.1056/NEJMoa070829.

Medical Therapy: Courage Trial

N Engl J Med 2008;359:677–87. http://www.nejm.org/doi/full/10.1056/NEJMoa072771.

Medical Therapy: Pentaerithrityl Tetranitrate

Eur Heart J. 2014;35:895–903. http://eurheartj.oxfordjournals.org/content/35/14/895.

NSAID Risk: AMI

Am J Med. 2014;127:53–60. http://www.sciencedirect.com/science/article/pii/S0002934313007717.

Optimal Medical Theapy and Outcomes

Am J Cardiol. 2015;116:671–7. http://www.ajconline.org/issue/S0002-9149(14)X0040-8.

PCI: Fractional Flow Reserve-Guided

N Engl J Med. 2014;371:1208–17. http://www.nejm.org/doi/full/10.1056/NEJMoa1408758.

PCI: QOL

Circulation. 1995;92:1710–9. http://circ.ahajournals.org/content/92/7/1710.full?sid=37277ff5-fc6a-4076-926b-80ddb1140218.

PCI Versus Optimal Medical Therapy

Circulation. 2013;127:769–81. http://circ.ahajournals.org/content/127/7/769.abstract.

Physical Activity

Eur Heart J. 2013;34:3286–93. http://eurheartj.oxfordjournals.org/content/34/42/3286.

Porcelain Aorta

Circulation. 2015;131:827–36. http://circ.ahajournals.org/content/131/9/827.extract?etoc.

Post-traumatic Stress Disorder

J Am Coll Cardiol. 2013;62:970–8. http://content.onlinejacc.org/article.aspx?articleID=1709455.

Post-traumatic Stress Disorder

Am J Cardiol. 2011;108:29–33. http://www.ncbi.nlm.nih.gov/pubmed/21530936.

RAAS Inhibitors: Outcomes

Eur Heart J. 2014;35:1760–8. http://eurheartj.oxfordjournals.org/content/35/26/1760.

Ranolazine: Terisa Trial

J Am Coll Cardiol. 2013;61:2038–45. http://content.onlinejacc.org/article.aspx?articleID=1666389.

Refractory Angina Pectoris: Outcomes

Eur Heart J. 2013;34:2683–8. http://eurheartj.oxfordjournals.org/content/34/34/2683.abstract.

Spinal Cord Stimulation

Am J Cardiol. 2003;9:951–5. http://www.sciencedirect.com/science/article/pii/S0002914903001103.

Statins

N Engl J Med. 2005;352:1425–35. http://www.nejm.org/doi/full/10.1056/NEJMoa050461#t=article.

Statins

Lancet. 2010;376:1670–81. http://www.sciencedirect.com/science/article/pii/S0140673610613505.

Statins: High-Dose Therapy

Circulation. 2013;127:2485–93. http://circ.ahajournals.org/content/127/25/2485.full.

ST2 Increase: Long-Term Predictor

Clin Chem. 2014;60:530–40. http://www.clinchem.org/content/60/3/530.full.

Troponin

N Engl J Med. 2015;373:610–20. http://www.nejm.org/doi/full/10.1056/NEJMoa1415921.

Weather: Effects of Temperature Extremes on Outcomes

Heart. 2013;99:195–203. http://heart.bmj.com/content/99/3/195.abstract.

Updates and More

https://clinicalguidecvd.com/sihd

Chapter 90
Stroke: Ischemic

Management Keys

PREHOSPITAL
Early recognition by patient/non-professional observers of sudden: [1]

Arm weakness
Dizziness
Facial weakness (facial droop)
Severe headache
Slurred speech
Visual loss

Call 911 when stroke suspected [2]
Prehospital recognition of possible stroke by EMS [See APPENDIX A]
Prehospital interventions/management

Establish IV line [5]
Maintain O_2 saturation >94 %
Hypotension: place head on stretcher flat/isotonic saline
Hypertension: consult with medical control if systolic BP >220 mmHg
Glucose <60 mg/dL: IV glucose [5]
No delay in transport for interventions
Obtain family/bystander information regarding:

V.E. Friedewald, *Clinical Guide to Cardiovascular Disease*,
DOI 10.1007/978-1-4471-7293-2_90,
© Springer-Verlag London 2016

Time of symptom onset (last time patient was normal) [3]
Seizure activity
Trauma
Medications/recent surgery

EMS transport to nearest Primary Stroke/Comprehensive
Stroke Center
EMS advance notification of hospital [4]

HOSPITAL
Timely emergency department care with same priority as
patients with AMI/serious trauma regardless of neurological deficit severity
Hospitalization for:

Observation for changes that might prompt added
treatment interventions
Observation/decrease likelihood of bleeding post-rtPA
Prevention of complications
Begin long-term treatment to prevent stroke
recurrence
Begin rehabilitation

Admit (consider) to neurocritical care unit for:

Severe neurological deficit
Large volume infarcts with potential for significant
cerebral edema
Significant comorbidities
Blood pressure difficult to control
Prior IV/intraarterial recanalization interventions

Perform complete CT to rule out hemorrhage before rtPA
administration [33]
Early fibrinolytic Rx within 4.5 h of last time patient
known to be well [28][31]
Strict adherence to guidelines/protocols for rtPA adminis-
tration/post-lysis management due to high (6 %) risk of
intracranial hemorrhage
Consider intra-arterial thrombectomy for select patient
subsets; this should not affect usage of rtPA [30][31]

Monitor for short/long-term complications

Early ambulation

Begin intensive speech/physical/occupational treatment as soon as patient able to participate

Lifestyle changes/medical treatment/appropriate revascularization for secondary prevention of recurrent stroke/other forms of atherosclerotic CVD

ICD-10 Code

I63.9

Alternate Names/Abbreviation

Cerebrovascular accident (CVA)

Wallenberg syndrome (Lateral medullary syndrome) [27]

Description/Etiology

Stroke: acute loss of neurological function due to abnormal brain tissue perfusion; two types:

Ischemic (87 %)

Hemorrhagic (13 %)

Classification:

Large-artery atherosclerosis

Basilar

Internal carotid

Other branches of circle of Willis

Vertebral

Vessel-vessel atheroembolism (eg, carotid to cerebral artery)

Cardiac embolism, including:

AF
Cardiac myxomas
Paradoxical from venous system through congenital
   shunt
Severe LV dysfunction
Valvular fibroelastomas

Small vessel disease, often associated with vascular
damage due to: [25]

DM
Dyslipidemia
Systemic Arterial Hypertension
Tobacco use

Stroke of other determined etiology, including:

Coagulopathies
Genetic disease
Metabolic disease
Vasculopathies

Stroke of undetermined etiology (diagnosis of exclusion)

Predisposing/Comorbid Conditions

ANKYLOSING SPONDYLITIS
AORTIC DISSECTION
ATRIAL FIBRILLATION [34]
ATRIOVENTRICULAR HEART BLOCK
CARDIOMYOPATHY – DILATED
CARDIOMYOPATHY – HYPERTROPHIC
CAROTID ARTERY STENOSIS
COCAINE
CORONARY ARTERY DISEASE
DIABETES MELLITUS
DYSLIPIDEMIA
FABRY DISEASE [MAY OCCUR AT YOUNG AGE]

FH: STROKE
GOUT
HEART FAILURE
HERPES VIRUS INFECTION [36]
HYPERCOAGULATION STATES
HYPERTENSION – SYSTEMIC ARTERIAL
INFECTIVE ENDOCARDITIS
MYXOMA – LEFT ATRIUM
MYXOMA – LEFT VENTRICLE
PERIPHERAL ARTERY DISEASE
PSORIASIS
RHEUMATIC DISEASES [37]
RHEUMATOID ARTHRITIS
SICKLE CELL DISEASE/TRAIT
SYSTEMIC LUPUS ERYTHEMATOSUS
TAKAYASU ARTERITIS
TOBACCO USE

Demography

Increased in persons:

Age >55 years
Blacks
Males

Pathophysiology

Ischemic stroke: obstruction/occlusion of:

Anterior cerebral artery

Frontal pole
Mesial frontal pole

Anterior cerebellar artery

Lateral pontine

Middle cerebral artery

> Parietal lobe
> Posterior frontal lobe
> Temporal lobe

Posterior cerebral artery

> Occipital lobe

Posterior inferior cerebellar artery [27]

> Lateral medulla

Vertebral artery [27]

> Lateral medulla
> Medial medulla

Signs/Symptoms [Appendix A]

BLOOD PRESSURE, ARTERIAL – INCREASED/ ELEVATED [15]
COGNITION – DEFECT, NS
COGNITION, COMMAND RESPONSE – DECR
CONSCIOUSNESS – ALTERED [DROWSY/ OBTUNDED]
CONSCIOUSNESS – LOSS, PROLONGED (COMA)
CONSCIOUSNESS – LOSS, SUDDEN (SYNCOPE) [38]
DIZZY/LIGHTHEADED/PRESYNCOPE [38]
EARS, BILAT, EARLOBE CREASE, DIAGONAL
EXTREM – NUMB, FOCAL
EXTREM, UNILAT, SENSORY – DECR/ABSENT
EXTREM, UPPER – ARM DRIFT [29]
EYES, GAZE – DECR/ABS (GAZE PALSY)
EYES, MOTION – DECR/PARALYZED (OPHTHALMOPLEGIA)
EYES, MOTION – JERKY (NYSTAGMUS)
EYES, VISION – DECR/LOSS
FACE – HORNER SYNDROME
FACE – PAIN (UNILATERAL)

FACE – SENSORY (PAIN/TEMP) – DECR/ABSENT
FACE, MUSCLES, UNILAT – WEAK/PARALYZED
  (FACIAL DROOPING)
FALL [38]
FEVER [14]
GAIT – UNSTEADY (ATAXIA)
HEADACHE
HICCUPS
HYPOTENSION   (BLOOD   PRESSURE   –
  DECREASED/LOW) [20] RARE
MENTATION – ATTENTION – IMPAIRED/ABSENT
MENTATION – CONFUSION [26]
MENTATION – DISORIENTED [26] [38]
MENTATION,   CALCULATING   –   ABSENT
  (ACALCULIA)
MENTATION,DECISION-MAKING – DECR/ABSENT
  (ABULIA) [ESP FRONTAL LOBE INVOLV]
MENTATION, READING – ABSENT (ALEXIA)
MENTATION, WRITING – ABSENT (AGRAPHIA)
MOOD – LETHARGIC [38]
MUSCLES – WEAK, FOCAL
MUSCLES – QUADRIPLEGIA [PONS INFARCT;
  PROGRESSIVE]
MUSCLES, MOVEMENT – UNCOORDINATED
  (ATAXIA)
MUSCLES, MOVEMENT – UNCOORDINATED
  (ATAXIA)
MUSCLES, MOVEMENT – UNCOORDINATED
  (DYSMETRIA) [38]
MUSCLES, UNILAT – WEAK/PARALYSIS
  (HEMIPARESIS/HEMIPLEGIA)
NAUSEA
SEIZURES [38] [ESP AT ONSET]
SPEECH – DISTURBED/ABSENT (DYSPHASIA/
  APHASIA)
SPEECH – INARTICULATE (DYSARTHRIA)
SWALLOWING – DIFFICULT (DYSPHAGIA)

TONGUE – WEAKNESS [ESP VERTEBRAL/ MEDULLA]
VOMITING (EMESIS)

Differentiation

CNS abscess [6]
CNS tumor [7]
Conversion disorder
Drug toxicity, including:

> Carbamazine
> Lithium
> Phenytoin

Electrolyte disturbance
Hypertensive encephalopathy [8]
Hypoglycemia [9]
Hyperglycemia
Meningitis/encephalitis
Migraine/auras
Multiple sclerosis exacerbation
Other causes of acute focal neurological deficits
Other causes of coma
Other causes of seizures
Peripheral Vertigo
Psychogenic [11]
Seizure
Sepsis
Subdural hemorrhage
Wernickes Encephalopathy [10]

Complications

Acute Pulmonary Embolism
AMI
Bleeding post-rtPA
Cerebral edema/brain herniation
Cognitive decline

Decubitus ulcer
DVT
GI ulcers/bleeding
Hemorrhagic transformation of infarct
Pneumonia/aspiration pneumonitis
Seizures
Spasticity
Stroke progression/expansion/recurrence

Laboratory

BLOOD, GLUCOSE – DECR (HYPOGLYCEMIA) [16]
[RARE]
BLOOD, GLUCOSE – INCR (HYPERGLYCEMIA)
[17][COMMON]

Imaging [12][13][33]

ART, BASILAR, FLOW – OBS [32]
ART, BASILAR, LESION – OBS [32]
ART, CAROTID, FLOW – OBS
ART, CEREBRAL, FLOW – OBS [32]
ART, CEREBRAL, LESION – OBS [32]
ART, VERTEBRAL, FLOW – OBS
ART, VERTEBRAL, LESION – OBS
BRAIN, CEREBRUM – ISCHEMIA/INFARCT
BRAIN, CEREBRUM, REGIONAL PERFUSION –
DECR/ABSENT

Other Tests

Brain angiography: superior to noninvasive imaging for:

Arterial narrowing at specific sites
Identifying nonatherosclerotic disease, including:

Dissection
Fibromuscular dysplasia
Moyomoya disease
Vasculitis

Planning surgical/endovascular procedures

Cardiac monitoring: continuous for at least 24 h

Treatment: Nonpharmacologic [24]

Endotracheal intubation:

When airway threatened
With mechanical ventilatory assist in management of
elevated intracranial pressure/malignant brain edema

IV fluids: [21]

Avoid hypervolemia
Glucose [16]
Maintenance fluids only unless hypovolemic, as excess
fluids may cause/exacerbate:

Brain ischemia
Renal insufficiency
Thrombosis

Patient position [19]

Non-hypoxic: supine
Hypoxic: upright
Risk for airway obstruction/aspiration, possible elevated intracranial pressure: head of bed elevated
$15°–30°$ (with frequent monitoring of airway, O_2,
neurological status)

Supplemental O_2: maintain pO_2 >94 % [18]

Treatment: Pharmacologic [24]

Anticoagulants: [23]

Unfractionated heparin
Low molecular weight heparins/danaparoid

Antiplatelet agents/anticoagulants – oral (contraindicated during first 24 h after IV rtPA)

ASA
Clopidogrel

Antiplatelet agents – IV: contraindicated during first 24 h after IV rtPA
Fibrinolysis – IV rtPA [22] [28][31]
Fibrinolysis – intra-arterial (eg, alteplase): consideration for patients ineligible for IV rtPA [22] [28] [31]
Thrombin inhibitors: alternative to anticoagulants

Dabigatran

Blood pressure control [15]
Hyperthermia: ASA/acetaminophen

Treatment: Surgical/Invasive [24]

Acute angioplasty/stenting: usefulness not established

Extracranial
Intracranial

Acute carotid endarterectomy: usefulness not established
Intra-arterial thrombectomy/mechanical clot disruption/ extraction: [30] [31] [35]

Merci Retrivel System
Penumbra System
Solitaire
Trevo

Prevention

Primary

Anticoagulation for patients with AF
ASA (high risk pts)
Carotid Artery Stenosis (asymp)

Aggressive treatment of all atherosclerotic risk factors
ASA unless contraindicated
Cartotid endarterectomy/angioplasty/stent considered in select patients

Hypertension control (with stricter control in patients with DM)
Lipid control (including statins for high risk patients, eg, those with CAD)
Physical activity
Tobacco cessation

Secondary

Risk factor reduction

Lifestyle
Medications

Anticoagulation for AF
Carotid revascularization for symptomatic Carotid Stenosis

Course

Most functional recovery occurs within 3 months
1-year mortality after first stroke:

Age 40–69 years: 14–24 %
Age >69 years: 22–27 %

Notes

[1] Effective/repetitive public education about these features is essential and proven effective

[2] EMS involvement results in shorter pre-hospital delays/earlier diagnostic testing (CT/MRI)

[3] Needed information for possible fibrinolytic therapy

[4] Shortens time to be seen by ER physician/brain imaging/increased use of IV rtPA alteplase

[5] Caution: avoid excess IV fluids

[6] Suspect in patients with:

> History of drug abuse
> Endocarditis
> Medical device implant with fever

[7] Suspect in patients with:

> Gradual symptom progression
> Other primary malignancy
> Seizure at onset

[8] Suspect in patients with:

> Cerebral edema
> Cortical blindness
> Delirium
> Headache
> Seizure
> Severe hypertension

[9] Suspect in patients with:

> Decreased level of consciousness
> DM
> Low serum glucose

[10] Suspect in patients with:

> Ataxia
> Confusion
> History of alcohol abuse
> Ophthalmoplegia

[11] Suspect in patients with:

> Inconsistent physical findings
> Lack of objective cranial nerve findings
> Neurological findings in nonvascular distribution

[12] Brain intracranial imaging studies performed to detect:

> Bleeding
> Cerebral hemodynamic status
> Degree of possible reversibility
> Fibrinolysis contraindications
> Infarct location
> Infarct size
> Infarct vascular distribution
> Large vessel occlusion
> Stroke severity

[13] Brain extracranial imaging studies performed to detect obstruction amenable to revascularization

[14] Hyperthermia present in about 1/3 and associated with poor neurological outcome; primary/secondary causes of fever should be sought, including:

> Infective Endocarditis
> Pneumonia
> Sepsis
> Urinary tract infection

[15] Increased arterial pressure common in acute stroke (>75 %), especially patients with history of hypertension; typically spontaneously decreases within 90 min of onset; extreme hypertension detrimental, causing encephalopathy, cardiac dysfunction, renal insufficiency

> Optimal BP during Acute Ischemic Stroke has not been established; ideal BP range likely depends on stroke subtype and individual patient comorbidities

[16] Hypoglycemia: rare in acute stroke and should be treated (when <60 mg/dL) as soon as detected as may cause autonomic/neurological symptoms/seizures/permanent brain damage

[17] Hyperglycemia: occurs in >40 % of patients (especially those with DM); due to nonfasting state/stress; associated with worse outcomes; no evidence that targeting specific glucose levels for treatment improves outcomes and aggressive treatment carries risk of hypoglycemia, which should be avoided

[18] Hypoxia: occurs in in >60 % of pts within 48 h of onset (100 % of pts with history of cardiac/pulmonary disease); due to:

> Aspiration
> Atelectasis
> Hypoventilation
> Partial airway obstruction
> Pneumonia

[19] Patient position affects:

> Cerebral perfusion pressure
> Intracranial pressure
> O_2 saturation
> MCA mean flow velocity

[20] Hypotension rare (<1 %)/suggests another cause, incl:

> Aortic Dissection
> Cardiac dysrhythmias
> Myocardial ischemia
> Shock

[21] Isotonic solutions preferable to minimize ischemic brain edema; relation between hydration/outcomes indefinite in acute stroke

[22] Data supporting relative efficacy of rtPA versus intra-arterial treatment lacking

[23] Efficacy uncertain in this setting; potential benefits for emergency use:

> Halt neurological worsening/improve neurological outcomes
> Prevent early recurrent embolization

[24] Many agents/procedures that have been tried and have uncertain efficacy/not recommended/investigational include:

> Albumin
> Hyperbaric O_2
> Hypervolemia/hemodilution
> Hypothermia
> Induced HTN
> Mechanical flow augmentation, including:
>
>> Willisian/leptomeningeal collaterals
>> Extracorpreal counterpulsation
>
> Near-infrared therapy
> Neuroprotective agents
>
>> Antiinflamatory agents
>> CCBs
>> Citicoline
>> Clomethiazole
>> Free-radical trapping agents
>> Hematopoietic growth factors
>> N-methyl-aspartate agents
>> Statins
>
> Surgical decompression
> Vasodilatation

[25] Especially lacunar infarcts (small size: <15 mm^2) typically located in deep structures, including:

> Basal ganglia
> Internal capsule
> Pons
> Thalamus

[26] Confusion/disorientation may be real or perceived due to expressive/receptive aphasia/visuospatial neglect abnormality

[27] Wallenberg Syndrome: due to obstruction of:

Vertebral artery – distal branches
Vertebral artery – superior lateral medullary artery
Posterior inferior cerebellar artery (less common than vertebral)

Signs/symptoms include:

Ataxia
Dysphagia
Facial pain/temporary sensory loss
Hemisensory pain/temporary loss (contralateral; all others ipsilateral)
Hiccups
Hoarseness
Horner syndrome
Nausea/vomiting
Nystagmus
Vertigo

[28] Dose: 0.9 mg/kg (max dose 90 mg) over 1 h; give first 10 % as bolus over 1 min

[29] Arm drift: patient closes eyes and extends both arms straight out for 10 s

Normal: both arms move the same, or both arms do not move at all
Abnormal: one arm either does not move, or one arm drifts down compared to the other

[30] Intra-arterial thrombectomy considerations (consult latest Guidelines for most current recommendations):

Documented occlusion in distal internal carotid/proximal cerebral artery
Relatively normal noncontrast head CT
Severe neurological deficit
Can be performed within 6 h of when patient last seen to be normal
Clearly benefits patients receiving rtPA before intra-arterial thrombectomy
rtPA should not be withheld if patient meets criteria

Benefit in patients who do not receive rtPA or have rtPA exclusions requires further study

Favorable results occur when

Performed in endovascular stroke center by coordinated multidisciplinary team that extends from prehospital stage to endovascular suite

Minimizes time to recanalization
Uses stent-retriever devices
Avoids general anesthesia

[31] rtPA highly effective in recanalizing smaller distal thrombi but dissolves proximal large thrombi in only 15–25 %: reason for considering added intra-arterial embolectomy in appropriate patients

[32] However, 19–39 % of acute ischemic strokes have no identifiable intracranial occlusion

[33] Avoid imaging that may delay stroke workflow

[34] Strokes related to AF have poorer outcomes than non-AF related stroke, including worse functional impairment, recurrence, death

[35] Mechanical thrombectomy meta-analysis (2015) conclusion: In acute ischemic stroke due to large artery occlusion, mechanical thrombectomy after usual care was associated with improved functional outcomes compared with usual care alone, and was found to be relatively safe, with no excess in intracranial hemorrhage. There was a trend for reduction in all-cause mortality with mechanical thrombectomy.

[36] Herpes viruses may trigger childhood ischemic stroke, even if infection is subclinical

[37] Including Rheumatoid Arthritis, Systemic Lupus Erythematosus, Ankylosing Spondylitis, Gout, Psoriasis

[38] Symptom associated with missed diagnosis of stroke

Appendix A: National Institutes of Health Stroke Scale

IA Level of consciousness

> 0 – Alert
> 1 – Drowsy
> 2 – Obtunded
> 3 – Coma/unresponsive

IB Orientation questions

> 0 – Answers both correctly
> 1 – Answers 1 correctly
> 2 – Answers neither correctly

IC Response to commands

> 0 – Performs both tasks correctly
> 1 – Performs 1 task correctly
> 2 – Performs neither

2 Gaze

> 0 – Normal horizontal movements
> 1 – Partial gaze palsy
> 2 – Complete gaze palsy

3 Visual fields

> 0 – No visual field defect
> 1 – Partial hemianopia
> 2 – Complete hemianopia
> 3 – Bilateral hemianopia

4 Facial movement

> 0 – Normal
> 1 – Minor facial weakness
> 2 – Partial facial weakness
> 3 – Complete unilateral palsy

5 Motor function (arm)

    a. Left
    b. Right
    0 – No drift
    1 – Drift before 5 s
    2 – Falls before 10 s
    3 – No effort against gravity
    4 – No movement

6 Motor function (leg)

    a. Left
    b. Right
    0 – No drift
    1 – Drift before 5 s
    2 – Falls before 5 s
    3 – No effort against gravity
    4 – No movement

7 Limb ataxia

    0 – No ataxia
    1 – Ataxia in 1 limb
    2 – Ataxia in 2 limbs

8 Sensory

    0 – No sensory loss
    1 – Mild sensory loss
    2 – Severe sensory loss

9 Language

    0 – Normal
    1 – Mild aphasia
    2 – Severe aphasia
    3 – Mute or global aphasia

10 Articulation

    0 – Normal
    1 – Mild dysarthria
    2 – Severe dysarthria

11 Extinction/inattention

    0 – Absent
    1 – Mild (loss 1 sensory modality lost)
    2 – Severe (loss 2 modalities lost)

Guidelines

AHA/ASA: guidelines for the early management of patients with acute ischemic stroke
Stroke.   2013;44:870–947.   http://stroke.ahajournals.org/content/44/3/870.long.

Patient Information

Images

http://www.mayoclinic.org/ischemic-stroke/img-20009031.

Medlineplus

ENGLISH

https://www.nlm.nih.gov/medlineplus/ischemicstroke.html.

ESPANOL

https://www.nlm.nih.gov/medlineplus/spanish/ischemicstroke.html.

CDC: Types of Stroke

http://www.cdc.gov/stroke/types-of-stroke.htm.

Stroke Awareness Foundation

http://strokeinfo.org/.

National Stroke Association

http://www.stroke.org/understand-stroke/what-stroke/ischemic-stroke.

Merck

http://www.merckmanuals.com/home/brain-spinal-cord-and-nerve--disorders/stroke-cva/ischemic-stroke.

Cedars-Sinai

http://www.cedars-sinai.edu/Patients/Programs-and-Services/Stroke-Program/Stroke-Resources/Acute-Ischemic-Stroke.aspx.

ASA

http://www.strokeassociation.org/STROKEORG/AboutStroke/TypesofStroke/IschemicClots/Ischemic-Strokes-Clots-UCM-310939-Article.jsp.

Mayo Clinic

http://www.mayoclinic.org/ischemic-stroke/img-20009031.

Professional Information

Review: Endovascular Intervention

Eur Heart J. 2015;36:2373–80. http://eurheartj.oxfordjournals.org/content/36/35/2373.

Review: Endovascular Intervention

Stroke. 2015;46:1447–52. http://stroke.ahajournals.org/content/46/6/1447.full.

Review: Stroke Prevention in Atrial Fibrillation

JAMA. 2015;313:1950–62. http://jama.jamanetwork.com/article.aspx?articleid=2293300.

Review: Thromboinflammation

Stroke. 2016;47:1165–72. http://stroke.ahajournals.org/content/47/4/1165.extract?etoc.

Alteplace Timing/Safety/Efficacy: Meta-analysis

Lancet. 2015;384:1929–35. http://www.sciencedirect.com/science/article/pii/S0140673614605845.

Air Travel

Stroke. 2016;47:1117–9. http://stroke.ahajournals.org/content/47/4/1117.abstract?etoc.

Aortic Valve Fibroelastoma

Tex Heart Inst J. 2015;42:131–5. http://thij.org/doi/full/10.14503/THIJ-14-4262.

Cancer: Young Adults

Stroke.2015;46:1601–6.http://stroke.ahajournals.org/content/46/6/1601.full.

Cincinnati Prehospital Stroke Assessment

Ann Emerg Med. 1999;33:373–8. http://www.annemergmed.com/article/S0196-0644(99)70299-4/abstract.

Cocaine Use/Risk

Stroke. 2016;115.011417. http://stroke.ahajournals.org/content/early/2016/03/10/STROKEAHA.115.011417.abstract.

Cognitive Decline Post-stroke

JAMA. 2015;314:41–51. http://jama.jamanetwork.com/article.aspx?articleid=2382979.

Depression: Nursing Assessment

Stroke. 2016;47:e1–3. http://stroke.ahajournals.org/content/47/1/e1.extract?etoc.

Diabetes Mellitus: Stroke Risk/Glycemic Control

J Am Coll Cardiol. 2016;67:239–47. http://content.onlinejacc.org/article.aspx?articleID=2481278.

Earlobe Crease

Am J Cardiol. 2015;116:286–93. http://www.ajconline.org/article/S0002-9149(15)01120-0/abstract.

Herpes Virus Infection in Childhood Ischemic Stroke

Circulation. 2016;133:732–41. http://circ.ahajournals.org/content/133/8/732.full.

Imaging for Endovascular Interventions

Stroke. 2015;46:1453–61. http://stroke.ahajournals.org/content/46/6/1453.full.

Intracranial Hemorrhage After Ischemic Stroke

Circ Outcomes. 2015;114.001606. http://circoutcomes.ahajournals.org/content/early/2015/07/07/CIRCOUTCOMES.114.001606.abstract.

Los Angeles Prehospital Stroke Screen

Stroke. 2000;31:71–6. http://stroke.ahajournals.org/content/31/1/71.full.

Mechanical Thrombectory Meta-analysis (2015)

J Am Coll Cardiol. 2015;66:2498–505. http://content.onlinejacc.org/article.aspx?articleID=2473752.

Misdiagnosis

Stroke. 2016;47:668–73. http://stroke.ahajournals.org/content/47/3/668.full.

Misdiagnosis in Patients with Peripheral Vertigo Having CT

Stroke. 2015;46:108–13. http://stroke.ahajournals.org/content/46/1/108. abstract.

Parenteral Fluids (Based on Cochrane Review)

Stroke. 2016;47:e6–7. http://stroke.ahajournals.org/content/47/1/e6.full.

Prehospital Stroke Recognition

Stroke. 2015;46:1513–7. http://stroke.ahajournals.org/content/46/6/1513. full.

Prevention: Atrial Fibrillation/Chronic Kidney Disease

Circulation. 2016; 133:1512–5. http://circ.ahajournals.org/content/133/15/1512.full.

Rheumatic Diseases: Risk

Stroke. 2016;115.012052. http://stroke.ahajournals.org/content/early/2016/02/25/STROKEAHA.115.012052.abstract.

Takayusu Arteritis (Case Report)

QJM. 2016:109:45–6. http://qjmed.oxfordjournals.org/content/109/1/45.

Updates and More

https://clinicalguidecvd.com/stroke

Chapter 91
Supraventricular Tachycardia: (SVT/Paroxysmal Supraventicular Tachycardia/ PSVT)

ICD-10 Code

I47.1

Alternate Names/Abbreviation

SVT (Supraventricular Tachycardia): three forms:

AVNRT: Atrioventricular Node Reentry Tachycardia (most common form)
AVRT: Atrioventricular Reentry Tachycardia [2]
AT: Atrial Tachycardia [20]

PSVT (Paroxysmal Supraventicular Tachycardia):

AVNRT
AVRT

V.E. Friedewald, *Clinical Guide to Cardiovascular Disease*, DOI 10.1007/978-1-4471-7293-2_91, © Springer-Verlag London 2016

Description/Etiology [21]

Supraventricular Tachycardia: nonspecific term describing atrial and/or ventricular rates >100 bpm at rest; mechanism involves cardiac tissue from His bundle or above; abrupt onset and cessation; duration lasts seconds-hours [1]

May occur in isolated form or associated with structural heart disease

Predisposing/Comorbid Conditions

HYPERMETABOLIC CONDITIONS
PREEXCITATION SYNDROMES
STRUCTURAL HEART DISEASE

Demography

All ages/populations
Onset of AVRT and AVNRT most often age <20 year
AVRT: males more often
AVNRT: females 2:1
AT: frequency increases with age

Pathophysiology

Two mechanisms: triggered and reentry
Triggered activity: impulse generation dependent on a preceding action potential

Early after-depolarization, which is promoted by:

Slow heart rate
Decreased outward currents
Increased outward currents

Delayed after-depolarizations

States of intracellular Ca^{++} overload

Reentry: due to abnormal conduction, and requires:

Slow conduction
Unidirectional block

Signs/Symptoms

ABDOMEN – BELCHING
ABDOMEN – FULLNESS
ABDOMEN – PULSATION, SENSE OF
CHEST – PAIN, EFFORT (ANGINA PECTORIS) [3]
CHEST – PALPITATIONS [15]
CONSCIOUSNESS – LOSS, SUDDEN (SYNCOPE) [4]
DIZZY/LIGHTHEADED/PRESYNCOPE
EXTREM, TEMP – DECR [6]
HEAD – PULSATIONS, SENSE OF
HEAD, SENSATION – FULLNESS
HEART, RATE – RAPID (TACHYCARDIA) [7]
HEART, S1, INTENSITY – INCR [DURING TACHY: AVNRT/AVRT]
HEART, S1, INTENSITY – VAR [DURING TACHY: AT]
HYPOTENSION   (BLOOD   PRESSURE   – DECREASED/LOW) [6]
MENTATION – WEAKNESS (MALAISE)
MOOD – ANXIOUS
MOOD, COMBATIVE
MOUTH, SALIVATION – INCR (PTYALISM)
NAUSEA
NECK, JVP, A WAVE – INCR/LARGE (CANNON WAVE) [[16] DURING TACHY: AVNRT/AVRT]
NECK, SENSATION – FULLNESS
NECK, SENSATION – PULSATIONS
SWEATING – INCR (DIAPHORESIS/HYPERHIDROSIS)
URINATION – INCR (POLYURIA)
VOMITING (EMESIS) [5]

Differentiation

Wide QRS Complex: VT
Narrow QRS Complex: Fascicular VT [18]

Complications

HF [8]
Tachycardia-Induced Cardiomyopathy

Laboratory

NS

ECG [13]

P WAVE – ABSENT
P WAVE – FOLLOWS QRS [17]
P WAVE – IMBEDDED WITHIN QRS [17]
P WAVE, MORPH – VAR/ABN
QRS – LONG, NS [9]
QRS – LVH PATTERN [9]
QRS – NORMAL [9]
QRS – RBBB/RBBB PATTERN [9]
RATE, ATRIAL – RAPID [11]
ST SEGMENT – DEPR [10] [12]
T WAVE – INVER, ABN [10] [12]

Imaging

NS/VAR WITH COMORBID

Other Tests

Ambulatory ECG monitoring
EP testing

Treatment: Nonpharmacologic: AVNRT [19]

Vagal stimulation [14]
Electrical cardioversion: always warranted in presence of
hemodynamic instability [22]

Treatment: Pharmacologic: AVNRT [19]

Adenosine [23]
Beta-blockers (oral) [25]
Amiodrone [26]
Diltiazem [24]
Verapamil [24]

Treatment: Surgical/Invasive [19]

RF ablation

Notes

[1] Usually does not include AF/Flutter or Multifocal Atrial
Tachycardia
[2] WPW
[3] May resemble classic angina pectoris, or may be true
angina due to precipitation of myocardial ischemia in
patients with co-existing CAD
[4] Onset; uncommon unless associated with Sinus Node
Dysfunction; occurs more often in older persons
[5] May terminate the event

[6] With prolonged episodes at very fast rates, especially with co-existing CVD

[7] 150–300 BPM; absolutely regular, unchanging with position, effort, breathing

[8] Especially when associated with structural heart disease

[9] QRS typically narrow in PSVT except in setting of BBB or antegrade preexcitation, requiring differentiation from VT; VT can have narrow complex QRS (fascicular VT) also requiring differentiation from PSVT

[10] May persist for days after cardioversion; not necessarily due to CAD

[11] Unaffected by vagal stimulation (eg, carotid massage)

[12] ST-T wave changes may occur both in presence or absence of CAD

[13] Many different ECG patterns may occur, dictated by location of originating site and conduction path

[14] **Vagal maneuvers** ***

For acute conversion of AVNRT, vagal maneuvers, including Valsalva and carotid sinus massage, can be performed quickly and should be the first-line intervention to terminate SVT. These maneuvers should be performed with the patient in the supine position. There is no "gold standard" for proper Valsalva maneuver technique, but in general, the patient raises intrathoracic pressure by bearing down against a closed glottis for 10–30 s, equivalent to at least 30–40 mmHg. Carotid massage is performed after absence of bruit has been confirmed by auscultation, by applying steady pressure over the right or left carotid sinus for 5–10 s. Another vagal maneuver based on the classic diving reflex consists of applying an ice-cold, wet towel to the face (85); in a laboratory setting, facial immersion in water at 10 °C (50 °F) has proved effective in terminating tachycardia, as well. One study involving 148 patients with SVT demonstrated that Valsalva was more successful than carotid sinus massage, and switching from one technique to the other resulted in an overall success rate of 27.7 %. The practice of applying pressure to the eyeball is potentially dangerous and has been abandoned.

[15] Palpitations with abrupt onset/termination and without clear trigger more often due to AVNT/AVRT; converse true for AT

[16] Cannon waves regular in AVNRT/AVRT; irregular in AT

[17] Short R-P tachycardia usually AVNRT/AVRT; long R-P tachycardia usually AT

[18] Conduction via specialized/rapid pathways

[19] Treatment should be determined by electrophysiology expert when possible, especially with drug therapy

[20] AT more often associated with underlying cardiac disease and has gradual onset

[21] **Definitions of supraventricular tachycardias** ***

Supraventricular tachycardia (SVT): An umbrella term used to describe tachycardias (atrial and/or ventricular rates in excess of 100 bpm at rest), the mechanism of which involves tissue from the His bundle or above. These SVTs include inappropriate sinus tachycardia, AT (including focal and multifocal AT), macroreentrant AT (including typical atrial flutter), junctional tachycardia, AVNRT, and various forms of accessory pathway-mediated reentrant tachycardias.

Paroxysmal supraventricular tachycardia (PSVT): A clinical syndrome characterized by the presence of a regular and rapid tachycardia of abrupt onset and termination. These features are characteristic of AVNRT or AVRT, and, less frequently, AT. PSVT represents a subset of SVT.

Atrial fibrillation (AF): A supraventricular arrhythmia with uncoordinated atrial activation and, consequently, ineffective atrial contraction. ECG characteristics include: (1) irregular atrial activity, (2) absence of distinct P waves, and (3) irregular R-R intervals (when atrioventricular conduction is present).

Sinus tachycardia: Rhythm arising from the sinus node in which the rate of impulses exceeds 100 bpm.

- **Physiologic sinus tachycardia**: Appropriate increased sinus rate in response to exercise and other situations that increase sympathetic tone.

- **Inappropriate sinus tachycardia:** Sinus heart rate >100 bpm at rest, with a mean 24-h heart rate >90 bpm not due to appropriate physiological responses or primary causes such as hyperthyroidism or anemia

Atrial tachycardia (AT)

- **Focal AT:** An SVT arising from a localized atrial site, characterized by regular, organized atrial activity with discrete P waves and typically an isoelectric segment between P waves. At times, irregularity is seen, especially at onset ("warm-up") and termination ("warm-down"). Atrial mapping reveals a focal point of origin.

- **Sinus node reentry tachycardia:** A specific type of focal AT that is due to microreentry arising from the sinus node complex, characterized by abrupt onset and termination, resulting in a P-wave morphology that is indistinguishable from sinus rhythm.

- **Multifocal atrial tachycardia (MAT):** An irregular SVT characterized by ≥3 distinct P-wave morphologies and/or patterns of atrial activation at different rates. The rhythm is always irregular.

Atrial flutter

- **Cavotricuspid isthmus–dependent atrial flutter:** typical: Macroreentrant AT propagating around the tricuspid annulus, proceeding superiorly along the atrial septum, inferiorly along the right atrial wall, and through the cavotricuspid isthmus between the tricuspid valve annulus and the Eustachian valve and ridge. This activation sequence produces predominantly negative "sawtooth" flutter waves on the ECG in leads 2, 3, and aVF and a late positive deflection in V1. The atrial rate can be slower than the typical 300 bpm (cycle length 200 ms) in the presence of antiarrhythmic drugs or scarring. It is also known as "typical atrial flutter" or "cavotricuspid isthmus–dependent atrial flutter" or "counterclockwise atrial flutter."

- **Cavotricuspid isthmus–dependent atrial flutter**: reverse typical: Macroreentrant AT that propagates around in the direction reverse that of typical atrial flutter. Flutter waves typically appear positive in the inferior leads and negative in V1. This type of atrial flutter is also referred to as "reverse typical" atrial flutter or "clockwise typical atrial flutter."

- **Atypical or non–cavotricuspid isthmus–dependent atrial flutter**: Macroreentrant ATs that do not involve the cavotricuspid isthmus. A variety of reentrant circuits may include reentry around the mitral valve annulus or scar tissue within the left or right atrium. A variety of terms have been applied to these arrhythmias according to the re-entry circuit location, including particular forms, such as "LA flutter" and "LA macroreentrant tachycardia" or incisional atrial re-entrant tachycardia due to re-entry around surgical scars.

  Junctional tachycardia: A nonreentrant SVT that arises from the AV junction (including the His bundle).

  Atrioventricular nodal reentrant tachycardia (AVNRT): A reentrant tachycardia involving two functionally distinct pathways, generally referred to as "fast" and "slow" pathways. Most commonly, the fast pathway is located near the apex of Koch's triangle, and the slow pathway inferoposterior to the compact AV node tissue. Variant pathways have been described, allowing for "slow-slow" AVNRT.

- **Typical AVNRT**: AVNRT in which a slow pathway serves as the anterograde limb of the circuit and the fast pathway serves as the retrograde limb (also called "slow-fast AVNRT").

- **Atypical AVNRT**: AVNRT in which the fast pathway serves as the anterograde limb of the circuit and a slow pathway serves as the retrograde limb (also called "fast-slow AV node reentry") or a slow pathway serves as the anterograde limb and a second slow pathway serves as the retrograde limb (also called "slow-slow AVNRT").

Accessory pathway: an accessory pathway is defined as an extranodal AV pathway that connects the myocardium of the atrium to the ventricle across the AV groove. Accessory pathways can be classified by their location, type of conduction (decremental or nondecremental), and whether they are capable of conducting anterogradely, retrogradely, or in both directions. Of note, accessory pathways of other types (such as atrio-fascicular, nodo-fascicular, nodo-ventricular, and fasciculoventricular pathways) are uncommon.

- **Manifest accessory pathway**: A pathway that conducts anterogradely to cause ventricular pre-excitation pattern on the ECG.

- **Concealed accessory pathway**: A pathway that conducts only retrogradely and does not affect the ECG pattern during sinus rhythm.

- **Pre-excitation pattern**: An ECG pattern reflecting the presence of a manifest accessory pathway connecting the atrium to the ventricle. Pre-excited ventricular activation over the accessory pathway competes with the anterograde conduction over the AV node and spreads from the accessory pathway insertion point in the ventricular myocardium. Depending on the relative contribution from ventricular activation by the normal AV nodal/His Purkinje system versus the manifest accessory pathway, a variable degree of pre-excitation, with its characteristic pattern of a short P-R interval with slurring of the initial upstroke of the QRS complex (delta wave), is observed. Pre-excitation can be intermittent or not easily appreciated for some pathways capable of anterograde conduction; this is usually associated with a low-risk pathway, but exceptions occur.

- **Asymptomatic pre-excitation (isolated pre-excitation)**: The abnormal pre-excitation ECG pattern in the absence of documented SVT or symptoms consistent with SVT.

- **Wolff-Parkinson-White syndrome**: Syndrome characterized by documented SVT or symptoms consistent with SVT in a patient with ventricular pre-excitation during sinus rhythm
  Atrioventricular reentrant tachycardia (AVRT): A reentrant tachycardia, the electrical pathway of which requires an accessory pathway, the atrium, atrioventricular node (or second accessory pathway), and ventricle.

- **Orthodromic AVRT:** An AVRT in which the reentrant impulse uses the accessory pathway in the retrograde direction from the ventricle to the atrium, and the AV node in the anterograde direction. The QRS complex is generally narrow or may be wide because of pre-existing bundle-branch block or aberrant conduction

- **Antidromic AVRT**: An AVRT in which the reentrant impulse uses the accessory pathway in the anterograde direction from the atrium to the ventricle, and the AV node for the retrograde direction. Occasionally, instead of the AV node, another accessory pathway can be used in the retrograde direction, which is referred to as pre-excited AVRT. The QRS complex is wide (maximally pre-excited).
  Permanent form of junctional reciprocating tachycardia (PJRT): A rare form of nearly incessant orthodromic AVRT involving a slowly conducting, concealed, usually posteroseptal accessory pathway.
  Pre-excited AF: AF with ventricular pre-excitation caused by conduction over ≥1 accessory pathway(s).

[22] **Synchronized cardioversion** ***

Should be performed for acute treatment in hemodynamically unstable patients with AVNRT when adenosine and vagal maneuvers do not terminate the tachycardia or are not feasible. Synchronized cardioversion is highly effective in terminating SVT (including AVRT and

AVNRT). Most stable patients with SVT respond to pharmacological therapy, with success rates of 80–98 % for agents such as verapamil, diltiazem, or adenosine. In some resistant cases, a second drug bolus or higher dose of initial drug agent is often effective. Nevertheless, in rare instances, drugs may fail to successfully restore sinus rhythm, necessitating synchronized cardioversion.

[23] **Adenosine** ***

Can be considered as both a therapeutic and diagnostic agent in narrow-complex tachyarrhythmias. It will acutely terminate AVNRT in approximately 95 % of patients and will unmask atrial activity in arrhythmias, such as atrial flutter or AT.

[24] **Diltiazem and verapamil** ***

Intravenous diltiazem and verapamil are particularly effective in converting AVNRT to sinus rhythm. These drugs should be used only in hemodynamically stable patients. It is important to ensure the absence of VT or pre-excited AF, because patients with these rhythms may become hemodynamically unstable and develop ventricular fibrillation if administered diltiazem or verapamil. Diltiazem or verapamil should also be avoided in patients with suspected systolic heart failure. Evidence for the effectiveness of beta blockers to terminate AVNRT is limited. In a trial that compared esmolol with diltiazem, diltiazem was more effective in terminating SVT (237). Nonetheless, beta blockers have an excellent safety profile, so it is reasonable to use them to attempt to terminate SVT in hemodynamically stable patients.

[25] **Oral beta-blockers** ***

Overall, there are no data specifically studying the effect of oral beta-blocker monotherapy for the acute termination of AVNRT. However, two studies have demonstrated success with the combination of oral diltiazem and propranolol to terminate AVNRT or AVRT. Oral beta blockers have an excellent safety profile, and administration (particularly in patients without intravenous access) can be performed in conjunction with vagal maneuvers.

[26] **Amiodarone** ***

Intravenous amiodarone may be considered for acute treatment in hemodynamically stable patients with AVNRT when other therapies are ineffective or contraindicated.

In a small cohort study, intravenous amiodarone was effective in terminating AVNRT. Long-term toxicity is not seen with intravenous amiodarone if given for a short period of time.

*** **Extracted verbatim from ACC/AHA/HRS 2015 Guideline for the Management of Adult Patients With Supraventricular Tachycardia: A Report of the American College of Cardiology/American Heart Association Task Force on Clinical Practice Guidelines and the Heart Rhythm Society.** J Am Coll Cardiol 2016;67:e27–e115

Guidelines

ACC/AHA/HRS 2015 guideline for the management of adult patients with supraventricular tachycardia: a report of the American College of Cardiology/American Heart Association Task Force on clinical practice guidelines and the Heart Rhythm Society.
J Am Coll Cardiol. 2016;67:e27–115. http://content.onlinejacc.org/article.aspx?articleID=2443667.

Patient Information

Images

http://www.nlm.nih.gov/medlineplus/ency/imagepages/18052.htm.
http://www.nlm.nih.gov/medlineplus/ency/imagepages/8810.htm.

Medlineplus

ENGLISH

http://www.nlm.nih.gov/medlineplus/ency/article/000187.htm.

ESPANOL

http://www.nlm.nih.gov/medlineplus/spanish/ency/article/000183.htm.

Cleveland Clinic

http://my.clevelandclinic.org/heart/disorders/electric/ventricular-tachycardia.aspx.

Mayo Clinic

http://www.mayoclinic.org/diseases-conditions/tachycardia/basics/definition/con-20043012.

Johns Hopkins

http://www.hopkinsmedicine.org/heart-vascular-institute/conditions-treatments/conditions/supraventricular-tachycardia.html.

Merck

http://www.merckmanuals.com/home/heart-and-blood-vessel-disorders/abnormal-heart-rhythms/paroxysmal-supraventricular-tachycardia-svt-psvt.

AHA

http://www.heart.org/HEARTORG/Conditions/Arrhythmia/AboutArrhythmia/Tachycardia-Fast-Heart-Rate-UCM-302018-Article.jsp#.

Stanford

https://stanfordhealthcare.org/medical-conditions/blood-heart-circulation/supraventricular-tachycardia.html.

Seattle Childrens Hospital

http://www.seattlechildrens.org/medical-conditions/heart-blood-conditions/supraventricular-tachycardia/.

Professional Information

Review

N Engl J Med. 2012;367:1438–48. http://www.nejm.org/doi/full/10.1056/NEJMcp1111259.

Review

N Engl J Med. 2006;354:1039–51. http://www.nejm.org/doi/full/10.1056/NEJMcp051145.

Review

Card Electrophy Clin. 2014;6:483–509. http://www.sciencedirect.com/science/article/pii/S1877918214000616.

Adenosine

Circulation. 1999;99:1034–40. http://circ.ahajournals.org/content/99/8/1034.full.

AVNRT

Circulation.   2010;122:831–40.   http://circ.ahajournals.org/content/122/8/831.long.

Perioperative Management

Contin Educ Anaesth Crit Care Pain. 2014. http://ceaccp.oxfordjournals.org/content/early/2014/06/07/bjaceaccp.mku018.

Postural Tachycardia Syndrome

Circulation.   2013;127:2336–42.   http://circ.ahajournals.org/content/127/23/2336.full.

Swallowing-Induced Atrial Tachycardia

Circulation.2014;130:e113–5.http://circ.ahajournals.org/content/130/13/e113.full.

Updates and More

https://clinicalguidecvd.com/svt

Chapter 92
Takayasu Arteritis

Management Keys

Prompt recognition, evaluation, and treatment [14]

ICD-10 Code

M31.4

Alternate Names/Abbreviation

Pulseless Disease

Description/Etiology

Chronic large vessel inflammatory vasculitis with protean manifestations secondary to multiorgan tissue hypoperfusion, mainly involving aorta and large branch arteries, including:

Brachiocephalic
Carotid
Coronary
Pulmonary artery and branches

V.E. Friedewald, *Clinical Guide to Cardiovascular Disease*, DOI 10.1007/978-1-4471-7293-2_92, © Springer-Verlag London 2016

Renal
Subclavian
Vertebral

Aortic arch most common area involved
Cause unknown; cell-mediated autoimmunity likely

Predisposing/Comorbid Conditions

ACUTE FEBRILE ILLNESS [1]
MYOCARDITIS

Demography

Females 8:1 (varies among reporting countries)
Age of onset 10–40 years
Most commonly reported in Japan, SE Asia, India, Mexico [10]

Pathophysiology

Vascular injury mainly involving arterial media/adventia, leading to aneurysm formation/secondary vascular stiffening and atherosclerosis, composed of:

Myointimal proliferation
Wall thickening
Luminal Stenosis
Destruction of wall tissue leading to aneurysm formation and secondary vascular stiffening and atherosclerosis

Vascular distribution varies among populations within different reporting countries

Signs/Symptoms [13]

ABDOMEN – PAIN, AFTER MEALS (ABDOMINAL ANGINA)
APPETITE – DECR (ANOREXIA) [1]

ARTERIAL PRESSURE – LE > RE
ARTERIAL PULSE, BRACHIAL, L – DECR/ABSENT
ARTERIAL PULSE, BRACHIAL, R – DECR/ABSENT
ARTERIAL PULSE, CAROTID – DECR/ABSENT
ARTERIAL PULSE, UE – ASYMMETRIC
ARTERIES – PAIN
ARTERY, CAROTID – PAIN
ARTERY, CAROTID – TENDER
ARTERY, MULTIPLE LOCATIONS – BRUITS [12]
BLOOD PRESSURE, ARTERIAL – INCREASED/
   ELEVATED
BOWEL MOVEMENTS – DIARRHEA
CHEST – PAIN [1]
CHEST – PAIN, EFFORT (ANGINA PECTORIS)
CHEST, LAT – PAIN, PLEURITIC [1]
CHEST, POST – PAIN, PLEURITIC [1]
CONSCIOUSNESS – LOSS, SUDDEN (SYNCOPE)
DIZZY/LIGHTHEADED/PRESYNCOPE [11]
EARS, HEARING – LOSS (DEAFNESS)
EXTREM, LOWER, BILAT – PAIN, EFFORT
   (CLAUDICATION)
EXTREM, UPPER, USE – PAIN
EYES, LENS – OPACITY (CATARACT) [2]
EYES, RETINA – CENTRAL VENOUS RETINOPATHY
EYES, RETINA – DETACHED
EYES, VISION – ABN, NS
EYES, VISION – DECR/LOSS
FACE, JAW – PAIN, CHEWING
FACE, JAW – WEAKNESS, CHEWING
FATIGUE
FEVER [1]
HEADACHE
HEART, LSB, MID – MURMUR, DIAS
JOINTS – PAIN (ARTHRALGIA) [1]
MOUTH, PALATE – ULCERATION
MUSCLES – PAIN (MYALGIA) [1]
MUSCLES, UNILAT – WEAK (HEMIPARESIS) [3]
MUSCLES, UNILAT – WEAK/PARALYSIS
   (HEMIPARESIS/HEMIPLEGIA) [3]
SEIZURES
SKIN, FACE – ATROPHY

SKIN, FACE – PIGMENTATION
SKIN, NOSE – ULCER
SPEECH – ABSENT (APHONIA)/LOSS (APHASIA)
SWEATING, NOCT – INCR (DIAPHORESIS, NOCT) [1]
WEIGHT – LOSS [1]

Differentiation

Bechets Disease
Infectious aneurysms [6]
Infective Endocarditis
Other congenital and acquired causes of aortic dilatation/
    aortic regurgitation [4]
Other causes of arteritis involving aorta [5]

Complications [7]

AMI [8]
Aortic Dissection
Aortic Regurgitation
Giant Cell Myocarditis
HF
Premature Atherosclerosis
Renal Failure
Renovascular Hypertension
Retinopathy/Blindness
Stroke – Ischemic
Sudden Death

Laboratory

BLOOD, C-REACTIVE PROTEIN (CRP) – INCR
BLOOD, ESR – INCR
BLOOD, HGB/HCT – DECR (ANEMIA)
BLOOD, IGG – INCR
BLOOD, WBC – INCR (LEUKOCYTOSIS)

ECG

N/NS ABN

Imaging [9]

AV, LEAFLETS – THICK
IVS, THICKNESS – INCR (SEPTAL HYPERTROPHY)
LV, WALL MOTION, SEG – DECR/AKINETIC
MV, LEAFLETS – THICK
MYOCARD – SCAR(S)

Other Tests

NS

Treatment: Nonpharmacologic

NS

Treatment: Pharmacologic [14]

Antihypertensives
Biologics (investigational)

Tocilizumab
Tumor necrosis factor-α antagonists

Corticosteroids

Treatment: Surgical/Invasive

Discrete stenotic angioplasty and/or artery bypass [15]

Prevention

NS

Course

Prognosis improving with earlier diagnosis and treatment interventions

Main cause of death: renovascular hypertension complications

Notes

[1] Acute episode
[2] Develop rapidly
[3] Transient
[4] Eg, Fibromuscular Dysplasia, Marfan Syndrome, Ehlers-Danlos Syndrome
[5] Eg, Giant Cell Arteritis, Ankylosing Spondylitis, Reiter Syndrome, Bechet Syndrome, Psoriatic Arthritis, Relapsing Polychondritis, Systemic Lupus Erythematosus
[6] Tuberculosis, Syphilis, Staph Aureus
[7] Aneurysm rupture rare
[8] Coronary involvement in 10–13 %, including obstruction of coronary ostia/main epicardial arteries and coronary artery aneurysms
[9] Imaging: main modality for diagnosis; list does not include findings due to vascular dilatation/stenosis; imaging abnormalities of myocardium may occur in absence of ischemic symptoms
[10] Reported as more common in rainy season
[11] Especially when looking upward/looking back/raising arms
[12] Including back, neck, chest, abdomen
[13] Clinical manifestations due to tissue ischemia secondary to arterial stenoses/thrombus formation

[14] 2010 Thoracic Aortic Disease Guidelines – Sec. 7.1: Recommendations for Takayasu Arteritis and Giant Cell Arteritis

Class I

1. Initial therapy for active Takayasu arteritis and active giant cell arteritis should be corticosteroids at a high dose (prednisone 40–60 mg daily at initiation or its equivalent) to reduce the active inflammatory state. (Level of Evidence: B)
2. The success of treatment of patients with Takayasu arteritis and giant cell arteritis should be periodically evaluated to determine disease activity by repeated physical examination and either an erythrocyte sedimentation rate or C-reactive protein level. (Level of Evidence: B)
3. Elective revascularization of patients with Takayasu arteritis and giant cell arteritis should be delayed until the acute inflammatory state is treated and quiescent. (Level of Evidence: B)
4. The initial evaluation of Takayasu arteritis or giant cell arteritis should include thoracic aorta and branch vessel computed tomographic imaging or magnetic resonance imaging to investigate the possibility of aneurysm or occlusive disease in these vessels. (Level of Evidence: C)

Class IIa

1. It is reasonable to treat patients with Takayasu arteritis receiving corticosteroids with an additional anti-inflammatory agent if there is evidence of progression of vascular disease, recurrence of constitutional symptoms, or re-elevation of inflammatory marker. (Level of Evidence: C)

[15] 2010 ACCF/AHA/AATS/ACR/ASA/SCA/SCAI/SIR/ STS/SVM Guidelines for the Diagnosis and Management of Patients with Thoracic Aortic Disease

Class I

3. Elective revascularization of patients with Takayasu arteritis and giant cell arteritis should be delayed until the acute inflammatory state is treated and quiescent. (Level of Evidence: B)

Guidelines

2014 ESC guidelines on the diagnosis and treatment of aortic diseases

Eur Heart J. 2014;35:2873–926. http://eurheartj.oxfordjournals.org/content/35/41/2873.

2010   ACCF/AHA/AATS/ACR/ASA/SCA/SCAI/SIR/STS/SVM guidelines for the diagnosis and management of patients with thoracic aortic disease.

Circulation. 2010;121:e266–369. http://circ.ahajournals.org/content/121/13/e266.full.

Patient Information

Images

http://www.nlm.nih.gov/medlineplus/ency/imagepages/1056.htm.

Medlineplus

ENGLISH

http://www.nlm.nih.gov/medlineplus/ency/article/001250.htm.

ESPANOL

http://www.nlm.nih.gov/medlineplus/spanish/ency/article/001250.htm.

Mayo Clinic

http://www.mayoclinic.org/diseases-conditions/takayasus-arteritis/
basics/definition/con-20028085.

ACR

http://www.rheumatology.org/I-Am-A/Patient-Caregiver/Diseases-
Conditions/Takayasus-Arteritis.

Johns Hopkins

http://www.hopkinsvasculitis.org/types-vasculitis/takayasus-
arteritis/.

Vasculitis Foundation

http://www.vasculitisfoundation.org/education/forms/
takayasus-arteritis/.

Merck

http://www.merckmanuals.com/home/bone-joint-and-muscle-disor-
ders/vasculitic-disorders/takayasu-arteritis.

Cleveland Clinic

https://my.clevelandclinic.org/services/heart/disorders/
hic-Takayasus-Arteritis.

Professional Information

History

Int J Rheum Dis. 2014;17:931–5. http://onlinelibrary.wiley.com/doi/10.1111/1756-185X.12576/abstract;jsessionid=5945BD18FE2027DB43EB1BCABAA9F81C.f03t04.

Review

Int J Cardiol. 2013;168:3–10. http://www.sciencedirect.com/science/article/pii/S0167527313000624.

Review

Lancet. 2000;356:1023–5. http://www.sciencedirect.com/science/article/pii/S014067360002701X#.

Acute HF (Case Report)

J Am Coll Cardiol. 2013;61:1302–1302. http://content.onlinejacc.org/article.aspx?articleID=1668123.

Biologics Threapy

Circulation.   2015;132:1693–700.   http://circ.ahajournals.org/content/132/18/1693.abstract.

Images: Abdominal Aorta/Renal Artery

Circulation. 1997;95:529. http://circ.ahajournals.org/content/95/2/529.long.

Images: Inferior AMI/Dilated Cardiomyopathy

J Am Coll Cardiol. 2014;63:e35–e35. http://content.onlinejacc.org/article.aspx?articleID=1838328.

Ischemic Stroke (Case Report)

QJM. 2016:109:45–6. http://qjmed.oxfordjournals.org/content/109/1/45.

Multimodality Imaging

Sem Arthr Rheum. 2013;42:401–12. http://www.sciencedirect.com/science/article/pii/S0049017212001783.

Myocarditis (Case Report)

Eur Heart J. 2015;36:2564. http://eurheartj.oxfordjournals.org/content/36/38/2564.extract?etoc.

Pathophysiology

Eur J Int Med. 2006;17:241–6. http://www.sciencedirect.com/science/article/pii/S0953620506000434#.

Updates and More

https://clinicalguidecvd.com/takayusu

Chapter 93
Tetralogy of Fallot

ICD-10 Code

Q21.3

Alternate Names/Abbreviation

TOF

Description/Etiology

Four components:

1. Subpulmonary infundibular stenosis
2. VSD
3. Aorta overriding VSD by 50 % of its diameter
4. RVH

Varying degrees of PV stenosis, supravalvular stenosis, and pulmonary artery branch stenosis may coexist

Secundum ASD present in about 10 % of patients

V.E. Friedewald, *Clinical Guide to Cardiovascular Disease*,
DOI 10.1007/978-1-4471-7293-2_93,
© Springer-Verlag London 2016

Clinical presentation – unrepaired adults:

> Rare in societies with access to surgical correction except among immigrants
> Mild defects (pink tetralogy)
> Loud precordial murmur

Clinical presentation – repaired adults

> Usually asymptomatic
> Hemodynamic abnormalities suggested by exertional limitations or dysrhythmias

Comorbid Conditions

ATRIAL SEPTAL DEFECT – SECUNDUM
ATRIOVENTRICULAR SEPTAL DEFECT
CORONARY ARTERY ANOMALIES
DIGEORGE SYNDROME
DOWN SYNDROME
NOONAN SYNDROME
PULMONARY ARTERY ANOMALIES
RIGHT AORTIC ARCH
VACTERL SYNDROME

Demography

Gender equal

Pathophysiology

Reduced pulmonary blood flow and R-L intracardiac shunting secondary to RVOT obstruction with:

> Widely varying degrees of RVOT obstruction
> Intracardiac R-L shunting causing cyanosis
> Severity of cyanosis depending upon severity of outflow obstruction as well as hemoglobin

Severity of outflow tract obstruction function of fixed valve/subvalvular/supravalvular and dynamic (heart rate) components

All factors combine to determine clinical severity

Signs/Symptoms [1]

BODY, POSTURE – SQUATTING
BREATHING – DIFF (DYSPNEA)
BREATHING – RAPID (TACHYPNEA)
CHEST, ANT – MURMUR, CONT
CHEST, LAT – MURMUR, CONT
CHEST, POST – MURMUR, CONT
CONSCIOUSNESS – LOSS, SUDDEN (SYNCOPE)
HEART, LSB, MID – MURMUR, SYS
HEART, LSB, UPPER – MURMUR, DIAS
HEART, LSB, UPPER – MURMUR, SYS
HEART, P2, INTENSITY – DECR/ABSENT
HEART, S1, SPLIT – NARROW/SINGLE
HEART, S2 – PALPABLE
NECK, STERNOCLAV JOINT, R – PULSATION
SKIN, COLOR – BLUE (CYANOSIS)

Differentiation

Pulmonary Valve Stenosis
VSD

Complications

AF/Flutter
AV Block
Branch PA Stenosis or Hypoplasia
HF
Progressive AR
Residual outflow obstruction

Residual Pulmonary Regurgitation
RV dysfunction
Sudden Death
Sustained VT

Laboratory

NS

ECG

P WAVE – TALL/PEAKED
QRS – RBBB/RBBB PATTERN [2]
QRS – RVH PATTERN

Imaging

AORTA, ARCH – R
AORTA, DESCEND – R
AV, FLOW – REGURG
IVS – DEFECT
PA, MAIN – CONCAVE
PUL, VASCULARITY – DECR
PV, FLOW – REGURG
RV, OUTFLOW – OBS
TV, FLOW – REGURG

Genomics

CSX
NKX2.5
TBX5

Other Tests

Exercise test for functional capacity and exertional arrhythmias
Cardiac catheterization

Treatment: Nonpharmacologic

NS

Treatment: Pharmacologic

NS

Treatment: Surgical/Invasive

Complete repair [4]
VSD closure
Relief of RVOT obstruction [3]

Course

Variable; most TOF repair occurs in infancy/childhood but lifetime care/follow-up required
Pulmonary valve replacement ultimately indicated in most post-repair adults
Post-repair: most common problem in adults is pulmonary regurgitation, often missed on clinical examination because murmur is short/quiet and frequently missed on echo as well

Notes

[1] Post-repair patients are usually asymptomatic in absence of RV enlargement/failure and arrhythmia, with these findings:

Soft RVOT ejection systolic murmur

Pulmonary regurgitation murmur: low-pitched, late diastolic

Absent P2

Diastolic AR murmur

Pansystolic murmur from VSD patch leak

RBBB if correction made before mid-1990s (transventricular repair)

[2] Especially post-transventricular repair

[3] Including infundibular muscle resection; patch augmentation; transannular patch; extracardiac conduit; pulmonary valvotomy; pulmonary valve resection

[4] In adults, may require pulmonary valve replacement

Guidelines

ACC/AHA 2008 guidelines for the management of adults with congenital heart disease

J Am Coll Cardiol. 2008;52:e143–263. http://content.onlinejacc.org/article.aspx?articleid=1188032#tab1.

ESC guidelines for the management of grown-up congenital heart disease (new version 2010)

Eur Heart J. 2010; 31:2915–57. http://eurheartj.oxfordjournals.org/content/ehj/31/23/2915.full.pdf.

Patient Information

AHA

Circulation.   2014;130:e26–9.   http://circ.ahajournals.org/content/130/4/e26.full.

Images

http://www.nlm.nih.gov/medlineplus/ency/imagepages/1056.htm.
http://www.nlm.nih.gov/medlineplus/ency/imagepages/18088.htm.

http://www.nlm.nih.gov/medlineplus/ency/imagepages/18134.htm.
http://www.cdc.gov/ncbddd/heartdefects/TetralogyOfFallot-gra
phic2.html.

Medlineplus

ENGLISH

http://www.nlm.nih.gov/medlineplus/ency/article/001567.htm.

ESPANOL

http://www.nlm.nih.gov/medlineplus/spanish/ency/article/001567.
htm.

Genetics Home Reference

http://ghr.nlm.nih.gov/glossary=tetralogyoffallot.

Cleveland Clinic

http://my.clevelandclinic.org/childrens-hospital/health-info/diseases-
conditions/heart/tetralogy-of-fallot-childrens-overview.aspx.

Mayo Clinic

http://www.mayoclinic.org/diseases-conditions/tetralogy-of-fallot/
basics/definition/con-20043262.

Texas Heart Institute

http://www.texasheart.org/HIC/Topics/Cond/tetralog.cfm.

Professional Information

Review

J Am Coll Cardiol. 2013;62:2155–66. http://content.onlinejacc.org/article.aspx?articleID=1748237.

Adult Tetralogy of Fallot Risk Stratification

Heart. 2014;100:185–7. http://heart.bmj.com/content/100/3/185.extract.

BNP/Risk Stratification in Repaired TOF

Heart published online first: 5 January 2015. http://heart.bmj.com/content/early/2015/01/05/heartjnl-2014-306897.extract.

Cardiac MRI: Review/Decision Support

Cardiovasc Magn Reson. 2011;13:9. http://www.jcmr-online.com/content/13/1/9/abstract.

Coronary Artery Disease

Am J Cardiol. 2009;103:1445–50. http://www.ajconline.org/article/S0002-9149(09)00473-1/abstract.

ICD Follow-Up

Circulation. 2008;117:363–70. http://circ.ahajournals.org/content/117/3/363.full?sid=d5f5835f-da5c-4dbf-951f-4b1e7beacd78.

Long-Term 40 Year Follow-Up

Circulation. 2014;130:1944–53. http://circ.ahajournals.org/content/130/22/1944.full.

Physiologic/Phenotypic Characteristics of Late Survivors

Circulation.   2013;128:1861–8.   http://circ.ahajournals.org/content/128/17/1861.full?sid=d5f5835f-da5c-4dbf-951f-4b1e7beacd78.

Predictors of Death/VT – Indicator Registry

Heart. 2014;100:247–53. http://heart.bmj.com/content/100/3/247.full.

Pregnancy

Am   Heart   J.   2011;161:307–13.   http://www.ncbi.nlm.nih.gov/pubmed/21315213.

Pulmonary Valve Replacement

Circulation.   2014;130:795–8.   http://circ.ahajournals.org/content/130/9/795.full.

Pulmonary Valve Replacement

Circulation.   2013;128:1855–7.   http://circ.ahajournals.org/content/128/17/1855.full.

Transcatheter Pulmonary Valve Replacement: FDA Approval of Melody Valve

http://www.fda.gov/MedicalDevices/ProductsandMedical Procedures/DeviceApprovalsandClearances/Recently-ApprovedDevices/ucm431866.htm.

Unilateral Rib Notching (Case Report)

J Am Coll Cardiol. 2013;61:e171–e171. http://content.onlinejacc.org/article.aspx?articleID=1673113.

Updates and More

https://clinicalguidecvd.com/tof

Chapter 94
Thromboangiitis Obliterans (Buerger Disease)

Management Keys

Discontinue tobacco use is definitive treatment; even a few cigarettes a day may cause disease progression

ICD-10 Code

I73.1

Alternate Names/Abbreviation

BUERGER DISEASE

Description/Etiology

Nonatherosclerotic inflammation of small/medium arteries, veins, and nerves, most often in extremities but may also involve cerebral, coronary, renal, mesenteric, and pulmonary arteries

Typical presentation due to ischemic symptoms caused by stenosis/occlusion of distal small arteries and veins

V.E. Friedewald, *Clinical Guide to Cardiovascular Disease*,
DOI 10.1007/978-1-4471-7293-2_94,
© Springer-Verlag London 2016

Involvement of both upper and lower extremities and size/location of affected vessels help distinguish from atherosclerosis

Symptoms typically begin in peripheral area of a single limb and often progress proximally and involve multiple extremities, often as intermittent claudication of feet, legs, hands, or arms

Critical limb ischemia causing rest pain, ulcerations, and digital gangrene, occur in patients with more advanced disease.

Raynaud's phenomenon is present in >40 % of patients and may be asymmetrical

Comorbid Conditions

PERIODONTAL DISEASE
SUPERFICIAL THROMBOPHLEBITIS [2]
TOBACCO USE [1]

Demography

Males more often affected
Onset age <45 years
Most prevalent in Near East and Far East countries

Pathophysiology

Three Phases:

1. Acute thrombus occlusion of lumen but not vessel wall
2. Progressive thrombus organization
3. Organized thrombus/vascular fibrosis without inflammation

Signs/Symptoms [5]

EXTREM – PAIN, SHOOTING (PARESTHESIAS)
EXTREM – RAYNAUD PHENOMENON
EXTREM, ARMS – PAIN, EFFORT/REST [4]
EXTREM, FEET – PAIN, EFFORT/REST [4]
EXTREM, HANDS – PAIN, EFFORT/REST [4]
EXTREM, LEGS – PAIN, EFFORT/REST [4]
JOINTS – PAIN (ARTHRALGIA) [3]
RAYNAUD PHENOMENON
SKIN, EXTREM – NECROSIS
SKIN, EXTREM – ULCERS
VEINS, SUPERFICIAL – HARD, CORDLIKE [2]
VEINS, SUPERFICIAL – NODULES [2]

Differentiation

ATHEROSCLEROTIC PERIPHERAL VASCULAR
   DISEASE
AUTOIMMUNE DISEASE
CARDIAC EMBOLI
DIABETES MELLITUS
THROMBOPHILIA

Complications

ABDOMINAL ARTERY OBSTRUCTION [6]
CEREBRAL ARTERY OBSTRUCTION [7]
CORONARY ARTERY OBSTRUCTION [8]
PREMATURE ATHEROSCLEROSIS
RENAL ARTERY OBSTRUCTION

Laboratory

NS

ECG

N/NS ABN

Imaging

NS/VAR WITH COMORBID

Other Tests

Angiography [10]
Angiography also may be indicated for excluding large
artery occlusion

Treatment: Nonpharmacologic

Tobacco cessation [9]
Exercise

Treatment: Pharmacologic

Prostanoids

Treatment: Surgical/Invasive

Revascularization [12]
Amputation [11]

Prevention

Total tobacco cessation/avoidance

Course

Variable with success of smoking cessation
Risk for tissue loss/extremity amputation may approach
40 % if tobacco use continued

Notes

[1] Invariable
[2] Migratory, tender; may precede Ischemia
[3] Monoarthritis; may precede onset of disease by years
[4] Intermittent claudication and rest pain
[5] LE more often involved, usually below popliteal artery
[6] Ischemia/infarction small intestine, colon, spleen, pancreas
[7] Stroke
[8] Myocardial Ischemia/Infarction
[9] Most important and definitive; must be 100 % cessation
[10] Occlusion of distal extremity arteries with corkscrew-shaped collateral arteries (Martinelli Sign)
[11] Often UE
[12] Surgical revascularization usually not feasible due to distal/diffuse nature of disease; however, select patents with severe ischemia and suitable distal target vessels may be candidates for bypass surgery

Guidelines

Management of patients with peripheral artery disease (compilation of 2005 and 2011 ACCF/AHA guideline recommendations)
J Am Coll Cardiol. 2013;61:1555–70. http://content.onlinejacc.org/article.aspx?articleid=1659662.
ESC guidelines on the diagnosis and treatment of peripheral artery diseases
Eur Heart J. 2011; 32:2851–906. http://eurheartj.oxfordjournals.org/content/ehj/32/22/2851.full.pdf.

Patient Information

Images

http://www.nlm.nih.gov/medlineplus/ency/imagepages/18089.htm.
http://www.nlm.nih.gov/medlineplus/ency/imagepages/8747.htm.

Medlineplus

ENGLISH

http://www.nlm.nih.gov/medlineplus/ency/article/000172.htm.

ESPANOL

http://www.nlm.nih.gov/medlineplus/spanish/ency/article/000172.htm.

Mayo Clinic

http://www.mayoclinic.org/diseases-conditions/buergers-disease/basics/definition/con-20029501.

Johns Hopkins

http://www.hopkinsvasculitis.org/types-vasculitis/buergers-disease/.

CDC

http://www.cdc.gov/tobacco/campaign/tips/diseases/buergers-disease.html.

NORD

https://rarediseases.org/rare-diseases/buergers-disease/.

UC Davis

https://www.ucdmc.ucdavis.edu/vascular/diseases/buergers-disease.
html.

Vasculitis Foundation

http://www.vasculitisfoundation.org/education/forms/buergers-
disease/.

Professional Information

Review/Update

Circulation.   2010;121:1858–61.   http://circ.ahajournals.org/con-
tent/121/16/1858.full.

Review

N Engl J Med. 2000;343:864–9. http://www.nejm.org/doi/full/10.1056/
NEJM200009213431207.

Corkscrew DSA Image

Circulation.   2007;116:e539–40.   http://circ.ahajournals.org/con-
tent/116/21/e539.full?sid=8bf135ab-ce19-4511-af6f-
078fbe47d1ba.

Lower Extremity Nonatherosclerotic PAD

Circulation.   2012;126:213–22.   http://circ.ahajournals.org/content/126/2/213.long.

Updates and More

https://clinicalguidecvd.com/throb

Chapter 95
Tricuspid Regurgitation

ICD-10 Code

I36.1 (Nonrheumatic)
I07.1 (Rheumatic)

Alternate Names/Abbreviation

TR
TRICUSPID VALVE INSUFFICIENCY

Description/Etiology

About 80 % of cases of significant TR are functional and related to tricuspid annular dilation and leaflet tethering in setting of RV remodeling due to pressure/volume overload.

Mild degrees of TR are common in persons with normal anatomical TV and are of no physiologic significance

Most cases of TR are clinically silent and noted incidentally on physical exam or part of echo study

Primary TV disorders as etiology:

Carcinoid
Catheter-related trauma (esp Endomyocardial biopsy)

V.E. Friedewald, *Clinical Guide to Cardiovascular Disease*, 1259
DOI 10.1007/978-1-4471-7293-2_95,
© Springer-Verlag London 2016

Congenital
Infective Endocarditis
Radiation
Rheumatic
TV Prolapse

Iatrogenic causes:

Blunt chest wall trauma
RV pacemaker/ICD leads

Functional TR (80 % of cases of significant TR): due to TV annulus dilatation and leaflet tethering associated with RV remodeling/volume overload

Stages:

A At risk of TR [9]
B Progressive TR [10]
C Asymptomatic, severe TR [11]
D Symptomatic severe TR [12]

Predisposing/Comorbid Conditions

[SEE ETIOLOGY]
AORTIC STENOSIS – VALVULAR [FUNCTIONAL TR]
ATRIAL FIBRILLATION [FUNCTIONAL TR]
MITRAL STENOSIS – ACQUIRED [FUNCTIONAL TR]
PULMONARY HYPERTENSION [FUNCTIONAL TR]

Demography

Variable according to associated conditions

Pathophysiology

Most TR cases functional due to tricuspid annular dilation and leaflet tethering in setting of RV remodeling due to pressure/volume overload

TV annulus:

Saddle-shaped ellipsoid that becomes planar and circular as it dilates in an anterior-posterior direction

Often does not return to its normal size and configuration after relief of RV overload.

Severe TR causes:

Increased RA size/pressure and systemic venous pressure

RV enlargement

Progressive TR from annular dilatation

Signs/Symptoms [1]

ABDOMEN – DISTENSION
ABDOMEN – FLUID (ASCITES)
APPETITE – DECR (ANOREXIA)
BREATHING – DIFF (DYSPNEA)
BREATHING – RAPID (TACHYPNEA)
CHEST – PALPITATIONS [3]
EXTREM, LOWER, BILAT – EDEMA
FATIGUE
HEART, LSB, LOWER – IMP, SYS
HEART, LSB, LOWER – MURMUR, DIAS
HEART, LSB, LOWER – MURMUR, SYS [2] [4]
HEART, LSB, LOWER – THRILL, SYS
HEART, S2, SPLIT – REVERSED (PARADOXICAL)
    [SEVERE; EARLY PV CLOSURE]
LIVER – ENLARGED (HEPATOMEGALY)
LIVER – PULSATION, SYS
NAUSEA

NECK, JVP, V WAVE – INCR/LARGE [2]
NECK, JVP, Y DESCENT – RAPID [2]
NECK, SENSATION – PULSATIONS
SPLEEN, SIZE – INCR (SPLENOMEGALY)

Differentiation

Other causes of RV volume overload/failure

Complications

Progression of TR
Chronic/significant increased systemic vascular resistance
    may predispose to:

Hepatic dysfunction
Hepatocellular carcinoma
Protein-losing enteropathy
Systemic venous varices

Laboratory [1]

BLOOD, BILIRUBIN – INCR
BLOOD, LIVER ENZYMES – INCREASED

ECG [1]

DYSRHYTHMIAS – ATRIAL (PACS/OTHERS)
P WAVE – TALL/PEAKED
PR INTERVAL – LONG <1ST DEGREE BLOCK
QRS, AXIS – R

Imaging [1] [6]

RA, CHAMBER, SIZE – INCR
RV, CHAMBER, SIZE – INCR
TV, ANNULUS, DIAM – INCR [5]
TV, FLOW – REGURG

Other Tests [1]

Stress test [7]
Cardiac catheterization [8]

Treatment: Nonpharmacologic [1]

NS

Treatment: Pharmacologic [1]

Diuretics

Treatment: Surgical/Invasive

Surgical correction [13]

Course

Variable per type/etiology

Notes

[1] Does not include findings or recommendations for functional TR associated abnormalities, eg, LV failure, PH

[2] Murmur may be absent even in severe TR, and jugular vein findings may be only detectable feature on physical exam

[3] Especially if AF present

[4] Increases with inspiration

[5] Correlates with TV regurgitant volume

[6] TTE (TEE when suboptimal) useful for:

> Distinguishing primary from functional TR
> Detecting left heart disease
> Estimating PA pressure

[7] Usually limited by left heart disease, but may be useful for detecting symptoms not recognized by patient in guiding earlier intervention

[8] May be indicated when TTE/TEE are inadequate; also to determine cause of PH, severity of TR, RV function

[9] Stage A:

> Primary
>
> > Mild rheumatic change
> > Mild prolapse
> > Other (eg, IE with vegetation, early carcinoid deposition, radiation)
> > Intra-annular RV pacemaker or ICD lead
> > Postcardiac transplant (biopsy related)
>
> Functional
>
> > Normal
> > Early annular dilation

[10] Stage B

> Primary
>
> > Progressive leaflet deterioration/destruction
> > Moderate-severe prolapse
> > Limited chordal rupture
>
> Functional
>
> > Early annular dilation
> > Moderate leaflet tethering

[11] Stage C

> Primary

>> Flail or grossly distorted leaflets

> Functional

>> Severe annular dilation (>40 mm or 21 mm/m^2)
>> Marked leaflet tethering

[12] Stage D

> Primary

>> Flail or grossly distorted leaflets

> Functional

>> Severe annular dilation (>40 mm or >21 mm/m^2)
>> Marked leaflet tethering

[13] Surgical correction of TR most often considered at time of MV or AV surgery; severe TR (primary or functional) may not improve after treatment of left heart valve lesions and reduction of RV afterload; thus, severe TR often should be corrected as part of index procedure

Guidelines

2014 AHA/ACC guideline for the management of patients with valvular heart disease
J Am Coll Cardiol. 2014;63:e57–185. http://content.onlinejacc.org/article.aspx?articleID=1838843.
Guidelines on the management of valvular heart disease (version 2012)
Eur Heart J. 2012;33:2478–80. http://www.escardio.org/guidelines-surveys/esc-guidelines/Pages/valvular-heart-disease.aspx.

Patient Information

Images

http://www.nlm.nih.gov/medlineplus/ency/imagepages/18091.htm.
http://www.nlm.nih.gov/medlineplus/ency/imagepages/18090.htm.

Medlineplus

ENGLISH

http://www.nlm.nih.gov/medlineplus/ency/article/000169.htm.

ESPANOL

http://www.nlm.nih.gov/medlineplus/spanish/ency/article/000169.htm.

Cleveland Clinic

http://my.clevelandclinic.org/heart/disorders/valve/tricuspid.aspx.

Mayo Clinic

http://www.mayoclinic.org/diseases-conditions/tricuspid-valve-disease/basics/definition/con-20036723.

Texas Heart Institute

http://www.texasheartinstitute.org/HIC/Topics/Cond/vtricus.cfm.

Merck

http://www.merckmanuals.com/home/SearchResults?query=Tricuspid+Regurgitation&icd9=424.2.

Professional Information

Review

Circulation.   2009;119:2718–25.   http://circ.ahajournals.org/content/119/20/2718.full.

Review

J Am Coll Cardiol. 2015;65:2331–6. http://content.onlinejacc.org/article.aspx?articleID=2297643.

Assessment: Functional TR

Eur Heart J. 2013;34:1875–85. http://eurheartj.oxfordjournals.org/content/34/25/1875.

Association with MV Disease

J Am Coll Cardiol. 2009;53:401–8. http://www.sciencedirect.com/science/article/pii/S0735109708036619#.

C-V Waves

N Engl J Med. 2013;369:e27. http://www.nejm.org/doi/full/10.1056/NEJMicm1103312.

C-V Waves

N Engl J Med. 2012;366:e5. http://www.nejm.org/doi/full/10.1056/NEJMicm1012843.

Heart Failure: Impact of TR on Survival

Eur Heart J. 2013;34:844–52. http://eurheartj.oxfordjournals.org/content/34/11/844.

Mammoth Right Atrium

J Am Coll Cardiol. 2014;63:e21–e21. http://content.onlinejacc.org/article.aspx?articleID=1827543.

Pacemaker/ICD Leads

Heart. 2014;100:960–8. http://heart.bmj.com/content/100/12/960.full.

Pacemaker/ICD Leads

J Am Coll Cardiol. 2005;45:1672–5. http://content.onlinejacc.org/article.aspx?articleid=1136588&resultClick=3.

Pacemaker Implant: Case Study

Circulation.   2014;130:e23–5.   http://circ.ahajournals.org/content/130/4/e23.full.

Post-mitral Valvuloplasty

Heart. 2013;99:91–7. http://heart.bmj.com/content/99/2/91.abstract.

Progression After MV Repair

Circulation.   2005;112:I453-7.   http://circ.ahajournals.org/content/112/9-suppl/I-453.full.pdf+html?sid=ec03751f-c1be-4d34-b47c-4b5cdf314436.

Secondary TR

J Am Coll Cardiol. 2012;59:703–10. http://content.onlinejacc.org/article.aspx?articleid=1201134&resultClick=3.

Surgical Outcomes (Severe TR)

Heart.   2013;99:181–7.   http://heart.bmj.com/content/99/3/181.abstract.

Transcatheter Mitraclip Repair

Eur Heart J. 2016 37: 849–53. http://eurheartj.oxfordjournals.org/content/37/10/849.abstract?etoc.

Trauma: TR/AMI

Circulation.   2014;129:e496–8.   http://circ.ahajournals.org/content/129/20/e496.full.

Valve Replacement: Transfemoral

J Am Coll Cardiol. 2013;61:1929–31. http://content.onlinejacc.org/article.aspx?articleID=1662642.

Updates and More

https://clinicalguidecvd.com/tr

Chapter 96
Tricuspid Valve Stenosis

Management Keys

Suspect this diagnosis in patients with MS who do not have symptoms of pulmonary congestion

Suspect non-rheumatic etiology in absence of other valvular disease

Treat clinically significant TS surgically because medical treatment relatively ineffective

ICD-10 Code

Rheumatic: I0.70
Congenital: Q22.4 (Tricuspid Atresia)

Description/Etiology

Most common cause: Rheumatic Heart Disease [1]

Characterized by diastolic pressure gradient between RA and RV; mean diastolic gradient >2 mmHg is diagnostic

Clinical manifestations far overshadowed by associated left-sided (especially MV) valve disease [10]

Usually accompanied by TR

TTE essential for diagnosis in most cases

V.E. Friedewald, *Clinical Guide to Cardiovascular Disease*,
DOI 10.1007/978-1-4471-7293-2_96,
© Springer-Verlag London 2016

Other causes:

> Anorectic Drugs [3]
> Carcinoid
> Congenital
> Infective Endocarditis
> Fabry Disease
> Systemic Lupus Erythematosus
> Whipple Disease

Predisposing/Comorbid Conditions

LEFT HEART VALVE DISEASE [2]
RHEUMATIC FEVER
TRICUSPID REGURGITATION

Demography

Rheumatic: Underdeveloped Countries
Females > Males

Pathophysiology

Obstruction to flow from RA to RV at level of TV orifice with resulting:

Decreased RA emptying
RA/IVC enlargement
Increased RA pressure
Decreased RV filling
Decreased cardiac output
Hepatic congestion
Peripheral edema

Severe TS: thickened, distorted, calcified leaflets

Signs/Symptoms [2] [10]

ABDOMEN – DISTENSION
ABDOMEN – FLUID (ASCITES)
ABDOMEN – FULLNESS
BODY, GROWTH – DECR
EXTREM, LOWER, BILAT – EDEMA
FATIGUE
HEART, LSB, LOWER – MURMUR, DIAS
HEART, LSB, LOWER – OPENING SNAP
HEART, LSB, LOWER – THRILL, DIAS
HEART, RSB, LOWER – IMP, PRESYS
LIVER – ENLARGED (HEPATOMEGALY)
LIVER – PULSATION, PRESYS
NECK, JVP – ELEV
NECK, JVP, A WAVE – INCR/LARGE (CANNON WAVE)
NECK, JVP, Y DESCENT – SLOW
NECK, SENSATION – FLUTTERING
SKIN – SWELLING, EDEMA (ANASARCA)

Differentiation

Ebstein Anomaly
Pacemaker lead obstruction [4]
Pulmonary Valve Stenosis
RA Myxoma [4]
RA Thrombus [4]
RV Myxoma [4]
Tricuspid Atresia

Complications

Infective Endocarditis
Pulmonary embolism

Laboratory

NS

ECG

DYSRHYTHMIAS – ATRIAL (PACS/OTHERS)
P WAVE – TALL/PEAKED [5]

Imaging [8] [11]

CARDIOMEGALY
RA, CHAMBER, SIZE – INCR
TV, FLOW – OBS
TV, FLOW – REGURG
TV, LEAFLET, SEPARATION, DIAS – DECR
TV, LEAFLETS – THICK
TV, MOTION, DIAS – DOMING
VEIN, AZYGOS, SIZE – INCR
VENA CAVA, SUP, SIZE – INCR

Other Tests

Cardiac catheterization [6]

Treatment: Nonpharmacological

NS

Treatment: Pharmacological

NS

Treatment: Surgical/Invasive [7] [9]

TV valvuloplasty/repair
TV replacement

Course

Highly variable according to etiology and severity of associated lesions, especially left heart involvement in rheumatic form

Notes

[1] Most common cause globally, but rare in developed countries
[2] In rheumatic disease, involvement of other valves, especially MS, often dominates clinical picture; described changes are only those of pure TS, which is rare
[3] Eg, ergotamine, methysergide, anorexians, pergolide
[4] In addition to directly obstructing flow, trauma from these sources may damage TV and cause valve stenosis
[5] Biphasic if MS present
[6] Hemodynamic assessment of TS:

Rarely performed for acquired disease but may be performed in select cases at time of invasive study for another indication, such as MS with PH

Direct assessment of absolute RA/RV diastolic pressure may be useful in determining TS contribution to clinical findings

Trans-tricuspid diastolic gradient is highly variable and is affected by heart rate, forward flow, and phases of the respiratory cycle; severe TS usually has mean pressure gradients >5–10 mmHg at HR of 70 bpm

[7] Surgery for severe TS:

> Most often performed at time of operation for left-sided valve disease, mainly rheumatic MS/MR
>
> If repair not adequate or feasible due to valve destruction or multiple levels of pathological involvement, replacement may be necessary
>
> Choice of prosthesis should be individualized
>
> Perioperative mortality rates are higher for mitral plus tricuspid versus either isolated mitral or tricuspid surgery alone.

[8] Other TTE findings indicative of severe TS:

> Mean pressure gradient >5 mmHg
>
> Pressure half-time = 190 ms
>
> Valve area = 1.0 cm^2 (continuity equation)
>
> RA/IVC enlargement.
>
> Assessment of TS severity with TTE is often technically limited; these values less well validated than those for MS

[9] 2014 AHA/ACC Guideline recommendations:

Tricuspid valve surgery is recommended for patients with severe TS at the time of operation for left-sided valve disease. *(Level of Evidence: C)*

Tricuspid valve surgery is recommended for patients with isolated, symptomatic severe TS *(Level of Evidence: C)*

Percutaneous balloon tricuspid commissurotomy might be considered in patients with isolated, symptomatic severe TS without accompanying TR. *(Level of Evidence: C)*

[10] Absence of symptoms of pulmonary congestion (eg, dyspnea) in presence of MS suggests TS

[11] CXR: dilated RA, normal size PA, clear lungs

Guidelines

2014 AHA/ACC guideline for the management of patients with valvular heart disease

J Am Coll Cardiol. 2014;63:e57–185. http://content.onlinejacc.org/article.aspx?articleid=1838843.

Guidelines on the management of valvular heart disease (version 2012)

Eur Heart J. 2012;33:2451–96. http://www.escardio.org/guidelines-surveys/esc-guidelines/Pages/valvular-heart-disease.aspx.

Patient Information

AHA

http://www.heart.org/HEARTORG/Conditions/More/HeartValveProblemsandDisease/Problem-Tricuspid-Valve-Stenosis_UCM_450390_Article.jsp#.Vzx4QfMUV1s.

Mayo

http://www.mayoclinic.org/diseases-conditions/tricuspid-valve-disease/home/ovc-20168105.

Merck

http://www.merckmanuals.com/home/heart-and-blood-vessel-disorders/heart-valve-disorders/tricuspid-stenosis.

Texas Heart Institute

http://www.mayoclinic.org/diseases-conditions/tricuspid-valve-disease/home/ovc-20168105.

Professional Information

Anatomic Appearance in Rheumatic Heart Disease

Br Heart J. 1957;19:211–6. http://europepmc.org/backend/ptpmcrender.fcgi?accid=PMC479617&blobtype=pdf.

Auscultatory Findings/RA Pressure Pulse

Am J Med. 1985;78:375–84. http://www.sciencedirect.com/science/article/pii/0002934385903274.

Cardiac Catheterization

Am Heart J. 1985;110:60–4. http://www.sciencedirect.com/science/article/pii/0002870385905150.

Diagnosis/Treatment

Br Heart J. 1964;26:354–79. http://europepmc.org/backend/ptpmcrender.fcgi?accid=PMC1018152&blobtype=pdf.

Diagnosis in Presence of Atrial Fibrillation

Circulation. 1966;33:26–33. http://circ.ahajournals.org/content/33/1/26.full.pdf.

Echo

Eur J Echocardiogr. 2009;10:1–25. http://ehjcimaging.oxfordjournals.org/content/10/1/1.

Hemodynamics

Br Heart J. 1971;33: 16–31. http://www.ncbi.nlm.nih.gov/pmc/articles/
PMC487135/.

Isolated TS

Circulation.   1971;44:729–32.   http://circ.ahajournals.org/con-
tent/44/4/729.full.pdf+html.

Percutaneous Balloon Valvuloplasty

Am J Cardiol. 1993;71:353–4. http://www.sciencedirect.com/science/
article/pii/000291499390808P.

Mechanical Valve Replacement

J Thorac Cardiovasc Surg. 2014;148:603–8. http://www.sciencedirect.
com/science/article/pii/S0022522313011409.

Updates and More

https://clinicalguidecvd.com/ts

Chapter 97
Ventricular Septal Defect: Congenital

Management Keys

Suspect VSD in asymptomatic patients or patients with dyspnea with pansystolic LSB or apical murmur

Use echo as primary diagnostic tool in patients with VSD, including determining morphologic type, shunt magnitude, associated defects

Perform device or surgical VSD closure by experienced operators in patients according to current Guideline recommendations

Consider vasodilator theapy for adults with VSDs with progressive/severe pulmonary vascular disease

Counsel for activity and pregnancy in patients with VSD

ICD-10 Code

Q21.0

Alternate Names/Abbreviation

VSD

V.E. Friedewald, *Clinical Guide to Cardiovascular Disease*,
DOI 10.1007/978-1-4471-7293-2_97,
© Springer-Verlag London 2016

Description/Etiology

Most common congenital heart defect at birth (3–3.5/1000 live births); high rate of spontaneous closure of small VSDs; incidence much less in adults

Anatomical types:

Type 1: lie in RVOT; spontaneous closure uncommon; 6 % of defects in non-Asian populations; up to 33 % occur in Asian patients

Type 2: perimembranous; almost 80 % of VSDs; defect is in membranous septum and adjacent to TV septal leaflet, which can become adherent to the VSD, forming a pouch or "aneurysm" of IVS; pouch limits L-R shunting and can cause partial or complete closure of defect; on LV side of septum, defect is adjacent to AV

Type 3: inlet VSD; located in lower part of RV and adjacent to TV; typically occurs in Down syndrome

Type 4: muscular VSD; located centrally (midmuscular), apically, or at margin of IVS and RV free wall; can be multiple; spontaneous closure common, low incidence in adults

Usually occurs as isolated lesion, but also associated with many other defects (see Predisposing/Comorbid Condtions)

Clinical presentation: Isolated VSD depends largely on defect size and PVR

Small defects ≤25 % size of aortic annulus diameter have small L-R shunts, no left ventricle volume overload, no PAH, and present as systolic murmurs

Moderate defects: >25 % but <75 % of aortic diameter, have small-moderate L-R shunts, mild-moderate LV volume overload, no/mild PAH; patients may remain asymptomatic or develop symptoms of mild HF; symptoms usually abate with medical treatment and time as VSD size decreases

Large defects: >75 % of aortic diameter usually have moderate-large L-R shunts, LV volume overload,

PAH; most adult patients with large VSDs have history of HF in infancy; rarely, do not develop large L-R shunts and do not have normal postnatal fall in PVR; can present with R-L shunting and Eisenmenger syndrome later in childhood or as young adults.

Predisposing/Comorbid Conditions

AORTIC REGURGITATION - CHRONIC
AORTIC STENOSIS - SUBVALVULAR
ATRIOVENTRICULAR SEPTAL DEFECT
BICUSPID AORTIC VALVE
COARCTATION OF AORTA
DIGEORGE SYNDROME
DOWN SYNDROME
NOONAN SYNDROME
PULMONARY STENOSIS
TETRALOGY OF FALLOT
TRANSPOSITION OF GREAT ARTERIES - CORRECTED
TREACHER COLLINS SYNDROME

Demography

No gender predilection

Pathophysiology

Varies according to anatomical type; shunt direction and magnitude determined by

PVR
Defect size
LV/RV systolic and diastolic function
Presence of RVOT obstruction

Usual shunt direction is L-R; when significant, can cause:

Increased pulmonary blood flow and pulmonary venous return

LA/LV volume overload and enlargement

Significant L-R shunt:

Ratio of pulmonary to systemic blood flow >1.5/1.0 and/or

LH chamber dilatatation

Progressive increase in PVR leads to PAH

Signs/Symptoms

BODY, GROWTH - DECR
BREATHING - DIFF (DYSPNEA)
BREATHING - DIFF, RECLINING FLAT (ORTHOPNEA)
CHEST, ANT, L - BULGE
CHEST, RIBS, LOWER - DEFORMED (HARRISON GROOVES)
EXTREM, LOWER, BILAT - EDEMA
FATIGUE
HEART, LSB, MID - MURMUR, SYS [1]
HEART, LSB, UPPER - IMP, SYS
HEART, LV, APEX - MURMUR, DIAS
HEART, LV, APEX - MURMUR, SYS [1]
HEART, LV, APEX - THRILL, SYS
HEART, LV, APEX, IMP - FORCEFUL/SUSTAINED
HEART, P2 – INCR [3]
JOINT, SHOULDER - PAIN
SKIN - FLUSHING
SKIN, COLOR - BLUE (CYANOSIS) [2]
SKIN, COLOR - PALE (PALLOR)
SPUTUM - BLOOD (HEMOPTYSIS)
SWEATING - INCR (DIAPHORESIS/HYPERHIDROSIS)

Differentiation

Atrioventricular septal defect
Double-outlet RV with normally related great arteries
Infundibular Pulmonary Stenosis
PDA
Subaortic stenosis

Complications

Dysrhythmias (especially post-repair)
Heart block (especially post-repair)
HF
Infective Endocarditis
Pneumonia
PAH
SCD

Laboratory

NS

ECG [4]

AV COND - 1ST DEGREE BLOCK
Q WAVE - ABN
QRS - BVH PATTERN
QRS - LVH PATTERN
QRS, AXIS - L
QRS, R WAVE - TALL

Imaging [7] [8]

ASSESS FOR ASSD ABNORMALITIES AND VSD LOCALIZATION/NUMBER OF DEFECTS
CARDIOMEGALY
IVS - DEFECT
IVS, FLOW ACROSS - BIDIRECTIONAL
IVS, FLOW ACROSS - LEFT TO RIGHT
LA, CHAMBER, SIZE - INCR [LARGE SHUNTS] [5]
LV, CHAMBER, SIZE - INCR [LARGE SHUNTS] [5]
PA, BRANCHES, SIZE - INCR
PA, MAIN, SIZE - INCR

Genomics

CSX
DTNA
NKX2.5
TBX5

Other Tests

Cardiac catheterization [9]

Treatment: Nonpharmacologic

Activity counseling [13]
Pregnancy counseling [14]

Treatment: Pharmacologic

Vasodilators [10]

Treatment: Surgical/Invasive

Device closure [12]
Surgical closure [11]

Course

Adults with no PAH have normal/close to normal life expectancy post-VSD closure

Notes

[1] Murmur features:

Determined by blood flow velocity across the defect
Loud/pansystolic with high pressure difference between LV and RV
Small defects loud; intensity can decrease in late systole as muscular contraction reduces defect size
As RV pressure increases, murmur shortens and becomes lower pitched

[2] With R-L shunt, indicates PAH
[3] Increased P2 indicates elevated PVR/PA pressure
[4] ECG may be normal with small shunts/no PAH
[5] L-R shunt magnitude across VSD reflected by LA/LA volume overload
[6] CMR: useful when inlet or apical VSD cannot be well seen on echo; also used to quantify AR severity and for LV size/function
[7] CXR: Small VSD – normal

Significant L-R shunt – LA and LV enlargement with increased pulmonary vascular markings
Significant PAH – no LV enlargement with prominent PA segment and decreased pulmonary vascular markings at lung periphery

[8] Echo mainstay of diagnosis, for:

> Number/location of defects
> Chamber sizes
> Ventricular function
> Presence or absence of aortic valve prolapse and/or regurgitation
> Presence or absence of RV or LV outflow obstruction
> Presence or absence of TR
> Estimation of RV systolic pressure from TR jet, VSD jet, and/or septal configuration should be a part of the study
> In adults with poor echo windows, TEE may be necessary

[9] ACC/AHA 2008 Guidelines: Recommendations for cardiac catheterization:

Class I

- Cardiac catheterization to assess the operability of adults with VSD and PAH should be performed in an ACHD regional center in collaboration with experts *(Level of Evidence: C)*

Class IIa

- Cardiac catheterization can be useful for adults with VSD in whom noninvasive data are inconclusive and further information is needed for management. Data to be obtained include the following:

  - Quantification of shunting. *(Level of Evidence: B)*
  - Assessment of pulmonary pressure and resistance in patients with suspected PAH. Reversibility of PAH should be tested with various vasodilators. *(Level of Evidence: B)*
  - Evaluation of other lesions such as AR and double-chambered right ventricle. *(Level of Evidence: C)*

- Determination of whether multiple VSDs are present before surgery. *(Level of Evidence: C)*
- Performance of coronary arteriography is indicated in patients at risk for coronary artery disease. *(Level of Evidence: C)*
- VSD anatomy, especially if device closure is contemplated. *(Level of Evidence: C)*

[10] ACC/AHA 2008 Guidelines: Recommendation for Medical Therapy

Class IIb

Pulmonary vasodilator therapy may be considered for adults with VSDs with progressive/severe pulmonary vascular disease *(Level of Evidence: B)*

[11] ACC/AHA 2008 Guidelines: Recommendations for Surgical Ventricular Septal Defect Closure

Class I

- Surgeons with training and expertise in CHD should perform VSD closure operations. *(Level of Evidence: C)*
- Closure of a VSD is indicated when there is a Qp/Qs (pulmonary–to–systemic blood flow ratio) of 2.0 or more and clinical evidence of LV volume overload. *(Level of Evidence: B)*
- Closure of a VSD is indicated when the patient has a history of IE. *(Level of Evidence: C)*

Class IIa

- Closure of a VSD is reasonable when net left-to-right shunting is present at a Qp/Qs greater than 1.5 with pulmonary artery pressure less than two thirds of systemic pressure and PVR less than two thirds of systemic vascular resistance. *(Level of Evidence: B)*
- Closure of a VSD is reasonable when net left-to-right shunting is present at a Qp/Qs greater than 1.5 in the presence of LV systolic or diastolic failure. *(Level of Evidence: B)*

Class III

- VSD closure is not recommended in patients with severe irreversible PAH. *(Level of Evidence: B)*

[12] ACC/AHA 2008 Guidelines: Recommendations for device closure

Class IIb

- Device closure of a muscular VSD may be considered, especially if the VSD is remote from the tricuspid valve and the aorta, if the VSD is associated with severe left-sided heart chamber enlargement, or if there is PAH. *(Level of Evidence: C)*

[13] ACC/AHA 2008 Guidelines: Recommendations for activity:

No activity restrictions are indicated for patients with small VSDs, no associated lesions, and normal ventricular function. If pulmonary vascular disease is present, activity is usually self-restricted, but patients should be advised against strenuous exercise or travel to altitudes above 5000 feet. Long-distance air travel should be approached with caution to avoid dehydration, with specific recommendation by an ACHD specialist concerning the need for supplemental oxygen

[14] ACC/AHA 2008 Guidelines Recommendations for pregnancy:

Class III

- Pregnancy in patients with VSD and severe PAH (Eisenmenger syndrome) is not recommended owing to excessive maternal and fetal mortality and should be strongly discouraged. *(Level of Evidence: A)*

Guidelines

ACC/AHA 2008 guidelines for the management of adults with congenital heart disease

J Am Coll Cardiol. 2008;52:e143–e263. http://content.onlinejacc.org/
    article.aspx?articleid=1188032#tab1.

**ESC guidelines for the management of grown-up congenital heart
    disease (new version 2010)**

Eur Heart. J 2010;31:2915–57. http://eurheartj.oxfordjournals.org/
    content/ehj/31/23/2915.full.pdf.

Patient Information

AHA

http://www.heart.org/HEARTORG/Conditions/CongenitalHeart
    Defects/AboutCongenitalHeartDefects/Ventricular-Septal-
    Defect-VSD_UCM_307041_Article.jsp#.Vz73T_MUV1s.

CDC

http://www.cdc.gov/ncbddd/heartdefects/ventricularseptaldefect.
    html.

MAYO

http://www.mayoclinic.org/diseases-conditions/ventricular-septal-
    defect/basics/definition/con-20024118.

Medlineplus

https://www.nlm.nih.gov/medlineplus/ency/article/001099.htm.

Stanford

http://www.stanfordchildrens.org/en/topic/default?id=ventricular-
    septal-defect-vsd-90-P01829.

Professional Information

Anatomical Types

Ann Thorac Surg. 2000;69:S25–S35. http://www.sciencedirect.com/science/article/pii/S0003497599012709.

Device Closure

J Am Coll Cardiol. 2004;43:1257–63. http://www.sciencedirect.com/science/article/pii/S0735109704000816.

Natural Course in Adolescents

Pediatr Cardiol. 1998;19:230–4. http://link.springer.com/article/10.1007%2Fs002469900291.

Pathophysiology

Circulation. 2008;117:1090–9. http://circ.ahajournals.org/content/117/8/1090.full.

Small VSDs in Adults

Eur Heart J. 1998;19:1573–82. http://eurheartj.oxfordjournals.org/content/19/10/1573.

Spontaneous VSD Closure after School Age

Pediatr Int. 2008;50:632–5. http://www.ncbi.nlm.nih.gov/pubmed/19261109.

Unrepaired Perimembranous VSDS in Adults

Am J Cardiol. 2010;105:404–7. http://www.sciencedirect.com/science/article/pii/S0002914909024187.

VSD Closure: Long-Term Followup

J Am Coll Cardiol. 2015;65:1941–51. http://www.sciencedirect.com/science/article/pii/S0735109715009043.

Updates and More

https://clinicalguidecvd.com/vsd

Chapter 98
Williams Syndrome

Management Keys

Careful routine monitoring, including four-extremity BPs, ECG (especially for QT interval), and close examination of peripheral vasculature

Take particular caution during invasive procedures

Avoid treating with RAAS inhibitors for Systemic Arterial Hypertension until Renal Artery Stenosis excluded

ICD-10 Code

Q78.8

Alternate Names/Abbreviation

WS
WILLIAMS-BEUREN SYNDROME
ELFIN FACIES SYNDROME
BEUREN SYNDROME
HYPERCALCEMIA-AORTIC STENOSIS

V.E. Friedewald, *Clinical Guide to Cardiovascular Disease*, 1295
DOI 10.1007/978-1-4471-7293-2_98,
© Springer-Verlag London 2016

Description/Etiology

Multisystem autosomal dominant developmental disorder caused by deletions of portions of Chromosome 7, involving one or more combinations of 25 genes

Phenotypic expressions include distinctive facial features, mental retardation, developmental delays, hypercalcemia, Supravalvular Aortic Stenosis, Systemic Aterial Hypertension, cerebellar abnormalities

CV defects:

Most common cause of death in patients with WS

Structural CV abnormalities occur in about 80 % of all WS patients

Present in up to 93 % of WS patients at age 1 year

Most consist of some form of arterial stenosis

Supravalvular AS most common CV abnormality (45–75 %), occurring in two forms:

Discrete, hourglass narrowing at sinotubular junction

Diffuse, long-segment stenosis of ascending aorta (associated with brachiocephalic arterial stenosis)

Familial cases rare

Predisposing/Comorbid Conditions

ANXIETY/ANXIETY DISORDER
AORTIC STENOSIS - SUPRAVALVULAR [1]
ATTENTION   DEFICIT   HYPERACTIVITY DISORDER
CARDIAC VALVE ABNORMALITIES [23]
CAROTID ARTERY STENOSIS
CELIAC DISEASE
CORONARY ARTERY DISEASE [22]
DIABETES MELLITUS [13]

DIVERTICULOSIS
HYPERCALCEMIA [15]
HYPERTENSION - SYSTEMIC ARTERIAL
HYPOTHYROIDISM [16]
INTRACARDIAC DEFECTS [24]
MENTAL RETARDATION
NEPHROCALCINOSIS
OSTEOPENIA
OSTEOPOROSIS
PHOBIC DISORDER
PULMONARY ARTERY STENOSIS [PERIPHERAL]
    [19]
PULMONARY STENOSIS - SUPRAVALVULAR
RENAL ARTERY STENOSIS
THORACIC AORTA STENOSIS
TYPE I CHIARI FORMATION

Pathophysiology

ELN gene mutation affects elastin, which comprises about
    50 % of dry weight of normal aorta
Elastin: characterized by high degree of reversible disten-
    sibility, including ability to deform significantly with
    small forces; in arterial system, this characteristic allows
    energy storage in form of arterial distension during sys-
    tole and subsequent release of stored energy via vascu-
    lar recoil during diastole (Windkessel effect), greatly
    improving CV system efficiency
In arteries, smooth muscle cells produce most elastin; some
    also produced by endothelial cells and adventitial
    fibroblasts

Signs/Symptoms [18]

ABDOMEN - BRUIT [27]
ABDOMEN - PAIN [2]

ABDOMEN, LLQ - HERNIA, INGUINAL
ANORECTUM - PROLAPSE
ARTERIAL PRESSURE, UE, SYS - R > L [6]
ARTERIAL PULSE PRESSURE - DECR [6]
ARTERIAL PULSE, CAROTID - R > L [6]
ARTERIAL PULSE, DOWNSLOPE - GRADUAL [6]
ARTERIAL PULSE, PEAK - SUSTAINED [6]
ARTERIAL PULSE, RISE - SLOW [6]
ARTERIAL PULSE, UE - ASYMMETRIC [6] [7]
ARTERY, CAROTID - BRUIT [29]
ARTERY, CAROTID - THRILL [6]
BACK, CURV - ANT (LORDOSIS)
BACK, CURV - LAT (SCOLIOSIS)
BEHAVIOR - HYPERACTIVE [5]
BEHAVIOR - OBSESSIVE-COMPULSIVE
BLOOD PRESSURE, ARTERIAL - INCREASED/
     ELEVATED
BODY, EQUILIBRIUM - DECR
BODY, HT - DECR
BOWEL MOVEMENTS - CONSTIPATION
BREATHING - DIFF (DYSPNEA) [6]
COGNITION - DEFECT, NS [11]
CONSCIOUSNESS - LOSS, SUDDEN, EFFORT
     (EFFORT SYNCOPE) [6]
DIZZY/LIGHTHEADED, EFFORT [6]
EARS, HEARING - FEAR, LOUD SOUNDS
     (PHONOPHOBIA)
EARS, HEARING - LOSS (DEAFNESS) [3]
EARS, HEARING - SENSATION, INCREASED
     (HYPERACUSIS)
EYES, IRIS - STELLATE
EYES, LACRIMAL DUCT - NARROW
EYES, MOTION - WANDERING (STRABISMUS)
EYES, PERIORBITAL - FULLNESS
EYES, VISION - DECR/LOSS [SUBTOTAL]
EYES, VISION, 3D - DECR (STEREOPSIS)
FACE, CHEEKS - PROMINENT [4]
FACE, CHIN - POINTED

FACE, FOREHEAD - BROAD/PROMINENT

FATIGUE [6]

FLANK - BRUIT [27]

HAIR, COLOR - GRAY, PREMATURE

HEADACHE [28]

HEART, LV, APEX, IMP - FORCEFUL/SUSTAINED [6]

HEART, LV, APEX, IMP - FORCEFUL/SUSTAINED [6]

HEART, RSB, UPPER - MURMUR, SYS [6][8]

HEART, S2, SPLIT - REVERSED (PARADOXICAL) [6]

HEART, S4 LV [6]

JOINTS - CONTRACTURES [9]

JOINTS, MOVEMENT, RANGE - INCR (HYPERMOBILITY)

LIPS - THICK

MENTATION - ATTENTION DEFICIT/ HYPERACTIVITY DIS

MENTATION, LEARNING, DEVELOPMENT - DECR [10]

MOOD - ANXIOUS

MOOD - DEPRESSED [12]

MOUTH, SMILE - WIDE

MUSCLES, TONE - DECR (HYPOTONIA)

NECK, JVP, A WAVE - INCR/LARGE (CANNON WAVE) [6]

NECK, SUPRASTERNAL NOTCH - THRILL, SYS [6]

NOSE - SHORT

NOSE - UPTURNED

PERSONALITY - EBULLIENT

PUBERTY, DEVELOPMENT - EARLY (PRECOCIOUS PUBERTY)

SKIN, TEXTURE - SOFT

SLEEP - DISTURBED (INSOMNIA)

SWEATING - INCR (DIAPHORESIS/ HYPERHIDROSIS) [6]

SYNDROME - RESTLESS LEGS
TEETH - MALOCCLUSION
TEETH - SMALL
TENDON, REFLEXES - INCR (HYPERACTIVE REFLEXES)
URINATION - BEDWETTING (ENURESIS)
URINATION - INCR (POLYURIA)
URINATION - URGENCY
WEIGHT - INCREASED/GAIN

Differentiation

Other syndromes that include physical/behavioral features and congenital heart disease, including:

Digeorge Syndrome
Noonan Synrome
Turner Syndrome
Fragile X Syndrome
Fetal Alcohol Syndrome

Complications [21]

AMI [14]
Dental Caries
Recurrent Otitis Media
Recurrent Urinary Tract Infection
Stroke
Sudden Death [25]

Laboratory [18]

BLOOD, CALCIUM - INCR [15]
BLOOD, GLUCOSE - INCR (HYPERGLYCEMIA) [13]
URINE, CALCIUM - INCR

ECG [18]

DYSRHYTHMIAS - VENTRICULAR (PVCS/OTHERS)
JT INTERVAL - LONG [33]
QRS - LVH PATTERN [6][26]
QRS - RBBB/RBBB PATTERN [26]
QT/QTC INTERVAL - LONG [32]
ST SEGMENT - DEPR [6]
T WAVE - INVER, ABN [6]

Imaging [CV ONLY] [18]

AORTA, ASCEND, SIZE - DECR [6]
AORTA, ASCEND, SYS - GRADIENT [6]
ART, CORONARY, SIZE - INCR/ANEURYSM
LV, MYOCARD, WALL THICKNESS - INCR
  (HYPERTROPHY) [6]

Genomics

BAZ1B
CLIP2
ELN
FZD9
GTF2I
GTF2IRD1
LIMK1
NCF1
STX1A

Other Tests

Ambulatory ECG monitoring (especially when QT
  prolonged)

Treatment: Nonpharmacologic [18]

Dental hygiene
Dietary calcium restriction

Treatment: Pharmacologic [18]

Antihypertensives (RAAS inhibitors contraindicated until
   RAS excluded)
Beta-blocker for QT prolongation
Oral hypoglycemics

Treatment: Surgical/Invasive [18][19][31]

Complex aorta patching for Supravalvular AS [30]
Transcatheter intervention for PS (when necessary) [19]
Reconstruction of coronary ostia
CABG

Prevention

Pregnancy counseling of affected persons

Course

Variable according to abnormalities

Notes

[1] >50 % of patients with Supravalvular AS have WS
[2] May occur without apparent cause
[3] Sensorineural; detected in adolescence and adults

[4] Young children: face described as "pixie-like", "cute", "elfin"

[5] Declines after childhood

[6] Features of Supravalvular AS

[7] With Supravalvular AS, due to Coanda effect: preferential blood flow into right brachiocephalic artery

[8] Crescendo-decrescendo; ejection click absent; radiates to right carotid artery

[9] Especially lower extremities

[10] Mean IQ approximately 55 (sometimes normal)

[11] Williams-Beuren syndrome cognitive profile: includes relative strengths in memory/language and weaknesses in spatial/motor skills; strength in facial recognition

[12] Usually not major; more often dysthymia

[13] >50 % have DM/abnormal glucose metabolism

[14] May occur due to coronary ostial stenosis, which can occur in absence of Supravalvular AS

[15] Usually mild, but may be moderate-severe elevation in infants/young children; usually resolves in childhood

[16] Usually subclinical

[17] Relates to hypertension

[18] Pathology highly variable and treatment individualized according to associated conditions; life-long supportive care with team approach often necessary

[19] Peripheral pulmonary stenosis often resolves spontaneously

[20] May be secondary to RAS or occur in its absence, related to NCF1 mutation

[21] Cardiovascular disease most common cause of death

[22] Due to coronary artery diffuse stenosis, aneurysm, ostial stenosis, AV inflow obstruction, sinotubular ridge, or combinations

[23] Valvular AS, MVP, MR; TV involvement rare; Ebstein Anomaly reported

[24] Especially VSD, usually muscular

[25] 25–100x risk in general population; cause uncertain in many cases

[26] 60 % RVH, 40 % LVH

[27] Common, often due to RAS
[28] May indicate intracranial stenosis
[29] May indicate brachiocephalic stenosis
[30] Angioplasty ineffective
[31] Periprocedural CV collapse reported in WS patients: particular caution indicated at these times
[32] Due to uncertain mechanism in WS, but may also be prolonged by use of CNS drugs for ADHD, anxiety, etc., including but not limited to: phenothiazines, haloperidol, tricyclic antidepressants, astemizole, ketoconazole, itraconazole, probucol, ketanserin, cisapride, papaverine, tacrolimus, arsenic trioxide
[33] JT interval rather than QT interval measure may be preferable in presence of prolonged QRS

Guidelines

ACC/AHA 2008 guidelines for the management of adults with congenital heart disease

J Am Coll Cardiol. 2008;52:e143–e263. http://content.onlinejacc.org/article.aspx?articleid=1188032#tab1.

ESC guidelines for the management of grown-up congenital heart disease (new version 2010)

Eur Heart J. 2010;31:2915–57. http://eurheartj.oxfordjournals.org/content/ehj/31/23/2915.full.pdf.

Patient Information

Images

https://www.nlm.nih.gov/medlineplus/ency/imagepages/17243.htm.

Medlineplus

ENGLISH

https://www.nlm.nih.gov/medlineplus/ency/article/001116.htm.

ESPANOL

https://www.nlm.nih.gov/medlineplus/spanish/ency/article/001116.htm.

Genetics Home REF

http://ghr.nlm.nih.gov/condition/williams-syndrome.

Williams Syndrome ASSN

http://williams-syndrome.org/ws.

Cleveland Clinic

http://my.clevelandclinic.org/disorders/genetic-disorders/hic-williams-syndrome.aspx.

NORD

https://rarediseases.org/rare-diseases/williams-syndrome/.

Professional Information

Review

N Engl J Med. 2010;362:239–52. http://www.nejm.org/doi/full/10.1056/NEJMra0903074.

Review

Circulation. 2013;127:2125–34. http://circ.ahajournals.org/content/127/21/2125.full.

Acquired Coarctation

Heart.   1998;80:205–6.   http://heart.bmj.com/content/80/2/205.
full#ref-1.

Adult Course of Supravalvular Aortic Stenosis

Eur Heart J. 2012. doi: 10.1093/eurheartj/ehs206. http://eurheartj.
oxfordjournals.org/content/early/2012/07/19/eurheartj.ehs206.
full.

Cognitive Profile

Brain Cogn. 2004;44:604–28. http://www.sciencedirect.com/science/
article/pii/S0278262600912326.

Cardiovascular Abnormalities

Am J Cardiol. 2010;105:874–78. http://www.sciencedirect.com/sci-
ence/article/pii/S0002914909027647.

Cardiovascular Abnormalities

J Pediatr. 2010;156:253–8. http://www.sciencedirect.com/science/arti-
cle/pii/S0022347609008403.

Diabetes Mellitus

Am J Med Genet C Semin Med Genet. 2010;154C:291–8. http://
www.ncbi.nlm.nih.gov/pmc/articles/PMC2882962/.

JT Interval

Am J Cardiol. 2010;106:1029–33. http://www.ncbi.nlm.nih.gov/pubmed/20854969.

Neuropsychiatric Review

J Child Psychol Psychiatry. 2008;49:576–608. http://onlinelibrary.wiley.com/doi/10.1111/j.1469-7610.2008.01887.x/full.

Updates and More

https://clinicalguidecvd.com/williams

Chapter 99
Wolff-Parkinson-White Syndrome

ICD-10 Code

I45.6

Alternate Names/Abbreviation

ACCELERATED AV CONDUCTION
PRE-EXCITATION AV CONDUCTION
PREEXCITATION SYNDROME
WPW

Description/Etiology

- Premature excitation of ventricular myocardium by impulse bypass of normal conduction pathway via accessory pathways [6], causing tachyarrhythmias in many affected persons [5]
- Patients with WPW typically present with palpitations or presyncope caused by an atrioventricular reciprocating tachycardia or, less commonly, a primary atrial tachycardia
- Persons with ECG preexcitation pattern may be asymptomatic [20]

V.E. Friedewald, *Clinical Guide to Cardiovascular Disease*,
DOI 10.1007/978-1-4471-7293-2_99,
© Springer-Verlag London 2016

Rapid conduction of AF over an accessory pathway resulting in VF rare but may be first manifestation

Accessory pathways thought to be an embryologic remnant

Also occurs in patients with myopathic and structural congenital heart disease, particularly Ebstein anomaly

Uncommonly, may coexist with cardiac rhabdomyoma, usually discovered in newborns, associated with tumors located at AV groove or septum, and believed caused by disruption of AV annulus electrical integrity rather than being true accessory pathways.

HCM may be associated with WPW, often associated with specific gene mutations

Comorbid Conditions

ATRIAL SEPTAL DEFECT - SECUNDUM
CARDIOMYOPATHY - DANON DISEASE
CARDIOMYOPATHY - DILATED
CARDIOMYOPATHY - HYPERTROPHIC
COARCTATION OF AORTA
EBSTEIN ANOMALY
GRAVES DISEASE
HYPERTHYROIDISM
LEBER HEREDITARY OPTIC NEUROPATHY [7]
MITRAL VALVE PROLAPSE
POMPE DISEASE
PRKAG2 SYNDROME
TETRALOGY OF FALLOT
TOTAL ANOMALOUS VENOUS RETURN
TRANSPOSITION OF GREAT ARTERIES - CORRECTED
TRICUSPID ATRESIA
TUBEROUS SCLEROSIS
VENTRICULAR SEPTAL DEFECT

Demography

All populations
Sometimes familial

Pathophysiology

Antegrade conduction of impulse via accessory pathway, initiating ventricular depolarization (manifest as delta wave on ECG) before arrival of normally conducted impulse

Accessory pathways make possible retrograde ventricular-atrial impulse conduction and resultant tachyarrhythmias

Ventricular septal dyskinesis reported in some persons (reversible with ablation)

Majority of WPW cases have normal cardiac anatomy

Signs/Symptoms

CHEST - PALPITATIONS
CONSCIOUSNESS - LOSS, SUDDEN (SYNCOPE)
DIZZY/LIGHTHEADED/PRESYNCOPE
HEART, RATE - RAPID (TACHYCARDIA)
HEART, RHYTHM - IRREG
HEART, S1, INTENSITY - INCR
HEART, S2, SPLIT - REVERSED (PARADOXICAL)

Differentiation

AMI
Fabry Disease [10]
LBBB or RBBB
PVT
RVH

Complications

Cardiac Arrest
Rapid AF
SCD [12]
VF

Laboratory

NS

ECG [11]

DELTA WAVE [2]
DYSRHYTHMIAS - ATRIAL (PACS/OTHERS) [5]
DYSRHYTHMIAS - VENTRICULAR (PVCS/OTHERS)
PR INTERVAL - SHORT [3]
QRS - LONG, NS [4]
ST-T WAVE - ABN, NS

Imaging

NS/VAR WITH COMORBID

Genomics

PRKAG2

Other Tests

Ambulatory ECG monitoring

EP testing [9]
Stress test

Treatment: Nonpharmacologic

NS

Treatment: Pharmacologic

NS

Treatment: Surgical/Invasive [9]

Pathway ablation
Antitachycardia atrial pacemaker

Course

Highly variable

Notes

[1] During tachyarrhythmia
[2] Type A: initial positive QRS deflection in V1-2
Type B: initial negative QRS deflection in V1-2
Type C: initial negative QRS deflection in lateral leads
[3] <0.12 SEC
[4] >0.10 SEC; configuration dependent on location of bypass tract
[5] PSVT; sudden AF may be serious
[6] Accessory pathway: an extranodal AV pathway that connects atrial myocardium to ventricle across the AV groove; accessory pathways include AV tracks, nodofas-

cicular tracts, and many other variations; most common insertion is into left lateral LV free wall

[7] Inherited disorder of mitochondria causing subacute blindness, mainly in young men; WPW may also affect maternal carriers without blindness

[8] For comorbid cardiac conditions

[9] Consult current Guidelines for detailed recommendations of EP testing and treatment for asymptomatic and symptomatic persons with preexcitation findings

[10] Short PR in absence of preexcitation characteristic of Fabry Disease; uncertain mechanism

[11] Preexcitation ECG pattern:

> Reflects presence of a manifest accessory pathway connecting the atrium to the ventricle
>
> Pre-excited ventricular activation over accessory pathway competes with anterograde conduction over AV node and spreads from accessory pathway insertion point in ventricular myocardium
>
> Variable degree of pre-excitation, with characteristic pattern of short P-R interval with slurring of the initial upstroke of the QRS complex (delta wave) may occur, depending on relative contribution from ventricular activation by normal AV nodal/ His Purkinje system versus the manifest accessory pathway
>
> Can be intermittent or not easily appreciated with pathways capable of anterograde conduction; usually associated with low-risk pathways, with exceptions

[12] Increased risk of SCD in WPW associated with:

> History of symptomatic tachycardia
> Multiple accessory pathways
> Shortest pre-excited R-R interval of <250 ms during AF
> First 2 decades of life

Guidelines

2015 ACC/AHA/HRS Guideline for the management of adult patients with supraventricular tachycardia: a report of the American College of Cardiology/American Heart Association Task Force on Clinical Practice Guidelines and the Heart Rhythm Society

J Am Coll Cardiol. 2016;67:e27–e115. http://www.sciencedirect.com/science/article/pii/S0735109715058404.

2012 PACES/HRS expert consensus statement on the management of the asymptomatic young patient with a Wolff-Parkinson-White (WPW, Ventricular Preexcitation) electrocardiographic pattern

Heart Rhythm. 2012;9:1006–1024. http://www.hrsonline.org/Practice-Guidance/Clinical-Guidelines-Documents/2012%20Management%20of%20the%20Asymptomatic%20Young%20Patient%20with%20a%20Wolff-Parkinson-White.

Patient Information

Images

http://www.nlm.nih.gov/medlineplus/ency/imagepages/8810.htm.

Genetics Home Reference

http://ghr.nlm.nih.gov/condition/wolff-parkinson-white-syndrome.

Cleveland Clinic

http://my.clevelandclinic.org/heart/disorders/electric/wpw.aspx.

Medline Plus

ENGLISH

http://www.nlm.nih.gov/medlineplus/ency/article/000151.htm.

ESPANOL

http://www.nlm.nih.gov/medlineplus/spanish/ency/article/000151.
htm.

MAYO Clinic

http://www.mayoclinic.org/diseases-conditions/wolff-parkinson-
white/basics/causes/con-20043508.

SADS Foundation

http://www.sads.org/What-is-SADS/Wolff-Parkinson-White-
Syndrome#.VYVRh2fJB1s.

Texas Heart Institute

http://texasheart.org/HIC/Topics/Cond/arrhycat.cfm.

Professional Information

Early Description

Am Heart J. 1930;5:685–704. http://www.sciencedirect.com/science/
article/pii/S0002870330900865.

Atrial Fibrillation

Am J Cardiol. 1992;70:A38–A43. http://www.sciencedirect.com/sci-
ence/article/pii/000291499291076G.

Ablation: Asymptomatic Patients

Card Electrophysiol Clin. 2012;4:281–5. http://www.sciencedirect.
com/science/article/pii/S1877918212000755.

Catheter Ablation/EP

Circulation.   2014;130:811–9.   http://circ.ahajournals.org/content/130/10/811.long.

Diagnosis in Emergency Department

Am Journal Emerg Med. 2009;27:878–88. http://www.sciencedirect.com/science/article/pii/S0735675708004701.

Malignant Arrhythmias

Circulation.   2012;125:661–8.   http://circ.ahajournals.org/content/125/5/661.long.

Natural History

Am J Cardiol. 2013;112:961–5. http://www.sciencedirect.com/science/article/pii/S0002914913012332.

Population Study: SCD

Circulation.   1993;87:866–73.   http://circ.ahajournals.org/content/87/3/866.abstract?ijkey=480a8af85ba8cfb030f29fe8c3f2ce878730cdb5&keytype2=tf-ipsecsha.

Registry: Prognosis/Ablation

Circulation.   2014;130:811–9.   http://circ.ahajournals.org/content/130/10/811.full.

Septal Dyskinesis

Circulation.   2014;130:e196–8.   http://circ.ahajournals.org/content/130/23/e196.full.

Tuberous Sclerosis

Arch Dis Child. 1998;78:159–62. http://adc.bmj.com/content/78/2/159. full.

Updates and More

https://clinicalguidecvd.com/wpw